OXFORD MEDICAL PUBLICATIONS
Delirium in Old Age

Delirium in Old Age

Editors:

James Lindesay
Department of Psychiatry, University of Leicester, UK

Kenneth Rockwood
Division of Geriatric Medicine, Dalhousie University, Halifax, Canada

Alastair Macdonald
Division of Psychiatry and Psychology, King's College, London, UK

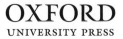

OXFORD
UNIVERSITY PRESS

OXFORD
UNIVERSITY PRESS

Great Clarendon Street, Oxford OX2 6DP

Oxford University Press is a department of the University of Oxford.
It furthers the University's objective of excellence in research, scholarship,
and education by publishing worldwide in

Oxford New York

Auckland Bangkok Buenos Aires Cape Town Chennai
Dar es Salaam Delhi Hong Kong Istanbul Karachi Kolkata
Kuala Lumpur Madrid Melbourne Mexico City Mumbai
Nairobi São Paulo Shanghai Taipei Tokyo Toronto

Oxford is a registered trade mark of Oxford University Press
in the UK and in certain other countries

Published in the United States
by Oxford University Press Inc., New York

© Oxford University Press, 2002

The moral rights of the author have been asserted

Database right Oxford University Press (maker)

First published 2002

A catalogue record for this title is available from the British Library

Library of Congress Cataloging in Publication Data

Delirium in old age / editors, James Lindesay, Kenneth Rockwood, Alastair Macdonald.

Includes bibliographical references.

1. Delirium in old age. I. Lindesay, James. II. Rockwood, Kenneth. III. Macdonald, Alastair.
RC520.7 .D45 2002   618.97'689 – dc21   2002072655

ISBN 0 19 263275 2

10 9 8 7 6 5 4 3 2 1

Typeset by Cepha Imaging Pvt Ltd, India
Printed in Great Britain
on acid-free paper by
Biddles Ltd, Guildford & King's Lynn

Foreword

Sharon K. Inouye

Delirium is a common, serious, and potentially preventable cause of morbidity and mortality for older persons. In fact, delirium represents the most frequent complication of hospitalization for the older population. Each year in the USA, delirium occurs during hospital stay in more than 2.3 million older patients, involving more than 17.5 million in-patient days and resulting in over US$4 billion (1994 US dollars) in hospital costs. Moreover, substantial additional costs accrue after hospitalization because of the increased need for institutionalization, rehabilitation, home care services, and medical and nursing follow-up care.

Despite its importance in terms of clinical, economic, and social considerations and despite considerable advances in the past decade, much remains unknown about delirium. This book provides a state-of-the-art update of delirium research: history, conceptualization, measurement, epidemiology, pathophysiology, assessment, diagnosis, causes, prevention, management, and education. What is presented, however, represents only the tip of the iceberg in terms of what remains to be elucidated about delirium. Chapter 11, which outlines a future research agenda, provides a wake-up call that we hope will heighten awareness to the importance of interdisciplinary research endeavours to address this critical area.

Delirium provides a valuable opportunity to understand better the functioning of the brain at a fundamental level. The description of delirium as 'acute brain failure' – involving multiple neural circuits, neurotransmitters, and higher cortical functions – suggests that understanding delirium may elucidate the essential underlying mechanisms of brain functioning. Thus, studying the pathophysiology of delirium (Chapter 4) should clearly represent a priority area for the advancement of brain research.

The importance of delirium, however, extends well beyond its assessment and management as a clinical syndrome. The Assessing Care of Vulnerable Elders (ACOVE) project has identified delirium as among the top three target conditions for quality of care improvement for vulnerable older adults. At least 40% of delirium is preventable, as demonstrated by the Yale Delirium Prevention Trial. Since it is often iatrogenic and closely linked to processes of care, delirium may serve as a useful marker for the quality of hospital care for older persons. In fact, delirium represents a prototypical case of failures in the system of hospital care, due to iatrogenesis, overmedication, failure to carry out proper geriatric assessment, reduction in skilled nursing staff, rapid pace of care, and poor attitudes towards care of elderly patients. Examining delirium provides an opportunity to improve the quality of hospital care for older persons more generally. The changes required to reduce delirium rates, however, would require large-scale shifts in local and national policies and approaches to care – including routine cognitive and functional assessment on admission, monitoring mental status as a 'vital sign', enhanced geriatric nursing and physician expertise at the bedside, case management services, improved provider education about delirium, and improved quality monitoring systems. Implementing these changes will impact not only on delirium, but will result in high-quality in-patient geriatric care and will likely reduce the incidence of other common geriatric syndromes as well, including functional decline, pressure ulcers, falls, and incontinence.

We hope that this volume will serve as a catalyst to rejuvenate attention and progress in delirium research and clinical care. All involved in the care of older persons – health-care providers, researchers, administrators, and policymakers – must work together to improve our health-care systems by addressing delirium, a priority area that is crucial to the health and quality of life for older persons.

Preface

In 1990, Oxford University Press published *Delirium in the elderly*, a slim volume that involved two of us (JL, AM) as co-authors. At that time, we commented that despite its importance, delirium was a neglected disorder in the medicine and psychiatry of old age, and relatively little was known about it. Twelve years on, we know rather more about delirium, but there is no evidence that we are getting any better at identifying and managing this disorder in clinical practice. Delirium is an important sign of serious illness, so its routine under-detection, even by clinicians experienced in the care of elderly people, is something of a puzzle. No one would fail to recognize that an altered mental state is alarming in a child, but amongst elderly people it often does not even merit comment in the health record.

Why this should be so is not clear. On the one hand, clinicians do not appear to engage effectively with their elderly, cognitively impaired patients. This disengagement, while unfortunate, is nevertheless understandable. For a long time it has been hard to argue, on medical grounds, with a nihilistic approach to cognitive impairment in old age. The absence of specific therapy, the rarity of truly reversible dementia, and the common mix of delirium with dementia have meant that, even if the former were distinguished from the latter, the happy textbook story of an acute, reversible cognitive problem simply did not hold. The clinical encounter usually starts with the history, where the patient speaks to the doctor and gives some hint about what is wrong, so it is easy to see how a physician might react to the prospect of an apparently disengaged patient, who does not even bother to make sense of his complaint, by himself not bothering with further inquiry and simply getting on with it. The increasing pace of high-technology medicine and the decreasing duration of hospital in-patient stays do not help in this regard, limiting as they do the opportunities for clinicians to engage with patients in a way that would encourage the recognition of delirium.

On the other hand, the problem can sometimes be one of over-engagement, where the clinician (often a novice, in our experience) will fill in both sides of the conversation. The mistake here is in reacting socially to the patient's inability to respond, by politely filling in the blanks and papering over the problem, rather than by recognizing that an inability to respond to simple inquiry requires more detailed queries, not more vague ones.

If it is hard for clinicians to escape a degree of blame, some of this must also rest with those charged with educating health professionals about brain function. Sadly, most have only the most rudimentary understanding about what happens in the brain outside the motor strip and its related pathways. Consequently, the faint recognition that a patient's cognitive function is not what it might be is too readily given the label of dementia, or a vague, non-localized 'stroke'.

That delirium is so poorly recognized also reflects adversely on delirium researchers. The past decade has seen significant growth in academic interest in this condition. However, any insights that they – we – have had to offer have evidently not been made plain or practical enough to be useful. And, as others have noted, we remain mired in descriptive studies that at best confirm what is known without advancing the field, and at worst add to the confusion with variable and imprecise terminology, or with unsupportable claims.

The aim of this book is to set out an agenda for improving this poor state of affairs. Our plan is to bring together what is known in a way that can be helpful to clinicians, and to meet the needs of researchers as an up-to-date and critical compendium of knowledge. Chapter 1 outlines the history of the delirium concept, which argues that the current diagnostic construct appears to be inefficient when applied to the ageing population of the modern world. Chapter 2 reviews the instrumentation of delirium from a critical perspective, and emphasizes the need for measures that capture the clinical phenomenon, and do not merely redefine delirium as a score on a psychometric test. As Robertsson usefully points out, different instruments exist for different purposes, and one important differentiating point is that of screening versus diagnostic and severity measures. Chapter 3 presents a review of the epidemiology of delirium, and specifically considers dementia as a risk for delirium, and *vice versa*. Chapter 4 reviews what is known about the neuropathophysiology of delirium, so that we might gain some systematic insights into the diverse clinical phenomena seen in clinical practice. Specific attention is given to delirium and the cholinergic system. Chapter 5 addresses the practical issues of patient assessment and diagnosis. Chapter 6 reviews the various physical and psychological causes of delirium in old age. Chapter 7 discusses the pharmacological and non-pharmacological management of delirium. Chapter 8 examines how delirium might be prevented from occurring in vulnerable patients. Together, these four chapters will provide clinicians with practical guidelines on patient management, to which all authors will contribute. Chapters 9 and 10 focus on problems of education: first, what do we tell patients' families, and second, how do we go about educating other health-care professionals? The final chapter presents a critical review of pressing issues in delirium, as well as an agenda for present action and future research.

We hope that this short book can be a part of ongoing efforts worldwide to advance the management of this common and serious problem. We invite the comments of interested readers, who may also consult this publication's website (http://www.oup.co.uk/isbn/0-19-263275-2) for electronic updates.

The Editors

Contents

Contributors *page xi*

1 The concept of delirium: historical antecedents and present meanings *1*
   Kenneth Rockwood and James Lindesay

2 The instrumentation of delirium *9*
   Barbro Robertsson

3 The epidemiology of delirium *27*
   James Lindesay, Kenneth Rockwood, and Daryl Rolfson

4 The neuropathophysiology of delirium *51*
   Paula Trzepacz and Roos van der Mast

5 Clinical assessment and diagnosis *91*
   Hannu Koponen, Kenneth Rockwood, and Colin Powell

6 The causes of delirium *101*
   Darryl Rolfson

7 The management of delirium *123*
   Edward Marcantonio

8 The prevention of delirium *153*
   Shaun O'Keeffe

9 The role of families, family caregivers, and nurses *187*
   Ingalill Rahm Hallberg

10 Education about delirium *205*
   Kenneth Rockwood

11 The future *213*
   James Lindesay, Kenneth Rockwood, and Alastair Macdonald

Index *223*

Contributors

Ingalill Halberg
Professor,
Department of Nursing,
Medical Faculty,
Lund University,
Sweden 2002

Hannu Koponen
Professor,
Department of Psychiatry,
University of Oulu,
FIN-90014,
Oulu,
Finland

James Lindesay
Professor of Psychiatry for the Elderly,
University of Leicester,
Leicester LE5 4PW, UK

Alastair Macdonald
Professor of Old Age Psychiatry,
Guy's, King's and St Thomas' Schools of
Medicine, Dentistry and Biomedical
Sciences, King's College, London
SE13 6J2, UK

Edward Marcantonio
Director of Quality and Outcomes
Research,
Hebrew Rehabilitation Center for the
Aged,
Department of Medicine,
1200 Center Street,
Roslindale, MA 02131, USA

Roos van der Mast
Director of Psychiatry Residency Training,
Mentrum Mental Health Care
Amsterdam,
37 2^e Constantijn Huygenstraat, NL-1054
AG, Amsterdam,
The Netherlands

Shaun O'Keeffe
Department of Geriatric Medicine,
Merlin Park Regional Hospital and
University College Hospital,
Galway, Ireland

Colin Powell
Dalhousie University,
5955 Veterans' Memorial Lane,
Room 2652,
Halifax, NS, B3H 2E1, Canada

Barbro Robertsson
Institute of Clinical Neuroscience,
Psychiatry Section,
Göteborg University,
Sahlgrenska University Hospital,
Mölndal, SE-431 80,
Sweden

Ken Rockwood
Dalhousie University,
5955 Veterans' Memorial Lane,
Room 1421,
Halifax, NS, B3H 2E1,
Canada

Daryl Rolfson
Assistant Professor,
University of Alberta,
1259 Glenrose Rehabilitation Hospital,
10230-111 Avenue,

Edmonton,
Alberta T5G 0B7,
Canada

Paula Trzepacz
Clinical Professor of Psychiatry and
Neurology,

University of Mississippi Medical School,
Adjunct Professor of Psychiatry,
Tufts University Medical School, and
Lilly Research Laboratories,
Indianapolis, IN,
USA

Chapter 1

The concept of delirium: historical antecedents and present meanings

Kenneth Rockwood and James Lindesay

Delirium has long been recognized as a problem of human cognition, and indeed was one of the first mental disorders to be described. Despite this long history, it remains to this day an elusive concept, resisting attempts to define it with any precision. As Lipowski (1980) has observed: 'it appears that clinicians by and large excel in observing and describing natural phenomena, but often display deplorable looseness in the use of words that are indispensable for labelling, classifying, and explaining what is observed and recorded.'

The history of describing delirium (L. *delirare* or 'out of the furrow', as characterized by Celsus) can be traced back to Hippocrates' Book of Epidemics (Lloyd 1950). Even early descriptions contrasted *phrenitis*, an acute and largely transient mental disorder seen in association with physical illness, and characterized by psychomotor agitation, insomnia, and disturbances of mood and perception, with *lethargus*, a disorder of somnolence, inertia, and reduced response to stimuli. Whether both types can be transposed to the modern view of delirium and its subtypes is not clear, but it is evident that writers both ancient and modern have papered over much of its clinical heterogeneity by calling all acutely disordered mental states 'delirium'. For example, it is likely that the earlier concept of *lethargus* included both those whom we would now recognize as having 'hypoactive delirium' and those that might be described as 'pre-terminal exhaustion' (Lipowski 1980). But what should we call the sometimes lingering, beclouded mental state seen in many people in the days to hours before death? Despite a long history of description, we still do not have consensus on this point (Casarett and Inouye 2001). Another difficulty has been the historical use of the term delirium to describe florid and raving insanity seen not just in association with physical illness or intoxication, but also with acute schizophrenia or manic episodes. As we shall see, the modern remedy to this problem (to distinguish between 'organic' and 'non-organic' mental syndromes) has not been entirely satisfactory.

Despite these descriptive and diagnostic difficulties, a number of features have been consistently described as core features of delirium throughout its long history. These include disturbance of consciousness, disturbance of thinking (cognition), rapid onset/ fluctuating course, and evidence of an external cause.

Alteration in the level of consciousness

Of all the features that make delirium distinct, disturbances of consciousness are amongst the most characteristic. Historically, this disturbance of consciousness has been described in three ways: as disruptions of the sleep–wake cycle; as part of the continuum between alertness and coma; and as a disorder of attention.

Insomnia and restless sleep have been noted as features of delirium from the time of Hippocrates, who also observed that 'when a delirium or raving is appeased by sleep, it is a good sign' (Lloyd 1950). Early attempts to induce restful sleep included both medicinal and environmental approaches. As has been noted elsewhere (Lindesay 1999), the potential hazard of the former approach has long been recognized: 'somniferous potions do noe small hurt, and sometimes they kill' (Barrough 1583).

Lipowski (1990) recalled to general attention that the anatomist and surgeon John Hunter explicitly linked delirium and sleep, and considered delirium as 'a dream arising from disease'. He further described delirium as 'a diseased dream arising from what may be called diseased sleep', resulting from the abnormally reduced awareness of the external world (Hunter 1835). Other pre-modern authors viewed delirium as a waking dream, or as a state intermediate between sleep and wakefulness (Lipowski 1990). These ideas on the relationship between delirium and sleep find resonance in the modern proposals of delirium as a disorder of wakefulness.

Delirium as a disorder of consciousness (albeit one falling short of coma) has a more recent history. In the early nineteenth century, Greiner (1817) introduced the term 'clouding of consciousness', which survived as an essential feature of delirium into DSM-III (American Psychiatric Association 1980). This term has been used to refer both to a quantitative level of reduced consciousness, and to an altered mental state with fragmentation of psychic experience and preoccupation with subjective events distorted by perceptual and affective disturbances (e.g. Jaspers 1963). Plum and Posner (1982) considered delirium to be an early step on the path to coma, and as a result of a defect in attention. Their hierarchy proceeds thus: *delirium* ('a floridly abnormal mental state characterized by disorientation, fear, irritability, misperception of sensus stimuli, and, often, visual hallucinations'), *obtundation*, *stupor*, and *coma*. Plum and Posner further noted that 'for all practical purposes the terms "clouding of consciousness" and "delirium" define equivalent alterations of arousal'.

Clouding of consciousness was dropped from the DSM-III diagnostic criteria for delirium on the grounds that it was so difficult to operationalize (Gottlieb *et al.* 1991). In DSM III-R (American Psychiatric Association 1987), delirium was conceptualized as an attentional disorder, although 'reduced level of consciousness' remained within the diagnostic criteria as a supportive element. To many clinical observers, however (including the present authors), it is the clouding of consciousness that is so characteristic of delirium that the diagnosis commonly can be made with confidence within seconds of entering the patient's room. Perhaps it was acknowledgement of this experience that resulted in the return of 'disturbance of consciousness (i.e. reduced clarity of awareness of the environment)' as an essential component of DSM-IV delirium (American Psychiatric Association 1994), and for the persistence of 'clouded consciousness' in the ICD-10 research criteria [World Health Organization (WHO) 1993].

In the present era, much still needs to be understood about the pathophysiology of delirium, but is seems likely that central cholinergic systems are implicated (Blass *et al.* 1981; Trzepacz 1999), which would explain why processes of alertness and wakefulness are deranged in this disorder. Perhaps the central issue in this regard is the historic problem of describing consciousness. If, with the philosopher John Searle, we understand consciousness to be an emergent property of brain activity ['mental phenomena are caused by neurophysiological processes in the brain and are themselves features of the brain' (Searle 1992)], then operationalization of its constituent features runs the risk of epiphenominalism, a trap into which DSM-III-R appears to have fallen, but which DSM-IV has the potential to avoid. This is not to dispute that the 'neurophysiological processes' are not hierarchially arranged and to some extent localizable (Stuss *et al.* 2001), but simply to note that we have yet to arrive at bedside testing for delirious patients where precision does not run the risk of speciousness.

Disturbance of thinking

Another aspect of the concept of delirium rooted in ancient times is that of disturbances of thinking. The term 'confusion' was introduced in the nineteenth century French and German literature to describe this aspect of the disorder (Berrios 1981). Confusion is generally understood as 'inability to think with one's customary clarity and coherence' (Lishman 1997). The disordered thinking seen in delirium has been variably conceptualized as resulting from impaired consciousness or from an inability to attend to internal intentional stimuli. Like many other aspects of delirium, this has not been studied systematically (Lipowski 1990).

The course of delirium

The course of delirium is another feature that has been characterized by writers since Hippocrates, who particularly have noted its general acute onset, transient and fluctuating course and variable outcome. In the modern era, transience has been held to differentiate delirium from dementia; previously it was held to distinguish delirium from other excited mental states, such as mania. As noted, the outcome of delirium was generally reported as either death (usually) or recovery. Recovery was generally understood to be complete, although even as early as 1583 Barrough remarked that if it resolves, delirium may be followed by loss of memory and reasoning power, a finding which has had recent substantiation in the modern literature (Rockwood *et al.* 1999), and which raises questions about the possible neurotoxic effect of a delirious episode upon the brain.

Delirium and external causation

The role of physical illness and toxins or infection was stressed by ancient authors, who particularly noted fever as an important determinant. Indeed, the first English medical dictionary describes mania as 'delirium without fever' (Quincy 1719). This relationship perhaps reached its apogee in Bonhoeffer (1912), who included delirium as one of the five related psychiatric syndromes (the others were 'excitement, twilight state, hallucinosis, and amentia') that could occur in association with systemic physical illness.

Controversies in conceptualizing delirium

Following Engel and Romano's 1959 study of neurophysiological changes in delirium, which helped usher in the modern understanding, several more systematic approaches to delirium were proposed. Engel and Romano also noted that most of their cases presented with psychomotor retardation rather than psychomotor agitation. In North America, there is been a persistent difference of opinion between neurologists and psychiatrists on how best to describe these variable phenotypes. In 1962, Victor and Adams proposed a classification of 'confusional states', including delirium, primary mental confusion and beclouded dementia. The latter, while not precisely described, did anticipate the most common form of delirium seen today. However, as an organizing principle, 'confusion' is cumbersome and of limited clinical utility; Lishman (1997) advises that the term is best avoided in nosology. 'Acute confusional state' nevertheless remains a popular synonym for delirium; the history of its description and usage suggests that it has been applied mainly to states of reduced alertness and psychomotor activity, in contrast to more florid presentations (Lipowski 1980). Neurologists have persisted for some time in favouring the term 'acute confusion' [for example, the behavioural neurologist Mesulam (1985) rejected 'delirium' as being 'too psychiatric']. They reserved 'delirium' for acute confusion with psychomotor agitation, the prototype of which is the syndrome of delirium tremens seen in association with acute withdrawal of alcohol or other addictive compounds. Such an approach, however, has been no more helpful than the earlier classifications. Similarly, the psychiatric concept of 'organicity' in mental disorders has also emphasized positive features, such as hallucinations, agitation and hyperactivity.

The modern conceptualization of delirium owes much to Lipowski's book on the topic, first published in 1980. Lipowski synthesized a great deal of the literature to that point, and proposed that the single term 'delirium' should be used to describe the spectrum of an acute mental disorder impairing consciousness which arises in association with medical illness, and which falls short of coma.

The most recent significant development in conceptualizing delirium has been the formulation of diagnostic criteria designed to bring some order to the 'terminological chaos' in this area. A landmark in this regard was DSM-III, which represented consensus expert opinion informing a rule-oriented approach to diagnosis. An important part of DSM-III was the distinction between organic mental syndromes and organic mental disorders. In the latter, a specific aetiology is held to be present. However, this distinction breaks down in the case of delirium, since the diagnostic criteria for this syndrome included the presence of a 'specific organic factor'. In DSM-III-R, the burden of 'organicity' had not entirely been shaken off, and this problem in characterizing delirium persisted until DSM-IV, when the concept of 'organic mental disorder' was abandoned, and the word 'syndrome' dropped. Delirium is considered to be due to a medical condition, to substance intoxication or withdrawal, or not otherwise specified. The latter allows for other causes, such as sensory deprivation, or even an abrupt change in environment, such as can be seen in patients with dementia who are institutionalized, or relocated from one area of a nursing home to another.

The parallel psychiatric diagnostic system to DSM is the International Classification of Diseases (ICD). Even in the most recent version, ICD-10, the concept of 'organic mental disorder' is retained, although it is noted that 'organic' means simply that the syndrome is so classified that it can be attributed to an independently diagnosable cerebral or systemic disease or disorder; and not that 'non-organic' disorders have no biological basis. Interestingly, the ICD-10 criteria for delirium do not specifically require the presence of an underlying medical condition (although its classification as an 'organic mental disorder' would seem to presume it). The ICD-10 criteria for delirium differ from those of DSM-IV in other respects, notably in the features held to be essential for the diagnosis, as opposed to those that are merely supportive. However, both systems regard a disorder of consciousness as essential, and neither attempts to disentangle the whole (consciousness) from its constituent parts (attention). They also agree that the historically core features of disturbances of thinking (cognition), rapid onset/fluctuation course, and evidence of cause are essential features. In the ICD-10 research criteria, psychomotor disturbance and sleep disturbance are also essential criteria, and DSM-IV requires either disturbed cognition or disturbed perception.

Lipowski (1980) proposed that delirium can present in distinct and different forms, as a hyperactive syndrome, as a hypoactive syndrome, or as a combination of the two. This widely accepted subtyping of delirium is supported by factor analytic studies (Trzepacz and Dew 1995; Camus *et al.* 2000a), but it is not recognized by the DSM-IV or ICD-10 diagnostic classifications, something that has hampered research into its aetiological, therapeutic and prognostic significance. Given that mixed states are common (Liptzin and Levkoff 1992), and that there appear to be few significant differences between them in terms of aetiology or outcome (O'Keeffe and Lavan 1999; Camus *et al.* 2000b), or on investigations such as EEG, the validity of the hyperactive/hypoactive subtypes still needs to be regarded with some caution (see Chapter 6). They may merely represent different severities of the disorder.

Delirium and dementia

A noteworthy intention of the modern diagnostic criteria has been to define the boundary between delirium and dementia. The latter is not just the other most common cause of global cognitive impairment in the modern world, but is also an important risk factor for delirium. Unfortunately, they do not appear to be particularly helpful in this regard. For example, disturbance of consciousness is described in Lewy body dementia, a condition that shares a number of features with delirium. Disturbance of cognition is clearly non-specific. Rapid onset may occur in vascular dementia, and a fluctuating course is seen both vascular and Lewy body dementias (McKeith *et al.* 1996). It is also well known that the cognitive function of patients with dementia may fluctuate during the course of the day (so-called 'sundowning'). The cause of delirium may not be apparent, particularly in elderly patients with significant pre-existing dementia (Lindesay 1999). Are there, then, any other features of delirium that might more reliably distinguish it from dementia?

It has been proposed that reversibility of cognitive dysfunction might be a useful discriminator, since patients with delirium are traditionally thought to recover to some extent if they do not die, whereas dementia is associated with progressive cognitive decline. Duration is noted as a feature in ICD-10, which states in its guidelines that the total duration of the condition is less than 6 months. Of course, it may be that not all delirium is reversible, and recent empirical studies suggest that delirium itself (Levkoff *et al.* 1992) or many delirium-related symptoms, especially memory impairment (Rockwood 1993) can persist for at least this long. However, this might also be the result of the contamination of study samples with cases of dementia meeting the criteria for delirium. Delirium defined in terms of reversibility of cognitive dysfunction is a relatively quiet disorder in elderly patients (Treloar and Macdonald 1997a, 1997b), associated with poor attention, incoherent speech, slow or vague thinking, fluctuating mental state, plucking at bedclothes and increased motor activity. It is not associated with florid symptoms such as delusions, hallucinations, aggression, and excitement. Of course, reversibility is not diagnostically helpful, since duration and outcome are not known at the onset of the disorder (Macdonald and Treloar 1996), but they may be useful criteria in future research into the phenomenology of delirium, and its relationship to the dementias often associated with it.

Conclusion

The concept of delirium has developed historically from the prototype of acute confusion with psychomotor agitation. While the modern view of delirium recognizes four core features (disturbance of consciousness, disturbance of cognition, limited course and external causation), their operationalization can produce a misleading picture of the most common manifestations of delirium in elderly people. As elderly people – especially those with dementia – are most likely to develop delirium, this is a serious impediment to good research and effective care. It may be that our current conceptualization of delirium, rooted as it is in centuries of observations on younger patients, will need further examination and revision if it is to be applicable to an ageing population with large numbers of elderly people with dementia. For now, existing research into delirium based upon current diagnostic criteria needs to be interpreted with some caution, given their limited ability to discriminate between delirium and dementia.

References

American Psychiatric Association. (1980). *Diagnostic and statistical manual of mental disorders*, 3rd edn. American Psychiatric Association, Washington, DC.

American Psychiatric Association. (1994). *Diagnostic and statistical manual of mental disorders*, 4th edn. American Psychiatric Association, Washington, DC.

American Psychiatric Association (1987). *Diagnostic and statistical manual of mental disorders*, 3rd edn. (revised). American Psychiatric Association, Washington, DC.

Barrough, P. (1583). *The Methode of Phisicke, conteyning the causes, signs, and cures of inward diseases in mans body from the head to the foote*. Vautrollier, London.

Berrios, G. E. (1981). Delirium and confusion in the 19th century: a conceptual history. *British Journal of Psychiatry*, **139**, 439–449.

Blass, J. P., Gibson, G. E., Duffy, T. E., and Plum, F. (1981). Cholinergic dysfunction: a common denominator in metabolic encephalopathies. In: *Cholinergic mechanisms* (eds G. Pepeu and H. Ladinsky). Plenum Press, New York.

Bonhoeffer, K. (1912). Die Psychosen im Gefolge von akuten Infectionen, Allgemeinekrankungen und inneren Erkrankungen. In: *Handbuch der Psychiatrie* (ed. G. L. Aschaffenburg). Deuticke, Leipzig.

Casarett, D. J. and Inouye, S. K. (2001). Diagnosis and management of delirium near the end of life. *Annals of Internal Medicine*, **135**, 32–40.

Camus, V., Burtin, B., Simeone, I., Schwed, P., Gonthier, R., and Dubos, G. (2000a). Factor analysis supports the evidence of existing hyperactive and hypoactive subtypes of delirium. *International Journal of Geriatric Psychiatry*, **15**, 313–316.

Camus, V., Gonthier, R., Dubos, G., Schwed, P., and Simeone, I. (2000b). Etiologic and outcome profiles in hypoactive and hyperactive subtypes of delirium. *Journal of Geriatric Psychiatry and Neurology*, **13**, 38–42.

Engel, G. L. and Romano, J. (1959). Delirium, a syndrome of cerebral insufficiency. *Journal of Chronic Diseases*, **9**, 260–277.

Gottlieb, G. l., Johnson, J., Wanich, C., and Sullivan, E. (1991). Delirium in the medically ill elderly: operationalizing the DSM-III criteria. *International Psychogeriatrics*, **3**, 181–196.

Greiner, F. C. (1817). *Der Traum und das fieberhafte Irreseyn*. Brockhaus, Altenburg.

Hunter, J. (1835). *The work of John Hunter, F. R. S.*, Vol. 1 (ed. J. F. Palmer). Longman, London.

Jaspers, K. (1963). *General psychopathology*, 7th edn, tr. J. Hoenig and M. Hamilton. Manchester University Press, Manchester.

Levkoff, S. E., Evans, D. A., Liptzin, B., *et al.* (1992). Delirium. The occurrence and persistence of symptoms among elderly hospitalized patients. *Archives of Internal Medicine*, **152**, 334–340.

Lindesay J. (1999).The concept of delirium. *Dementia and Geriatric Cognitive Disorders*, **10**, 310–314.

Lipowski, Z. J. (1980). *Delirium*. Charles C. Thomas, Springfield, IL.

Lipowski, Z. J. (1990). *Delirium: acute confusional states*. Oxford University Press, New York.

Liptzin, B. and Levkoff, S. E. (1992). An empirical study of delirium subtypes. *British Journal of Psychiatry*, **161**, 843–845.

Lishman, A. (1997). *Organic psychiatry*. Blackwell, Oxford.

Lloyd, G. F. R. (ed.) (1950). *Hippocratic writings*. Blackwell, Oxford.

Macdonald, A. J. D. and Treloar, A. (1996). Delirium and dementia: are they distinct? *Journal of the American Geriatrics Society*, **44**, 1001–1002.

McKeith, I.G., Galasko, D., Kosaka, K. *et al.* (1996). Consensus guidelines for the clinical and pathologic diagnosis of dementia with Lewy bodies (DLB): report of the consortium on DLB international workshop. *Neurology*, **47**, 1113–1124.

Mesulam M. M. (1985). *Principles of behavioral neurology*. F. A. Davis Company, Philadelphia.

O'Keeffe, S.T. and Lavan, J.N. (1999). Clinical significance of delirium subtypes in older people. *Age and Ageing*, **28**, 115–119.

Plum, F. and Posner, J. B. (1982). The diagnosis of stupor and coma. *Contemporary Neurology Series*, edition 3.

Quincy, J. (1719). *Lexicon physico-medicum*. Bell, Taylor and Osborn, London.

Rockwood K. (1993) The occurrence and duration of symptoms in elderly patients with delirium. *Journal of Gerontology*, **48**, M162–M166.

Rockwood K., Cosway S., Carver D., Jarrett P., Stadnyk K., and Fisk J. (1999). The risk of dementia and death after delirium. *Age and Ageing*, **28**, 551–556.

Searle, J. R. (1992). *The rediscovery of them*. MIT Press, Cambridge, MA.

Stuss DT, Piction TW, and Alexander MP. (2001). Consciousness, self-awareness, and the frontal lobes. In: *The Frontal Lobes and Neuropsychiatric Illness* (eds S. P. Salloway, P. F. Malloy, and J. D. Duffy), pp. 101–109. American Psychiatric Publishing, Inc., Washington, DC.

Treloar, A. and Macdonald, A. (1997a). Outcome of delirium: part 1. Outcome of delirium diagnosed by DSM-III-R, ICD-10 and CAMDEX and derivation of the Reversible Cognitive Dysfunction Scale among acute geriatric in-patients. *International Journal of Geriatric Psychiatry*, **12**, 609–613.

Treloar, A. and Macdonald, A. (1997b). Outcome of delirium: part 2. Clinical features of reversible cognitive dysfunction – are they the same as accepted definitions of delirium? *International Journal of Geriatric Psychiatry*, **12**, 614–618.

Trzepacz P. T. (1999). Update on the neuropathogenesis of delirium. *Dementia and Geriatric Cognitive Disorders*, **10**, 330–334.

Trzepacz, P. T. and Dew, M. A. (1995). Further analyses of the Delirium Rating Scale. *General Hospital Psychiatry*, **17**, 75–79.

Victor, M. and Adams, R. D. (1962). The acute confusional states. In: *Principles of internal medicine* (eds T. R. Harrison *et al.*). McGraw-Hill, New York.

Worcester, W. L. (1889). Delirium. *American Journal of Insanity*, **46**, 22–27.

World Health Organization (1993). *The ICD-10 classification of mental and behavioural disorders. Diagnostic criteria for research*. World Health Organization, Geneva.

Chapter 2

The instrumentation of delirium

Barbro Robertsson

Systematic observation and recording of behaviour and symptoms are important and necessary both in clinical practice and in research. In clinical practice, assessment instruments facilitate the detection of certain symptoms that may indicate an underlying brain disorder. Such instruments may also generate communicable symptom characterizations that are useful in the diagnostic process, in planning for the care of the patient, in evaluating the effect of interventions, and in education.

In delirium research there is a need for easy methods for identifying patients with delirium, for specified operationalizations of diagnostic criteria, and for methods of measuring severity of the disorder, preferably methods that generate numerical values. Systematic collection of information on behaviour is required, for instance for the diagnostic work-up. Systematic measurement of severity of the disorder is required, for instance for evaluation of treatment efficacy. Different kinds of instruments are needed for different purposes in the evaluation of delirium: screening instruments, diagnostic instruments, and instruments for measuring severity of delirium for evaluation of treatment efficacy.

Diagnostic manuals

The most commonly used standardized instruments for evaluation of delirium in clinical practice and research are the sets of diagnostic criteria in the current versions of the *Diagnostic and Statistical Manual of Mental Disorders* (DSM-IV) (American Psychiatric Association 1994) and the *International Classification of Diseases* (ICD-10)(World Health Organization 1993). The history and development of the different versions of these manuals are discussed in Chapter 1. These sets of criteria are summaries or syntheses of expert opinion and experience, and may be considered as assessment instruments in themselves. They constitute definitions and specifications of delirium, i.e. they are operationalizations of the concept of delirium.

Requirements

The most important requirement for these definitions or operationalizations is that they describe what we actually mean by delirium, in all its manifestations. Furthermore, they must be easily understandable and have sufficient precision. They must be applicable to the target group, including medically ill elderly individuals with impaired mental and psychomotor function. It must be possible to apply them at times and in situations where patients with suspected delirium are found. They must be useful in distinguishing delirium from dementia, depression, and psychosis. They have to 'balance the need to define a pure group for research purposes with the need to include cases of clinical interest' (Liptzin *et al.* 1991).

Advantages

As discussed in Chapter 1, these internationally accepted sets of diagnostic criteria have several advantages. They constitute guidelines for systematic diagnosis and contribute to clarity and consistency of approach in the diagnostic process worldwide. They facilitate communication and comparisons of research results across studies. One example in the field of delirium research is a study of postoperative delirium in elderly patients conducted in Taiwan by a Chinese research group (Chan and Brennan 1999). The patients were diagnosed according to DSM-IV and therefore the findings can easily be compared with findings from similar studies elsewhere.

Limitations

There are also limitations to this approach to diagnosis. These elaborated sets of criteria for delirium may give us a false impression of precision. In fact, a certain amount of subjective interpretation, operationalization, and application is unavoidable when using them. This is often no great problem in clinical practice. There may be problems, however, when two different sets of criteria are applied 'strictly'. In one study, different numbers of patients and partly different patients were identified as delirious by DSM-III and ICD-10 (Liptzin *et al.* 1991). According to the investigators, the DSM-III criteria were the most inclusive and the ICD-10 research criteria were 'overly restricted'. On the other hand, when the DSM-IV criteria were applied retrospectively to a group of patients diagnosed as delirious according to the third revised revision of the same manual (DSM-III-R), the investigators stated that 'in no case would the diagnosis have changed' (Rolfson *et al.* 1999).

These criteria are guidelines only, and the operationalizations, for example in DSM-IV, are often insufficiently specified. It is not quite clear how to employ these criteria for disturbances such as attentional deficits, cognitive change, and perceptual disturbances, especially in patients with other concurrent disorders. Furthermore, the degree of impairment necessary for a diagnosis is not specified. How to distinguish between delirium and dementia is not quite clear in all cases. Demented patients with delirium will not always be detected by the DSM-IV criteria. 'The utility of these criteria depends on the ability of clinicians and researchers to employ them consistently and in a variety of settings', and in research it must at least be described how and by whom the diagnostic criteria were applied (Gottlieb *et al.* 1991). On the other hand, every further specification implies restrictions. 'Delirium is a clinical diagnosis, some disagreement is common' (Rockwood *et al.* 1994). No set of criteria can yet take the place of experienced clinicians.

Delirium – a richly varied syndrome

The definition of delirium and the development of diagnostic criteria for delirium are complicated by the fact that delirium is a richly varied syndrome, which often coexists with other mental or somatic disorders with various symptoms. Furthermore, symptoms fluctuate between minutes and between days. There are no known biological markers for the syndrome and therefore the diagnosis must rely on clinical symptoms. Similar symptoms appear in other mental disorders, for instance psychosis, depression, and dementia. Delirium is common in dementia. It is more common in late-onset Alzheimer's disease and vascular dementia than in early-onset Alzheimer's disease and frontal lobe dementia (Robertsson *et al.* 1998). The symptoms of these dementia disorders vary, and superimposed delirium manifests itself differently. The differential diagnosis between dementia and delirium will thus vary with the presenting symptoms of dementia. Language disturbance will be harder to detect in a patient with sensory aphasia. Attentional deficits will be hard to distinguish from the disturbed motivation and concentration difficulties seen in frontal lobe dementia or from the slowness of thought seen in subcortical vascular dementia. The difficulties in distinguishing between dementia and delirium tend to increase with the severity of the dementia. In severe dementia the boundaries between dementia and delirium are almost erased.

Auxiliary instruments

The DSM and ICD criteria for delirium can be regarded as the first step of defining and operationalizing the concept of delirium. On many occasions and in many settings these criteria are not sufficient to identify patients with delirium and follow the course of the disorder. Other means of assistance are needed to more carefully investigate mental function and improve diagnostic efficiency both in clinical practice and in research. Instruments such as tests, questionnaires, structured interviews, observer's rating scales, checklists, and visual analogue scales are some types of instruments used. Instruments can be classified in a number of ways: for example, the size, appearance, and structure of the scale; the user; the purpose; and the degree of participation by the patient.

Scale structure

The number of items of a scale does not always determine the duration of the assessment or the workload imposed on the patient and the rater. The structure of the scale is more important. Every item is a small scale in itself and items and their scale points can be more or less well defined. Tests, in this context, are scales that include exact instructions on how to present each question or task for the patient, and how to score the patient's answer to a specific test item or his/her performance on a special task. Low test scores do not necessarily reflect cognitive impairment; they may be attributable to hearing or visual impairment, speech disabilities, or aphasia. Thus, cognitive tests need to be supplemented with other instruments or judgements. Scales may comprise a list of questions to the patient or a list of observations that the rater should make, or both. Simple items rate one aspect of behaviour, whereas more complex items require several questions to the patient and observation of his/her behaviour in diverse situations before they can be scored. Some items have only two scale steps, for instance present/not present. Other items have several more or less well-defined scale steps with points that usually have numbers to be used for scoring. Many scales mix different types of items.

Validity and reliability

The validity and reliability of an instrument are, among other things, functions of the scale design, the structure of items and scale points, and the training and experience of the rater. As there are many different ways to calculate these measures of trustworthiness, it is often hard to compare different scales in this respect. Sometimes validity and reliability may partly be in contrast to each other. A scale with simple test items, exact instructions on how to put the questions to the patient, and how to score any answer may have excellent reliability but be less valid in measuring delirium in an elderly patient with multiple disorders. Another rating scale with vaguely defined scale steps may be valid in the hands of experienced geriatric psychiatrists but unreliable when used by less trained raters. On the other hand, good reliability is a prerequisite of good validity.

Use in clinical practice

The role of assessment instruments in clinical practice is manifold. As delirium is a common mental disorder in old age, it occurs in many different settings: emergency departments, postoperative care, general medical departments, psychiatric units, nursing homes, and in the community. The patient's rehabilitation and well-being in any setting is, among other things, dependent on whether delirium is detected and properly treated or not. Available time, resources, experience, and ability to notice changes in mental status vary in the different settings. In geriatric care with doctors and nurses used to mentally impaired elderly patients, there may be excessive tolerance of behavioural disturbances, especially in demented patients. These behavioural disturbances may be symptoms of delirium. Assessment instruments can be good reminders of what should be looked for in order to detect the symptoms of delirium. In an emergency department the detection of cases of delirium increased markedly after a very simple mental checklist had been added to the routinely used assessment instruments (Elie *et al.* 2000).

Both screening and diagnostic instruments are useful in clinical practice. Screening instruments are less comprehensive, take less time to administer, and mostly require less experience of the rater. They should have good sensitivity, but may have less specificity for delirium. Scales for rating severity are of value when following the course of delirium and evaluating the effects of actions taken.

Psychiatrists usually have their favourite formal brief cognitive test when examining mental status. A short interview of the patient, test scores, observation of the patient doing the test, and an interview with the staff or a relative of the patient are often the basis for the diagnosis of delirium in clinical practice. This presupposes, however, sufficient time, resources and experience. Physicians less experienced in psychiatry and geriatrics may need instruments for the simple screening of all vulnerable patients. Patients positive on the screening test can then be examined further. A rating scale or a symptom checklist and a brief cognitive test are indispensable as a part of all status examinations of elderly patients. The results of the formal assessment or testing must be interpreted and balanced against other sources of information.

Special instruments have been developed by and for nurses. It has been claimed that other instruments lack 'necessary clinical nursing utility', whereas one such special instrument 'addresses a phenomenon of direct clinical nursing relevance' (Vermeersch 1990). Furthermore, 'standard mental status screening instruments which require a patient to respond to specific questions or commands, are limited in their usefulness for bedside assessment of acutely ill older patients…observation of a patient's behaviour has been the core of nursing assessment of mental status, but this is often not systematic or consistent' (Neelon *et al.* 1996). It has also been found that nurses often fail to notice cognitive disorders, and that notes on patients with cognitive impairment even could be more positive with words such as 'oriented' and positive terms related to self-care and social interaction (Palmateer and McCartney 1985). Nurses sometimes fail to make notes on behaviour that is not considered sufficient to act on or does not require specific interventions (Vermeersch 1990). Nurses are more trained in understanding behaviour as a response to a social situation than in regarding it as a symptom of a disorder, or in 'putting behaviour together' into a syndrome. As no single behaviour is sufficient for the diagnosis of delirium, nurses will need guidelines on what to look for. When disruptive behaviour is recorded without taking the whole picture into account, the notes will be misleading and the patient may receive wrong treatment. Nurses are possibly more experienced in making the patient feel as comfortable as possible than in exposing the patient to intricate examination questions. Nevertheless, nurses should be able to make formal assessments of cognitive function (Foreman *et al.* 1996).

Use in research

The requirements for assessment instruments for delirium to be used in research are somewhat different from those intended for clinical practice. The demand for reproducibility in research necessitates that diagnosis and assessments of patients are made according to structured methods with known validity and reliability. In small studies, the investigator may see all intended patients and make a diagnosis using the DSM-IV or ICD-10 criteria, or any other diagnostic instrument. In more extensive studies research assistants or nurses screen intended patients and the physician sees selected patients to make the diagnosis. In large research studies, involving hundreds of patients in multiple research centres, research assistants rather than the investigator him/herself will see the patients and register symptoms of delirium and collect information from other sources using structured instruments. The investigator will then make the diagnosis according to settled criteria without seeing the patient. In still another model, research assistants or nurses by themselves make the diagnosis with the help of structured instruments.

Screening and diagnostic instruments contain items such as presumed cause of the disorder, onset, and course of symptoms. They are not appropriate for assessing severity of delirium or evaluating the efficacy of intervention. Special assessment instruments have been developed for these purposes. Scales measuring severity of delirium contain items for symptoms that contribute, preferably to the same extent, to the severity; the scores can then be added up to a total delirium score. With repeated measurements this score can also be used to evaluate treatment efficacy.

Choosing a scale

Before choosing an assessment instrument for a special clinical or research situation, several questions need to be asked:

- Who is going to use the scale?
- For what purpose?
- How much participation from the patient is required?
- How much time will the assessment take?
- How much training of the rater is needed?
- How much interpretation of behaviour is needed?

Screening and diagnostic instruments

The following selection of assessment instruments has been guided by the author's opinion of their usefulness in different settings. There are a number of other scales for delirium evaluation. For the interested reader, there are two comprehensive reviews of various types of assessment instruments for delirium that describe more scales and more scale characteristics than those presented here. The sensitivity and specificity of 12 diagnostic scales have been summarized by Trzepacz (1994), and Smith *et al.* (1995) have examined 20 delirium evaluation instruments for validity, reliability, and ease and speed of administration in delirious patients.

Brief cognitive tests

Among the best-known brief cognitive tests used as instruments for delirium evaluation are the Mini-Mental State Examination (MMSE) (Folstein *et al.* 1975; Katzman *et al.* 1983), the Short Portable Mental Status Questionnaire (SPMSQ) (Pfeiffer 1975; Katzman *et al.* 1983), the Mental Status Questionnaire (MSQ) (Kahn *et al.* 1960;

Katzman *et al.* 1983), the Blessed Orientation-Memory-Concentration Test (Katzman *et al.* 1983), the Trail Making Test (Katzman *et al.* 1983; Lezak 1983), and the Clock Drawing Test (Katzman *et al.* 1983; Sunderland *et al.* 1989). These are quite easy to administer, and include precise instructions on how to score the patient's answers to the individual specific test questions or his/her performance on special tasks. They assess different aspects of cognitive function and generate a score that is considered to be a marker for cognitive impairment. This impairment may be a symptom of delirium, dementia, or any other mental disorder influencing cognitive function. Thus these instruments are used for screening for cognitive impairment, but they may also provide information for the diagnostic process or when completing observation rating scales.

The Delirium Rating Scale (DRS)

The DRS was developed as 'an adjunct to the DSM-III diagnostic criteria for delirium' (Trzepacz *et al.* 1988). The DRS comprises ten items: temporal onset of symptoms, perceptual disturbances, hallucination type, delusions, psychomotor behaviour, cognitive status during formal testing, physical disorder, sleep–wake cycle disturbance, lability of mood and variability of symptoms. Items of inattention and disorganized thinking, which are usually regarded as essential features of delirium, are not included, 'because of vague and varying definitions of these terms' (Trzepacz 1994). Items are rated on 2-, 3-, or 4-point scales. The scale is intended for use in conjunction with standardized cognitive tests chosen by the rater. Scores on the DRS items are summed to give a total score ranging from 0 to 32. The recommended cut-off score for the DRS is 12 points (Trzepacz 1999). The scale is recommended for use both clinically and in research. It was originally intended to be used by psychiatrists, but its sensitivity and specificity have been shown to be equally high when used by physicians and non-doctors (Rosen *et al.* 1994; Trzepacz *et al.* 1998).

DRS has been used in phenomenological studies of subtypes of delirium (Rockwood 1993; Meagher *et al.* 1996), in a study of symptoms in at-risk patients (DiMartini *et al.* 1991), in studies of outcome (Wada and Yamaguchi 1993; Rudberg *et al.* 1997), and in intervention studies (Rockwood *et al.* 1994; Meagher *et al.* 1996; Uchiyama *et al.* 1996; Sipahimalani and Masand 1998). When repeated measurements are needed, an adapted scale, omitting items of onset, fluctuation, and cause, has been used by some researchers (Koolhoven *et al.* 1996; Uchiyama *et al.* 1996). The DRS has been translated from English into at least seven languages. The scale has been revised (DRS-R-98), to enhance its use as a severity rating scale (Trzepacz 1999). A recent validation study has found this revision to have good sensitivity, specificity, inter-rater reliability, and internal consistency (Trzepacz *et al.* 2001).

Since the items are of widely differing nature, the total score does not seem quite meaningful as a measure of severity. It has been suggested that the total score should be regarded as a measure of the 'diagnostic certainty' rather than as a measure of severity of the disorder (Smith *et al.* 1995).

The Confusion Assessment method (CAM)

The CAM (Inouye *et al.* 1990) is a screening instrument that was devised to 'enable nonpsychiatrically trained clinicians to identify delirium quickly and accurately in both clinical and research settings'. It has two versions with nine and four items, respectively. The first version consists of nine operationalized DSM-III-R criteria. Four features – acute onset and fluctuating course, inattention, disorganized thinking, and altered level of consciousness – are considered 'cardinal elements' of the DSM-III-R criteria and constitute the CAM algorithm. Presence of both the first and the second criteria and of either the third or the fourth criterion are required for a diagnosis of delirium. If only the algorithm is used, CAM is a rapid and easily administered diagnostic instrument.

For the clinical setting, the designer of CAM has recommended that all patients with a diagnosis of delirium according to this instrument should receive further evaluation to confirm the diagnosis. She also points out that delirium superimposed on dementia is a particularly complex problem. 'Greater specification or alternate diagnostic criteria may be required for this group'.

In research, the CAM has been used to study the occurrence of delirium in various different settings (Patten *et al.* 1997; Elie *et al.* 2000; Gagnon *et al.* 2000). It has been used to diagnose delirium in a number of studies of risk factors for delirium (Marcantonio *et al.* 1994, 1998, 2000; Fisher and Flowerdew 1995; Inouye and Charpentier 1996; Inouye 1998; Lynch *et al.* 1998; Brauer *et al.* 2000), in pathogenetic studies (Flacker *et al.* 1998; Mussi *et al.* 1999), in studies aimed at improving recognition of delirium and preventing misdiagnosing in emergency department patients (Lewis *et al.* 1995; Elie *et al.* 2000), in studies of advanced cancer patients (Gagnon *et al.* 2000) and of medically ill elderly patients (Farrell and Ganzini 1995). In most cases, the CAM seems to be the only diagnostic instrument used, but in some cases a structured interview (Marcantonio *et al.* 1994; Lewis *et al.* 1995) or other instruments, for instance the Delirium Symptom Interview (Patten *et al.* 1997) and the Confusion Rating Scale (Gagnon *et al.* 2000), were used to record symptoms.

In most studies, the CAM has been administered by physicians, but nurses and 'study personnel' have also been reported as raters (Marcantonio *et al.* 1994; Rockwood *et al.* 1994; Fisher and Flowerdew 1995; Rolfson *et al.* 1999). The nurses' CAM interview in a study by Fischer and co-workers (Fisher and Flowerdew 1995) had high sensitivity. On the other hand, Rockwood *et al.* (1994) and Rolfson *et al.* (1999) found that the CAM performed poorly as a screening instrument for delirium when administered by non-physicians. They concluded that there is a need for training in the use of the CAM, especially by non-physicians. Nurses showed a superior ability to record features of delirium but seemed to be less trained in regarding behaviour as symptoms of a mental disorder. This is probably a more general problem, which cannot be attributable to the design of the CAM.

The CAM is probably the most useful, rapid and easily administered screening instrument for delirium in different settings, provided that it is handled by a rater who knows how to assess cognitive function. Validations of the scale in other languages are now being published (e.g. Fabbri *et al.* 2001).

The Delirium Assessment Scale (DAS)

The DAS (O'Keeffe 1994), developed to 'determine the severity of delirium symptoms', has three parts:

- questions to the patient
- observations of behaviour and
- questions to nursing and medical staff.

The first part contains 15 test items, principally from the MMSE and Digit Span, which cover orientation, memory, and attention, and one question to the patient about perceptual disturbances. In the second part, psychomotor activity, coherence of speech, fluctuations of symptoms, and global accessibility are rated. In the last part, the investigator is asked to rate psychomotor activity, fluctuations of symptoms, and sleep–wake cycle pattern. Several of the items in the observation part have scores ranging from 0 to 3, and are derived from the Brief Psychiatric Rating Scale (Overall and Gorham 1962) or from instruments adapted by Gottlieb *et al.* (1991), whereas other items are original. Several test items of attentiveness are included, but scores on attentiveness are not included in the summation, merely taken into account when making the global judgement. In a later study, the designer showed a significant correlation between global judgement of attention and scores on attention (O'Keeffe and Gosney 1997).

The Saskatoon Delirium Checklist (SDC)

The SDC was developed 'from the DSM-III criteria for delirium to give numerical rating score (40 = unimpaired and 0 = maximal delirium)' (Miller *et al.* 1988). Nine of the DSM-III criteria are rated according to how often each symptom is observed (never, very rarely, sometimes, usually, and always: scored 4–0). In an additional item, physical cause of the symptoms is rated. The scale is thus diagnostic and the scores indicate the certainty of the diagnosis rather than the severity of delirium. In the original study, the scale was used to establish differences in mental status between patients given low doses of scopolamine and those given placebo as pre-surgery medication (Miller *et al.* 1988). In another study, the scale was used to examine the incidence of postoperative delirium after cardiac surgery (Hofste *et al.* 1997). No studies of its validity or reliability have yet been published.

The Delirium Symptom Interview (DSI)

The DSI (Albert *et al.* 1992) is an extensive operationalization of the DSM-III criteria. It contains about 60 questions for the patient to answer, among them questions about his/her subjective experience of symptoms, and around 50 items where the rater's observation of behaviour is the basis for scoring. Scores range from 0 to 4 (e.g. no, mild, moderate, and severe, or never, rarely, sometimes, and frequently) in most of the observational items. Scores are not used as numerical values, and no sum is calculated. A comprehensive manual with exact instructions on how to score is available. The interview can be administered by non-clinicians, even lay interviewers. In combination with other data, it can, for instance, be used by researchers in large-scale epidemiological studies to define cases of delirium (Levkoff *et al.* 1992). Even if the scale was developed from DSM-III criteria, it can probably be adapted to any classification system. It has been used in connection with the DSM-III-R (Levkoff *et al.* 1992), in connection with the CAM (Patten *et al.* 1997; Flacker *et al.* 1998; Marcantonio *et al.* 2000), and in identifying delirium subtypes (Liptzin and Levkoff 1992). The disadvantages of relying on the patient's answers to structured direct questions to interpret his/her behaviour are partly counterbalanced by the presence of observational items.

The Organic Brain Syndrome (OBS) scale

The delirium subscale of the OBS scale is another instrument for the registration of symptoms of delirium by research assistants. In contrast to the DSI, it is an observer-rated scale with 39 items (Jensen *et al.* 1993). Scores range from 0 to 3 according to severity and/or frequency of behaviour. It has been used in studies of the prevalence of delirium in different care settings (Sandberg *et al.* 1998) and in studies of postoperative delirium (Edlund *et al.* 1999). In these studies, symptoms registered by research assistants were the basis for delirium diagnoses according to DSM-III and DSM-III-R criteria. The validity and inter-rater reliability of the OBS scale have not been reported.

The Confusion Rating Scale (CRS)

The CRS was developed for use by nurses as a screening instrument for finding cases with suspected delirium (Williams *et al.* 1988). The scale has one observational item for each of four domains:

- disorientation to place, time or recognition of persons;
- communication unrelated/inappropriate to the situation or unusual for the person, or lack of communication;
- behaviours inappropriate to the situation; and
- the presence of illusions of hallucinations.

Observable behaviour is rated as not present, present but mild, or present and pronounced (0–2) during each of the nurse's eight-hour shifts, giving a score of 0–8 for each shift. One study suggested that a total score of at least two indicates that a patient is screen-positive (Gagnon *et al.* 2000). In this study, patients positive on screening with the CRS received further diagnostic evaluation. Used by trained nurses, the CRS may be useful as a clinical screening instrument. It could be seen as 'guidelines on what to look for' (Williams *et al.* 1988), though it does not take into account symptoms of disturbed attention and consciousness or fluctuations in symptoms. It has been estimated to be 'the only delirium screening instrument that does not require patient participation, and can easily be integrated into routine care' (Gagnon *et al.* 2000). The low cut-off point was used to maximize the sensitivity of the scale.

Clinical Assessment of Confusion-A (CAC-A)

Another observation rating scale developed for use by nurses is the CAC-A (Vermeersch 1990). It contains 25 items comprising five dimensions: cognition, general behaviour, motor activity, orientation, and psychotic behaviour. Each symptom is rated as present or not present and each item has a weight of 2, 3, or 4. Scores are summed and the maximum total score is 77. As is pointed out by the designer of the scale, raters may have problems with how to record intermittent behaviour or variations in severity. None of the symptoms rated is actually specific to delirium. The CAC-A cannot distinguish between dementia and delirium. Thus other sources of information are necessary to assess delirium. The scale has been used as a screening instrument (Culp *et al.* 1997) and in revised form in a study of postoperative delirium (Rateau 2000).

The Neecham Confusion Scale (NCS)

The NCS (Neelon *et al.* 1996) was developed for use by nurses for rapid assessment, especially of early behavioural and physiological cues of symptoms of delirium. It has three subscales – processing, behaviour, and physiological control – each with three items. The items in the processing subscale are attention, ability to follow command, and orientation. The items of behaviour are appearance, motor and verbal behaviour. The third subscale assesses physiological stability in vital functions, oxygen saturation stability and urinary continence control. Scores range from 0 to 2, 4 or 5 in the items of the processing and behaviour subscales and from 0 to 2 in the items of the physiological control subscale. Scores are summed up for the whole scale and a maximum of 30 can be reached. Zero indicates most severe confusion and 30 normal function. A cut-off score of 24 has been suggested for confusion. The observer's rating of cognitive processing on items of attention and recognition is almost unique to this scale. In many scales, rating of attention is omitted because of the vague and varying definition of terms.

The items of physiological control make the scale limited in its application. For example, in many clinical settings it is not practicable to measure oxygen saturation. The scale has been used in studies of postoperative delirium (Jagmin 1998) and of the incidence of delirium in general hospitals (Wakefield 1996; Crawley 1998).

Scales measuring severity

The Confusional State Evaluation (CSE)

The CSE was developed as an instrument for assessing delirium severity, particularly in elderly people (Robertsson *et al.* 1997). In addition, the instrument could be used to measure changes of symptoms over time to evaluate the effects of interventions. It should primarily be regarded as a tool for measuring the severity of the disorder, not as a diagnostic tool replacing the judgment of an experienced and skilled clinician. It is an observer-rated scale, comprehensive enough to cover all important symptoms and brief enough for the ratings to be completed in a maximum of half an hour by a trained nurse, psychologist, or physician. It is applicable to delirium in demented patients, as well as to an acute confusional state in previously mentally unimpaired people (Robertsson 1999).

The CSE contains 22 items, 12 of which measure 'key symptoms' (disorientation to person, time, space, and situation, thought and memory disturbances, disability to concentrate, distractibility, perseveration, impaired contact, paranoid delusions, and hallucinations). The sum of the scores from these items gives the 'confusion score'. Seven items deal with symptoms occurring frequently with delirium: irritability, emotional lability, wakefulness disturbance, increased psychomotor activity, reduced psychomotor activity, mental uneasiness and disturbance of the sleep–wake pattern. Three items relate to the duration and intensity of the episode of delirium.

All the items are defined in an introductory note stating how to assess and what to assess. The items of the scale have been created to identify the particular impairment in mental functioning that is introduced by confusion rather than by dementia. For instance, disorientation to time refers primarily to the awareness of the time of day rather than the actual year, month, or date. There are five well-defined scale steps for each item with undefined half-steps in between.

The CSE is designed for used by trained nurses, physicians, and psychologists. It is essential that the rater have a good knowledge of dementia and delirium in the elderly. Detailed instructions, as well as training sessions with patients before the clinical use of the rating scale, are necessary. Inter-rater reliability and validity of the CSE have been studied and found to be satisfactory. Sensitivity to change over time and symptom profiles have also been studied (Robertsson *et al.* 1997). Study of the application of the CSE in pharmacological studies following patients daily and weekly is currently in progress.

The Memorial Delirium Assessment Scale (MDAS)

The MDAS (Breitbart *et al.* 1997) has 10 items rating awareness, orientation, short-term memory, digit span, attention, thinking, perception, delusion, psychomotor activity, and sleep–wake cycle. Each item has four well-defined scale points (0–3) indicating none, mild, moderate, and severe disturbance. Three items are test items: disorientation, short-term-memory impairment, and impaired digit span. Scores on the other items are based on the rater's own observations of the patient's behaviour. The scores on all items are summed to make up a delirium index of symptom severity. The scale has been used in terminally ill cancer patients to assess severity of delirium (Lawlor *et al.* 2000). In the development of the scale it was used by experienced psychiatrists.

The Delirium Index (DI)

The DI (McCusker *et al.* 1998) is an instrument for evaluation of the severity of delirium. It comprises seven items, which are operationalizations of seven of nine items from the CAM, which in turn are operationalizations of the items in the DSM-III-R. The symptoms to be rated are inattention, disorganized thinking, altered level of consciousness, disorientation, memory impairment, perceptual disturbances, and psychomotor agitation or retardation. The scale is to be used in conjunction with the MMSE and at least the first five items of MMSE constitute the basis for the ratings on DI. Each item is rated on a four-point scale (0–3). Scores are summed and total scores range from 0 to 21. When items 1, 2, 4, and 5 are not assessable for a patient, the score on item 3 will be applied to all these items. This procedure considerably detracts from the validity of the scale.

In studies of reliability and validity, nurses, an occupational therapist, and geriatric psychiatrists used the scale satisfactorily after training (McCusker *et al.* 1998). This indicates that the scale may have a broad field of application. It is intended to monitor changes in severity over time in patients previously diagnosed with delirium.

The Delirium Severity Scale (DSS)

The DSS was developed to meet the requirements of 'an instrument to monitor delirium severity'. It 'would reflect the patient's clinical state at the time of the assessment, be repeatable over relatively short time periods, and be easy enough for use by a variety of health care professionals' (Bettin *et al.* 1998). It consists of two standard cognitive tests, Forward Digit Span and Similarities, selected from 13 tests as the most sensitive to changes in delirium severity. The maximum score for the current version of Forward Digit Span is 24 and the maximum score for Similarities is 35. The validity and reliability of the DSS were studied in non-demented patients with no aphasia, no history of mental illness and no significant hearing or visual impairment (Bettin *et al.* 1998). The DSS was shown to be a reliable and valid instrument in detecting changes in delirium symptoms in these patients and to have minimal floor and ceiling effects. However, the usefulness of the scale is limited, as the validity of the tests seems to presuppose a relatively healthy patient with almost no functional impairment other than delirium.

Recommendations

In clinical practice as well as in research, a combination of two or more instruments for assessing delirium is recommended. A brief cognitive test, a diagnostic tool and a severity scale may supply most demands. A protocol with three different instruments for diagnosing delirium, NCS, CAM, and MMSE, is proposed by Rapp *et al.* (2000) for use by nurses in clinical practice. The MMSE is not used for screening for delirium but provides information that enables the user to complete the CAM and NCS. When assessment of severity of delirium also is requested, a combination of CAM, MMSE, and CSE would be sufficient.

References

Albert, M. S., Levkoff, S. E., Reilly, C., *et al.* (1992). The delirium symptom interview: an interview for the detection of delirium symptoms in hospitalized patients. *Journal of Geriatric Psychiatry and Neurology*, 5, 14–21.

American Psychiatric Association. (1994). *Diagnostic and statistical manual of mental disorders*, 4th edn. American Psychiatric Association, Washington, DC.

Bettin, K. M., Maletta, G. J., Dysken, M. W., Jilk, K. M., Weldon, D. T., Kuskowski, M., and Mach, J. R., Jr (1998). Measuring delirium severity in older general hospital inpatients without dementia. The Delirium Severity Scale. *American Journal of Geriatric Psychiatry*, 6, 296–307.

Brauer, C., Morrison, R. S., Silberzweig, S. B., and Siu, A. L. (2000). The cause of delirium in patients with hip fracture. *Archives of Internal Medicine*, 160, 1856–1860.

Breitbart, W., Rosenfeld, B., Roth, A., Smith, M. J., Cohen, K., and Passik, S. (1997). The Memorial Delirium Assessment Scale. *Journal of Pain Symptom Management*, 13, 128–137.

Chan, D. and Brennan, N. J. (1999). Delirium: making the diagnosis, improving the prognosis. *Geriatrics*, 54, 28–30, 36, 39–42.

Crawley, E. J. and Miller, J. (1998) Best practice. Acute confusion among hospitalized elders in a rural hospital *MEDSURG Nursing*, 7, 199–206.

Culp, K., Tripp-Reimer, T., Wadle, K., *et al.* (1997). Screening for acute confusion in elderly long-term care residents. *Journal of Neuroscience Nursing*, 29, 86–88, 95–100.

DiMartini, A., Pajer, K., Trzepacz, P., Fung, J., Starzl, T., and Tringali, R. (1991). Psychiatric morbidity in liver transplant patients. *Transplant Proceedings*, 23, 3179–3180.

Edlund, A., Lundström, M., Lundström, G., Hedqvist, B., and Gustafson, Y. (1999). Clinical Profile of delirium in patients treated for femoral neck fractures. *Dementia and Geriatric Cognitive Disorders*, 10, 325–329.

Elie, M., Rousseau, F., Cole, M., Primeau, F., McCusker, J., and Bellavance, F. (2000). Prevalence and detection of delirium in elderly emergency department patients. *Canadian Medical Association Journal*, 163, 977–981.

Fabbri, R. M., Moreira, M. A., Garrido, R., and Almeida, O. P. (2001) Validity and reliability of the Portuguese version of the Confusion Assessment Method (CAM) for the detection of delirium in the elderly *Arg Neuropsiquiatr*, 59, 175–179.

Farrell, K. R. and Ganzini, L. (1995). Misdiagnosing delirium as depression in medically ill elderly patients. *Archives of Internal Medicine*, 155, 2459–2464.

Fisher, B. W. and Flowerdew, G. (1995). A simple model for predicting postoperative delirium in older patients undergoing elective orthopedic surgery. *Journal of the American Geriatrics Society*, 43, 175–178.

Flacker, J. M., Cummings, V., Mach, J. R., Jr, Bettin, K., Kiely, D. K., and Wei, J. (1998). The association of serum anticholinergic activity with delirium in elderly medical patients. *American Journal of Geriatric Psychiatry*, 6, 31–41.

Folstein, M. F., Folstein, S. E., and McHugh, P. R. (1975). 'Mini-Mental State'. A practical method for grading the cognitive state of patients for the clinician. *Journal of Psychiatric Research*, **12**, 189–198.

Foreman, M. D., Fletcher, K., Mion, L. C., and Simon, L. (1996). Assessing cognitive function. *Geriatric Nursing*, **17**, 228–232 (quiz: 233).

Gagnon, P., Allard, P., Masse, B., and DeSerres, M. (2000). Delirium in terminal cancer: a prospective study using daily screening, early diagnosis, and continuous monitoring. *Journal of Pain Symptom Management*, **19**, 412–426.

Gottlieb, G. L., Johnson, J., Wanich, C., and Sullivan, E. (1991). Delirium in the medically ill elderly: operationalizing the DSM-III criteria. *International Psychogeriatrics*, **3**, 181–196.

Hofste, W. J., Linssen, C. A., Boezeman, E. H., Hengeveld, J. S., Leusink, J. A., and de-Boer, A. (1997). Delirium and cognitive disorders after cardiac operations: relationship to pre- and intraoperative quantitative electroencephalogram. *International Journal of Clinical Monitoring and Computing*, **14**, 29–36.

Inouye, S. K. (1998). Delirium in hospitalized older patients: recognition and risk factors. *Geriatric Psychiatry and Neurology*, **11**, 118–125 (see also: Discussion, pp 157–158).

Inouye, S. K. and Charpentier, P. A. (1996). Precipitating factors for delirium in hospitalized elderly persons. Predictive model and interrelationship with baseline vulnerability. *Journal of the American Medical Association*, **275**, 852–857.

Inouye, S. K., van Dyck, C., Alessi, C. A., Balkin, S., Siegal, A. P., and Horwitz, R. I. (1990). Clarifying confusion: the confusion assessment method. A new method for detection of delirium: see comments. *Annals of Internal Medicine*, **113**, 941–948.

Jagmin, M. G. (1998). Postoperative mental status in elderly hip surgery patients. *Orthopedic Nursing*, **17**, 32–42.

Jensen, E., Dehlin, O., and Gustafson, L. (1993). A comparison between three psychogeriatric rating scales. *International Journal of Geriatric Psychiatry*, **8**, 215–229.

Kahn, R. L., Goldfarb, A. I., Pollack, M., and Peck, A. (1960). Brief objective measures for the determination of mental status in the aged. *American Journal of Psychiatry*, **117**, 326–328.

Katzman, R., Brown, T., Fuld, P., Peck, A., Schechter, R., and Schimmel, H. (1983). Validation of a short Orientation-Memory-Concentration Test of cognitive impairment. *American Journal of Psychiatry*, **140**, 734–739.

Koolhoven, I., Tjon, A. T. M. R., and van der Mast, R. C. (1996). Early diagnosis of delirium after cardiac surgery. *General Hospital Psychiatry*, **18**, 448–451.

Lawlor, P. G., Nekolaichuk, C., Gagnon, B., Mancini, I. L., Pereira, J. L., and Bruera, E. D. (2000). Clinical utility, factor analysis, and further validation of the memorial delirium assessment scale in patients with advanced cancer: assessing delirium in advanced cancer. *Cancer*, **88**, 2859–2867.

Levkoff, S. E., Evans, D. A., Liptzin, B., *et al.* (1992). Delirium. The occurrence and persistence of symptoms among elderly hospitalized patients. *Archives of Internal Medicine*, **152**, 334–340.

Lewis, L. M., Miller, D. K., Morley, J. E., Nork, M. J., and Lasater, L. C. (1995). Unrecognized delirium in ED geriatric patients. *American Journal of Emergency Medicine*, **13**, 142–145.

Lezak, M. D. (1983). *Neuropsychological assessment.* Oxford University Press, New York.

Liptzin, B. and Levkoff, S. E. (1992). An empirical study of delirium subtypes. *British Journal of Psychiatry*, **161**, 843–845.

Liptzin, B., Levkoff, S. E., Cleary, P. D., *et al.* (1991). An empirical study of diagnostic criteria for delirium. *American Journal of Psychiatry*, **148**, 454–457.

Lynch, E. P., Lazor, M. A., Gellis, J. E., Orav, J., Goldman, L., and Marcantonio, E. R. (1998). The impact of postoperative pain on the development of postoperative delirium. *Anesthesia and Analgesia*, **86**, 781–785.

Marcantonio, E. R., Goldman, L., Mangione, C. M., *et al.* (1994). A clinical prediction rule for delirium after elective noncardiac surgery. *Journal of the American Medical Association*, **271**, 134–139.

Marcantonio, E. R., Goldman, L., Orav, E. J., Cook, E. F., and Lee, T. H. (1998). The association of intraoperative factors with the development of postoperative delirium. *American Journal of Medicine*, **105**, 380–384.

Marcantonio, E. R., Flacker, J. M., Michaels, M., and Resnick, N. M. (2000). Delirium is independently associated with poor functional recovery after hip fracture. *Journal of the American Geriatrics Society*, **48**, 618–624.

McCusker, J., Cole, M., Bellavance, F., and Primeau, F. (1998). Reliability and validity of a new measure of severity of delirium. *International Psychogeriatrics*, **10**, 421–433.

Meagher, D. J., O'Hanlon, D., O'Mahony, E., and Casey, P. R. (1996). The use of environmental strategies and psychotropic medication in the management of delirium. *British Journal of Psychiatry*, **168**, 512–515.

Miller, P. S., Richardson, J. S., Jyu, C. A., Lemay, J. S., Hiscock, M., and Keegan, D. L. (1988). Association of low serum anticholinergic levels and cognitive impairment in elderly presurgical patients. *American Journal of Psychiatry*, **145**, 342–345.

Mussi, C., Ferrari, R., Ascari, S., and Salvioli, G. (1999). Importance of serum anticholinergic activity in the assessment of elderly patients with delirium. *Journal of Geriatric Psychiatry and Neurology*, **12**, 82–86.

Neelon, V. J., Champagne, M. T., Carlson, J. R., and Funk, S. G. (1996). The NEECHAM Confusion Scale: construction, validation, and clinical testing. *Nursing Research*, **45**, 324–330.

O'Keeffe, S. T. (1994). Rating the severity of delirium: the delirium assessment scale. *International Journal of Geriatric Psychiatry*, **9**, 551–556.

O'Keeffe, S. T. and Gosney, M. A. (1997). Assessing attentiveness in older hospital patients: global assessment versus tests of attention. *Journal of the American Geriatrics Society*, **45**, 470–473.

Overall, J. and Gorham, D. (1962). The Brief Psychiatric Rating Scale. *Psychological Reports*, **10**, 799–812.

Palmateer, L. M. and McCartney, J. R. (1985). Do nurses know when patients have cognitive deficits? *Journal of Gerontological Nursing*, **11**, 6–7, 10–12, 15–16.

Patten, S. B., Williams, J. V., Haynes, L., McCruden, J., and Arboleda-Florez, J. (1997). The incidence of delirium in psychiatric inpatient units. *Canadian Journal of Psychiatry*, **42**, 858–863.

Pfeiffer, E. (1975). A short portable mental status questionnaire for the assessment of organic brain deficit in elderly patients. *Journal of the American Geriatrics Society*, **23**, 433–441.

Rapp, C. G., Wakefield, B., Kundrat, M., *et al.* (2000). Acute confusion assessment instruments: clinical versus research usability. *Applied Nursing Research*, **13**, 37–45.

Rateau, M. R. (2000). Confusion and aggression in restrained elderly persons undergoing hip repair surgery. *Applied Nursing Research*, **13**, 50–54.

Robertsson, B. (1999). Assessment scales in delirium. *Dementia and Geriatric Cognitive Disorders*, **10**, 368–379.

Robertsson, B., Karlsson, I., Styrud, E., and Gottfries, C. G. (1997). Confusional State Evaluation (CSE): an instrument for measuring severity of delirium in the elderly. *British Journal of Psychiatry*, **170**, 565–570.

Robertsson, B., Blennow, K., Gottfries, C. G., and Wallin, A. (1998). Delirium in dementia. *International Journal of Geriatric Psychiatry*, **13**, 49–56.

Rockwood, K. (1993). The occurrence and duration of symptoms in elderly patients with delirium. *Journal of Gerontology*, **48**, M162–M166.

Rockwood, K., Cosway, S., Stolee, P., *et al.* (1994). Increasing the recognition of delirium in elderly patients. *Journal of the American Geriatrics Society*, **42**, 252–256.

Rolfson, D. B., McElhaney, J. E., Jhangri, G. S., and Rockwood, K. (1999). Validity of the confusion assessment method in detecting postoperative delirium in the elderly. *International Psychogeriatrics*, **11**, 431–438.

Rosen, J., Sweet, R. A., Mulsant, B. H., Rifai, A. H., Pasternak, R., and Zubenko, G. S. (1994). The delirium rating scale in a psychogeriatric inpatient setting. *Journal of Neuropsychiatry and Clinical Neuroscience*, **6**, 30–35.

Rudberg, M. A., Pompei, P., Foreman, M. D., Ross, R. E., and Cassel, C. K. (1997). The natural history of delirium in older hospitalized patients: a syndrome of heterogeneity. *Age and Ageing*, **26**, 169–174.

Sandberg, O., Gustafson, Y., Brännström, B., and Bucht, G. (1998). Prevalence of dementia, delirium and psychiatric symptoms in various care settings for the elderly. *Scandinavian Journal of Social Medicine*, **26**, 56–62.

Sipahimalani, A. and Masand, P. S. (1998). Olanzapine in the treatment of delirium. *Psychosomatics*, **39**, 422–430.

Smith, M. J., Breitbart, W. S., and Platt, M. M. (1995). A critique of instruments and methods to detect, diagnose, and rate delirium. *Journal of Pain Symptom Management*, **10**, 35–77.

Sunderland, T., Hill, J. L., Mellow, A. M., *et al.* (1989). Clock drawing in Alzheimer's disease. A novel measure of dementia severity. *Journal of the American Geriatrics Society*, **37**, 725–729.

Trzepacz, P. T. (1994). A review of delirium assessment instruments. *General Hospital Psychiatry*, **16**, 397–405.

Trzepacz, P. T. (1999). The Delirium Rating Scale. Its use in consultation-liaison research. *Psychosomatics*, **40**, 193–204.

Trzepacz, P. T., Baker, R. W., and Greenhouse, J. (1988). A symptom rating scale for delirium. *Psychiatry Research*, **23**, 89–97.

Trzepacz, P. T., Mulsant, B. H., Amanda Dew, M., Pasternak, R., Sweet, R. A., and Zubenko, G. S. (1998). Is delirium different when it occurs in dementia? A study using the delirium rating scale. *Journal of Neuropsychiatry and Clinical Neuroscience*, **10**, 199–204.

Trzepacz, P. T., Mittal, D., Torres, R., Kanary, K., Norton, J., and Jimerson, N. (2001). Validation of the Delirium Rating Scale-revised-98: comparison with the delirium rating scale and the cognitive test for delirium. *J. Neuropsychiatry Clin Neurosci*, **13**, 229–242.

Uchiyama, M., Tanaka, K., Isse, K., and Toru, M. (1996). Efficacy of mianserin on symptoms of delirium in the aged: an open trial study. *Progress in Neuropsychopharmacological and Biological Psychiatry*, **20**, 651–656.

Vermeersch, P. E. (1990). The clinical assessment of confusion. *Applied Nursing Research*, **3**, 128–133.

Wada, Y. and Yamaguchi, N. (1993). Delirium in the elderly: relationship of clinical symptoms to outcome. *Dementia*, **4**, 113–116.

Wakefield, B. J. R. (1996). In *Prevalence, incidence, risk factors and short-term outcomes for hospitalized elderly patients experiencing acute confusion*. Doctoral-dissertation; research, The University of Iowa, p. 207.

Williams, M. A., Ward, S. E., and Campbell, E. B. (1988). Confusion: testing versus observation. *Journal of Gerontological Nursing*, **14**, 25–30.

World Health Organization (1993). *The ICD-10 classification of mental and behavioural disorders. Diagnostic criteria for research*. World Health Organization, Geneva.

Chapter 3

The epidemiology of delirium

James Lindesay, Kenneth Rockwood, and
Darryl Rolfson

The purposes of epidemiological research are to describe and define disorders; to provide prevalence and incidence rates to inform service development and evaluation; and to identify aetiological factors. To date, most epidemiological studies of delirium in old age have been carried out in medical and surgical in-patients, and have focused on estimating its prevalence and incidence in these settings, identifying significant risk factors, and evaluating its impact upon outcomes. The picture that emerges from these studies is not a consistent one; in particular, the estimated prevalence and incidence rates vary considerably between studies. This is due to a number of conceptual and methodological issues that need to be borne in mind when interpreting these data: case definition, case finding, selection bias, and differences in the populations being studied.

Case definition

The conceptual and definitional difficulties associated with delirium have been a significant obstacle to all forms of research into this disorder. The development of rule-oriented diagnostic criteria such as the *International Classification of Diseases* (ICD-10; World Health Organization 1992) and the *Diagnostic and Statistical Manual of Mental Disorders* (DSM-III, DSM-III-R, DSM-IV: American Psychiatric Association 1980, 1987, 1994) over the last two decades has provided a basis for the reliability (if not validity) of diagnosis and for a degree of comparability between studies. However, there are some important differences between these classifications so far as the essential criteria for delirium are concerned, and they do not always agree regarding case definition (Lipsitz *et al.* 1991). Within the DSM and ICD diagnostic systems, the diagnostic criteria for delirium have changed significantly over time, so studies using one version will not be directly comparable with those using another. These diagnostic systems are all more restrictive than clinical diagnosis, and study populations using these criteria will tend to exclude patients with emerging, resolving or partial delirium syndromes (Levkoff *et al.* 1992). Another problem is that they do not yet provide criteria for distinguishing between delirium and the recently described condition of Lewy body dementia (McKeith *et al.* 1996; Ballard and McKeith 1998). Regarding the hyper-active and hypoactive subtypes of delirium [for which the case has been made that out-comes are different (O'Keeffe 1999)], current diagnostic systems do not distinguish between these, and consequently there is little evidence available on relative frequency.

That a study has used a system of diagnostic criteria to identify cases of delirium does not of itself guarantee diagnostic consistency or reproducibility; as Johnson *et al.* (1990) point out, researchers also need to be explicit about how they have applied these criteria, either by describing the observations used to establish whether or not they were met, or by the use of one of the structured assessment instruments that have been validated against them. On their own, brief standardized assessments of cognitive function, such as the Mini-Mental State Examination (MMSE) (Folstein *et al.* 1975) are not specific for delirium, and patients who screen positive for cognitive impair-ment on these need to receive a more detailed diagnostic assessment (see Chapter 2).

Case finding

Differences in case-finding procedures are another significant source of variability between studies. Those that rely on medical and nursing records for their patient infor-mation will be subject to recording bias. Because the level of awareness by medical and nursing staff of delirium in their elderly patients is low (Cameron *et al.* 1987; Bowler *et al.* 1994; Rockwood *et al.* 1994), this method is likely to underestimate the rates of this disorder. Direct patient assessment provides more accurate and complete data, but even this procedure is usually dependent on staff observations of the fluctuation of symptoms and the sleep–wake cycle over the 24-hour period. The provision of struc-tured recording sheets may help to reduce this source of bias.

To establish incidence rates of delirium, it is necessary to carry out repeated assess-ments, with completeness of ascertainment being a function of the frequency of the assessments; the longer the interval between assessments, the more likely it is that tran-sient episodes will be missed. Another potential source of variability in case finding is the professional background of the assessor; medically qualified researchers may collect more accurate symptom data than lay staff, although this issue can be addressed by ensuring appropriate training and experience. It is unlikely that the methodology of the large-scale cross-sectional psychiatric epidemiological population survey will be efficient at estimating the prevalence of a relatively transient and fluctuating dis-order such as delirium. However, some population prevalence data for this disorder have been reported by the US Epidemiologic Catchment Area (ECA) study (Folstein *et al.* 1991).

Effective case finding does, however, obviate the problem of under-recognition. That many health-care professionals fail to recognize delirium is a remarkable feature of modern hospital care, as discussed at various points in this book (Chapter 8). Under-recognition remains an important obstacle to research and to clinical care. A particularly important paper in this regard is that of Elie and colleagues (2000).

Working at St Mary's Hospital Centre in Montreal, Canada, the authors found that, notwithstanding delirium being common in elderly patients in the emergency department, and despite it being an independent prognostic indicator, and physicians being prompted to note whether it was present, the sensitivity of the standard emergency department assessment was only 35.3%. The specificity was 98.5%. Perhaps one of the most remarkable features of this study was the setting: St Mary's has been at the centre of a large number of delirium studies, including important intervention trials in patients with delirium (Cole *et al.* 1991, 1994). That under-recognition should persist in such an environment suggests that the problem is not a trivial one.

From the standpoint of interpreting epidemiological studies, two points are evident. Without an active case-finding strategy, studies of the epidemiology of delirium are likely to be biased. This will be based both on under-recognition of the syndrome and on selection bias favouring more evident cases. The former is likely to give a conservative bias: i.e. to underestimate the strength of the exposure, given that under-recognition will mean that exposed cases are likely to be misassigned as unexposed. The effect of the latter is unclear, but confounding seems likely, with factors that favour recognition also favouring more (or less) favourable outcomes. Delirium with psychomotor agitation may be such an instance.

In addition, screening hospital populations for evidence of delirium can lead to underestimation of the deleterious effects of delirium, particularly if better recognition prompts better care and thus is associated with better outcomes (this seems likely, see Chapter 8). Vigour in treating delirious patients should be taken as implicit in any reports in which the investigator has a role in the clinical management of the patients under study.

Selection bias

Studies in apparently similar patient groups, such as general medical in-patients, operate different inclusion and exclusion criteria, and these can have a significant impact on the prevalence and incidence rates of delirium reported. For example, while these studies tend to focus on elderly patients, the precise age range included differs widely, from 20 years and above (Anthony *et al.* 1982) to 70 years and above (Gillick *et al.* 1982; Johnson *et al.* 1990). Even in studies with similar age cut-offs there may be very different proportions of younger and older patients. Some studies exclude in-patients that are predicted to be less unwell, such as short-stay admissions for specific diagnostic studies, or at predictably high risk of delirium, such as admissions from nursing homes or for terminal care (e.g. Francis *et al.* 1990; Johnson *et al.* 1990). If the case-finding method depends on assessment at or within a defined period after admission, weekend admissions, within-hospital transfers and brief admissions may be excluded (e.g. Francis *et al.* 1990; Johnson *et al.* 1990). Studies may exclude those patients that are difficult to assess because of sensory impairments, speech and language problems, inability to speak English, or severe dementia (e.g. Rogers *et al.* 1989; Francis *et al.* 1990;

Pompei *et al.* 1994). Some studies of postoperative patient groups exclude all subjects with pre-existing cognitive impairment (e.g. Hole *et al.* 1980; Berggren *et al.* 1987). Similarly, extremely ill patients may be excluded because they cannot be assessed, or because their families refuse consent to participation in the study (Levkoff *et al.* 1991). Clearly, excluding patients with known risk factors for delirium will result in an underestimate of its frequency.

Study setting

Studies have attempted to estimate the frequency of delirium in a wide range of in-patient settings and specific patient groups: general medical, geriatric, neurological, surgical (orthopaedic, cardiothoracic, gastrointestinal), psychiatric consultation-liaison, and psychogeriatric. A few studies have also examined the prevalence of delirium in non-hospital settings such as nursing homes, and in the community population. It is likely that the rates of delirium in these groups will differ both because of selection artefacts and their specific risks of developing the disorder. However, it is difficult to quantify these differences because of the lack of comparability between studies. Related factors include the geographical location of the study and the date that it was carried out. The range, quality, and style of service provision for elderly patients varies from country to country and also over time, and data from studies done in different health systems or a long time ago will be of limited applicability to the here and now. To date, no study has attempted any formal cross-national or cross-cultural comparisons of the rates and expression of delirium in institutional or community populations.

The prevalence and incidence of delirium in various settings

Community

Epidemiological investigations of delirium in the general population are few and far between. An early Californian study estimated the incidence of delirium in people over 60 years of age to be 53 per 100,000 (Freedman *et al.* 1965). More recently, prevalence rates for delirium in the community population have been reported by the Eastern Baltimore Mental Health Survey, which formed part of the multi-site ECA study in the USA, and had a small over-sample of elderly subjects (Folstein *et al.* 1991). It had a two-stage design involving a clinical review (including physical examination) of all screen-positive subjects and a random sample of those who were screen-negative (Folstein *et al.* 1985). Non-response rates were high and sample sizes small; only six cases of DSM-III delirium were identified, all aged over 55 years. There was a marked increase in the estimated weighted prevalence rate of delirium with age: 0.4% of those aged 18 years and over; 1.1% of those aged 55 years and over; and 13.6% of those aged 85 years and over. These figures are likely to be an underestimate, for the methodological reasons discussed above, but they suggest that delirium is less prevalent in the community than in hospital populations. However, the rate of 13.6%

in the over-85s is comparable with some prevalence estimates in elderly in-patient studies (see below). The factors associated with delirium in this study were polypharmacy, visual impairment, diabetes, and structural brain disease. In a recent community study of non-demented people aged 85 years and older (Rahkonen *et al.* 2001), 10% were found to have had an episode of delirium requiring medical attention over a 3-year period. Delirium was associated with a new diagnosis of dementia over this period, and with high systolic blood pressure.

The prevalence of delirium in community populations will also be affected by factors that determine the movement of delirious individuals into and out of other settings, such as hospitals and nursing homes. On the one hand, delirious subjects are prone to being removed from the community sample frame by death and hospital admission (Jacoby and Bergmann 1986). On the other, it is possible that shorter hospital admissions as a result of cost-containment practices may result in an increase of the community prevalence of delirium. The rates of delirium in recently discharged elderly in-patients are not known; nor are the outcomes associated with this. Admission-prevention strategies such as Hospital at Home schemes, and other intensive home support services may also keep delirious patients in the community. In a Swedish study of psychiatric disorders in elderly people (aged 75 years and over) in various care settings, Sandberg *et al.* (1998) found the prevalence of delirium in a home medical care group to be 34%, compared to 46% in emergency hospital care.

Hospital in-patients

It is not surprising that most epidemiological research in delirium has focused on in-patient populations. They are at increased risk of developing the disorder, and it is associated with clinically and economically important adverse outcomes. Inouye (1999) has estimated that in the USA, delirium complicates the hospital admissions of over 2.3 million persons each year, involving over 17.5 million in-patient days at a cost of over $4 billion to the Medicare budget (1994 prices). This does not include the cost of extra treatment and care at home and in institutions following discharge. The epidemiology of delirium in in-patient groups has been reviewed by several authors (Platzer 1989; Smith and Dimsdale 1989; Francis and Kapoor 1990; Johnson *et al.* 1990; Levkoff *et al.* 1991; Francis 1992; Fisher and Gilchrist 1993; O'Keeffe and Ni Chonchubhair 1994; Dyer *et al.* 1995; Van der Mast and Roest 1996; Bucht *et al.* 1999). All comment on the wide variability of the findings, and the various methodological and other explanations for this.

Medical and geriatric in-patients

Some of the highest rates of delirium to have been reported in elderly in-patients come from the earliest studies in this area. Flint and Richards (1956) found 'acute confusion' to be present in 42% of elderly general medical admissions, similar to the rate of 40% found by Robinson (1956) in neurological in-patients over 60 years. In a study of patients admitted to a geriatric unit, Bedford (1959) estimated the prevalence of 'acute confusional states' to be as high as 80%. With some exceptions, more recent studies using similar diagnostic criteria have reported lower prevalence rates, in the order of 10–20% (Table 3.1). Some studies report prevalence rates of delirium at the point of hospital admission, and some for the admission period as a whole, which contributes to the variability of the findings. Some have specifically estimated the incidence of delirium during the hospital stay, with results varying from 3.3% in a relatively young patient sample (Cameron *et al.* 1987) to 53.2% in a more elderly group that included both medical and surgical patients (Chisholm *et al.* 1982). Most recent studies report incidence rates in the order of 5–10% (Table 3.1). Interpretation of trends over time is difficult because of the methodological differences and difficulties, particularly the changing diagnostic criteria for delirium; if there has been a fall in the prevalence of delirium in elderly medical hospital admissions over the second half of the twentieth century, it may be due to changes in health care for this age group in the developed societies where most of this research has been carried out. However, it may merely reflect the introduction of relatively strict diagnostic criteria. The incidence rates of delirium following admission suggest that elderly medical in-patients are still a significantly vulnerable group.

Liptzin and Levkoff (1992) have studied the relative frequency of hypoactive and hyperactive delirium subtypes in their series of elderly general hospital admissions. Of the delirious patients, 15% had a hyperactive delirium, 19% had a hypoactive delirium, 52% met their criteria for both subtypes ('mixed'), and 14% met criteria for neither. Similar frequencies are reported by O'Keeffe and Lavan (1997) in a series of admissions to a geriatric unit: 21% with hyperactive delirium, 29% with hypoactive delirium, 40% with both syndromes, and 7% with neither.

Surgical in-patients

Studies in elderly surgical in-patient populations have for the most part focused on the incidence of postoperative/post-anaesthetic delirium in various patient groups, and following various operative and anaesthetic procedures (Table 3.2). There is no consistent definition of postoperative delirium; one review of the literature has defined it as delirium occurring within 30 days of an operation (Dyer *et al.* 1995), which some might consider rather too long. It is also apparent that not all operative procedures carry the same risk. Some, such as cardiothoracic surgery and repair of hip fracture, are consistently associated with higher rates of postoperative delirium, either because of the nature of the surgical intervention or because of the frailty of the patient groups involved. Delirium following cardiac surgery has received considerable attention. In a review of 44 studies of post-cardiotomy delirium carried out between 1963 and 1987, Smith and Dimsdale (1989) concluded that its incidence over this period was relatively constant at around 30% with no discernible trends over time; however, differences may have been obscured by changing definitions of post-cardiotomy delirium over the

Table 3.1 The frequency of delirium in medical in-patients

Study	No.	Age (years)	Delirium (%) Prevalence	Incidence
Flint & Richards (1956)	574	60+	42	
Bedford (1959)	5000	65+	80	
Hodkinson (1973)	588	65+	24	11.0
Bergmann & Eastham (1974)	100	65+	16	
Seymour et al. (1980)	71	70+	15	
Gillick et al. (1982)	173	70+	29.9	
Chisolm et al. (1982)	99	60+	5	53.2
Anthony et al. (1982)	97	20+	10	
Erkinjuntti et al. (1986)	2000	55+	15	
Erkinjuntti et al. (1987)	282	65+	21	
Cameron et al. (1987)	133	All ages	14	3.3
Rockwood (1989)	80	65+	16	10.4
Johnson et al. (1990)	235	70+	16	5.0
Francis et al. (1990)	229	70+	16	7.3
Gottlieb et al. (1991)	235	70+	20	5
Ramsay et al. (1991)	116	72+	20	
Jitapunkul et al. (1992)	184	82 (mean)	22	
Levkoff et al. (1992)*	325	65+	11	31.3
Kolbeinsson & Jonsson (1993)	331	70+	14	
Rockwood et al. (1993)	168	65+	18	7.0
Inouye et al. (1993) [†]	107	70+		25.2
	174	70+		16.7
Pompei et al. (1994)*	432	65+	15	
Pompei et al. (1994)*	323	70+	26	
Bowler et al. (1994)	153	60+	11	
Inouye & Charpentier (1996) [†]	196	70+		17.9
	312	70+		15.1
O'Keeffe & Lavan (1997)	315	82 (mean)	18	24.0
Rudberg et al. (1997)	432	65+	15	
Feldman et al. (1999)	61	70+	18	
Martin et al. (2000)*	156	65+		17.9
Uwakwe (2000)*	104	60+	10	

*Both medical and surgical patients.

[†]Two cohorts.

Table 3.2 The frequency of post-operative delirium in surgical in-patients (incidence rates unless otherwise stated).

Study	No.	Age (years)	Delirium (%)
General surgery			
Millar (1981)	100	65+	14
Seymour & Pringle (1983)	258	65+	10
Marcantonio et al. (1994)	1341	50+	9
Orthopaedic: hip fracture			
Williams et al. (1985)	170	65+	52
Furstenberg & Mezey (1987)	98	60+	33
Berggren et al. (1987)	57	64+	44
Gustafson et al. (1988)	111	65+	42
Magaziner et al. (1990)	536	65+	23
Marcantonio et al. (2000)	126	65+	41
Brauer et al. (2000)	571	69–101	5 (prevalence: 9.5%)
Galanakis et al. (2001)	37	60+	40
Orthopaedic: elective			
Hole et al. (1980)	60	All ages	12
Rogers et al. (1989)	46	65+	26
Williams-Russo et al. (1992)	51	68 (mean)	41
Fisher & Flowerdew (1995)	80	60+	18
Dai et al. (2000)	701	65+	5 (also urological)
Galanakis et al. (2001)	68	60+	15
Cardiothoracic			
Rubinstein & Thomas (1970)	36	20–69	31
Tune et al. (1981)	29	29–75	34
Calabrese et al. (1987)	59	40+	7
Okita et al. (1998)	52	70+	25
Rolfson et al. (1999)	71	71 (mean)	32
Gastrointestinal			
Kaneko et al. (1997)	36	70+	36

period reviewed. In a more recent study of patients undergoing myocardial revascularization, the reported incidence of delirium was 6.8% (Calabrese *et al.* 1987); this difference may be due to the fact that this study used more stringent diagnostic criteria (DSM-III) than any of the earlier studies (Levkoff *et al.* 1991). There is a wide spectrum of intellectual impairment following cardiac surgery. In a study of cognitive function following elective coronary bypass surgery (Shaw *et al.* 1986), 79% of the patients were impaired on one or more of the psychometric tests, and 24% on three or more. The cognitive functions most commonly affected were psychomotor speed, attention and concentration, new learning ability, and auditory short-term memory. Only 8% of the patients were significantly disabled by their cognitive impairment.

Surgery following hip fracture is also associated with a high incidence of postoperative delirium in elderly patients (Table 3.2), even in groups where those with pre-existing dementia have been excluded (e.g. Berggren *et al.* 1987). Surgery for hip fracture is usually an emergency procedure, and the patients are usually frailer and less well prepared than those undergoing elective orthopaedic procedures, where patients are more highly selected and the rates of postoperative delirium are lower (Table 3.2). One-third of the femoral neck fracture patients studied by Gustafson *et al.* (1988) and 46% of those studied by Brauer *et al.* (2000) were delirious prior to surgery. In their study of non-demented hip fracture patients, Berggren *et al.* (1987) found that the major factor significantly associated with postoperative delirium was the use of anti-cholinergic drugs. A previous history of depression was also associated, but this may have been a proxy for anticholinergic drug use as the majority of the depressed patients were also taking drugs with anticholinergic effects. Anticholinergic drug use has been associated with postoperative delirium more generally (Tune *et al.* 1981), and in hip fracture patients it may contribute to both the fall and the subsequent delirium (Lipowski 1989; Vetter and Ford 1989).

The rates of postoperative delirium following other surgical procedures have been less intensively studied, but in general they appear to be lower than those associated with cardiac and emergency orthopaedic operations. In a study of elderly general surgical patients, Millar (1981) found a rate of 14%, and a similar rate of 17% has been reported following gastrointestinal surgery in this age group (Kaneko *et al.* 1997) (Table 3.2). In a review of 20 studies of patients undergoing extraction of cataracts, the incidence of delirium varied from 0.3 to 15.9% (Summers and Reich 1979). A recent study has reported an incidence rate of 5.1% for this patient group (Milstein *et al.* 2000); factors associated with developing delirium were older age and more frequent use of benzodiazepine premedication.

Psychiatric in-patients

In contrast to medical and surgical in-patients, the frequency of delirium in elderly psychiatric admissions has been much less extensively researched. An early study of elderly patients admitted to the psychiatric receiving ward of a county general hospital found that 46% had an 'acute brain disorder'; this was co-morbid with a 'chronic brain disorder' in 71% of cases (Simon and Cahan 1963). Alcohol, drugs, and malnutrition were the commonest causes identified. More recently, Koponen *et al.* (1989) identified 13% meeting DSM-III criteria for delirium in a series of new admissions to a psychogeriatric unit. An unknown number of cases of delirium secondary to alcohol withdrawal were excluded. Most of the delirious patients had been admitted from other medical in-patient units, where they were not manageable because of their disturbed behaviour; over half of the cases of delirium in this study were described as hyperactive. A Canadian study of a mental-hospital-based psychogeriatric service for patients with severe behavioural disturbances identified delirium in 17% of patients, including 7% in whom it was the sole psychiatric diagnosis (Rockwood *et al.* 1991).

Some data are also available on the diagnostic breakdown of hospital in-patients referred to psychiatric liaison-consultation services. In a retrospective case-note review of 1966 psychiatric referrals from general hospital in-patients, the frequency of DSM-II acute brain syndrome was 20.8% (Henker 1979). A study of 150 referrals from a surgical department found that 20.7% met DSM-III criteria for delirium (9.8% of the referrals aged under 60 years and 43.8% of those aged over 60 years) (Golinger 1986). In a similar review of 793 referrals to a general hospital liaison-consultation service, 12.6% met DSM-III criteria for delirium (Sirois 1988). In samples such as these, there is likely to be referral bias towards hyperactive delirium with prominent symptoms and disturbed behaviour; in one series of delirious patients referred to a neuropsychiatric unit, nearly 80% had a hyperactive delirium (Kobayashi *et al.* 1992).

Other hospital settings

Some in-patient groups are at a particularly high risk of developing delirium, for example, those on intensive care units (ICUs) and those receiving terminal care. Pochard *et al.* (1995) found the incidence of delirium in ICU patients following discharge from mechanical ventilation to be 77% (mean age 51.6 years). A prospective cohort study of cancer patients admitted to hospital for terminal care found that 20% were delirious on admission, and among those who were not, the subsequent incidence of the disorder was 33%. Delirious patients were on significantly higher doses of parenteral morphine (Gagnon *et al.* 2000). Another study of in-patients with advanced cancer found a rate of delirium on admission of 42% and a subsequent incidence of 45% (Lawlor *et al.* 2000). Terminal delirium occurred in 88% of those who died. Approximately half of the delirious episodes were reversible, with reversibility being associated with opioids and other psychotropic medication, and with dehydration.

Another setting where delirious elderly patients are commonly encountered is the accident and emergency department. A study of elderly attendees at a US emergency department found that delirium was present in 24%, and that this was, not surprisingly, associated with a higher likelihood of hospital admission (Naughton *et al.* 1995). In another study, the prevalence was 12% (Hustey *et al.* 2000), and in only 46% was the delirium documented, estimates similar to Elie *et al.*

Nursing homes

The elderly residents of nursing homes and other long-term care settings are an important group at increased risk of developing delirium. They are physically frail, and have high rates of other psychiatric disorders, notably dementia and depression. They are liable to be receiving considerable quantities of medication, including psychotropic drugs. Hospital admissions from institutional care settings have higher rates of delirium than admissions from home (Levkoff *et al.* 1992; Marcantonio *et al.* 2000). There have been several studies of psychiatric disorders in these settings, but few provide reliable estimates of the rates of delirium in these populations. In one study of a random sample of elderly residents of an 'intermediate care' facility, Rovner *et al.* (1986) found 6% to be suffering from drug-induced delirium. A further 24% were demented and experiencing hallucinations and delusions, and a proportion of these were probably also delirious. Sabin *et al.* (1982) found that 25% of cognitively impaired nursing home residents had potentially reversible conditions. In the study of Swedish care settings previously cited (Sandberg *et al.* 1998), the rate of delirium in nursing homes was 58%, and in homes catering for a less disabled group it was 35%. In the nursing homes, the majority of the cases of delirium were co-morbid with dementia. Overall, the rates of delirium found in this study were high, but their estimate for nursing homes is similar to that of another Swedish study that reported rates of delirium in nursing homes and old people's homes of 62% and 32%, respectively (Dehlin *et al.* 1985). It is likely that many of the cases of delirium in these settings go unrecognized by care staff; in a series of residents referred to an on-site psychiatric liaison-consultation service to a nursing home in the USA, only 6% received a diagnosis of delirium (Bienenfeld and Wheeler 1989).

Risk factors for delirium

In a recent review, Inouye (1999) identified 14 studies published since 1980, which had identified independent risk factors for delirium using either multivariate statistics or methods of stratification. As she points out, the risk factors studied include both predisposing and precipitating factors, and it is not usually possible to identify the relationship between them. This chapter reviews the important predisposing factors; precipitating factors will be discussed in Chapter 6.

Age

The association between delirium and increasing chronological age in adulthood is apparent in both community and in-patient studies, with the very elderly being at greatest risk (e.g. Gustafson *et al.* 1988; Rockwood 1989; Folstein *et al.* 1991). However, it is not clear to what extent age itself acts as a risk factor, independently of other age-associated conditions, such as dementia, physical ill health and sensory impairment. In one multivariate analysis of risk factors for delirium, age (80 years +) was independently associated with delirium, with an odds ratio of 5.22 (Schor *et al.* 1992). However, this association has not been replicated in other studies (Francis *et al.* 1990; Inouye *et al.* 1993).

Chronological age is a discrete and universally available variable, making it attractive in the measurement of risk factors. However, its documented independent association with delirium should be viewed with some caution. Frailty, or the notion of physiological age, may better capture this association. Unlike chronological age, frailty has been more difficult to conceptualize and measure. With the recent development and validation of instruments which allow for its measurement (Rockwood *et al.* 1999; Rolfson *et al.* 2000), the independent association with chronological age may be replaced by frailty in future delirium cohorts. As a biological process, ageing is characterized by the progressive loss of adaptability, with reduction in functional reserves and the ability to accommodate and recover from physiological insults. Age-related changes in the metabolism of drugs may put some elderly patients at greater risk of developing toxic levels with apparently therapeutic doses, and the sensitivity of the brain to the psychoactive effects of drugs may also change with age. Factors such as these may contribute to an increased vulnerability to developing delirium as we get older; however, it is important to bear in mind that there is considerable variation between elderly individuals in the extent to which their physiology and drug-handling capacity alters with age.

Sex

Independent associations with gender have also been demonstrated. Male gender carries a relative risk of 1.9 (Elie *et al.* 1998). Three studies have reported an association between delirium and male gender (Schor *et al.* 1992; Williams-Russo *et al.* 1992; Fisher and Flowerdew 1995). Levkoff *et al.* (1992) found an independent relationship between male gender and delirium in an institutional but not in a community setting. Male gender may be a marker for alcohol abuse, which has also been identified as a risk factor for delirium in a few studies (Williams-Russo *et al.* 1992; Pompei *et al.* 1994; Marcantonio *et al.* 1994), and is commoner in men than women aged over 65 years (Myers *et al.* 1984).

Education

One study (Galankis *et al.* 2001) has reported an association between lower educational level and increased risk of delirium following hip surgery, suggesting that limited educational attainment may be a risk factor.

Dementia

Of the age-associated disorders, dementia is the condition that is most commonly identified as a risk factor for delirium (e.g. Erkinjuntti *et al.* 1986; Gustafson *et al.* 1988; Rockwood 1989; Francis *et al.* 1990; Schor *et al.* 1992; Marcantonio *et al.* 2000). Elie *et al.* (1998) combined the results of 12 of 15 trials that had shown any association, resulting in a combined relative risk of 5.2 [95% confidence interval (CI) 4.2–6.3]. In a cohort of 175 individuals with dementia, Robertsson *et al.* (1998) found that the 'degree of dementia' was an independent predictor of delirium. Although chronological age alone was not associated with delirium, late-onset Alzheimer's disease and vascular dementia appeared to have a stronger association with delirium than did early-onset Alzheimer's disease and frontotemporal dementia. Lerner *et al.* (1997) found that more functional impairment in Alzheimer's disease was associated with a higher incidence of delirium. However, this effect did not remain after correcting for multiple comparisons. Similarly, no association could be identified between behavioural disturbances in Alzheimer's disease and the risk of delirium.

Other neurological disorders, such as Parkinson's disease and stroke, are also associated with an increased risk of delirium (Cameron *et al.* 1987; Gustafson *et al.* 1988; Henon *et al.* 1999), probably the result of both increased cerebral vulnerability and the effects of drug treatments for these conditions. In such cases, the non-threatening hallucinations that sometimes accompany the disease itself must be distinguished from the symptom complex of delirium in which there is acute temporal onset and fluctuation, psychomotor agitation and new, unpleasant psychotic disturbances.

Other psychiatric disorders

There is disagreement about the effect of depression and anxiety as a risk factor for postoperative delirium. Millar (1981) found no association between 'postoperative intellectual impairment' and preoperative depression, past psychiatric history, or family psychiatric history in general surgical patients. Similarly, Simpson and Kellett (1987) found no association between preoperative anxiety and postoperative delirium following hip replacement. However, as mentioned above, Gustafson *et al.* (1987), Berggren *et al.* (1988) and Galankis *et al.* (2001) have reported a relationship between depression and postoperative delirium in their studies of hip fracture patients, perhaps because antidepressant use may specifically contribute to falls and subsequent hip fracture. Pompei *et al.* (1994) also found depression to be predictive of delirium in their study of elderly medical and surgical patients. The systematic review by Elie *et al.* (1998) reported that history of depression is associated with a increased risk of delirium of approximately 1.9 (CI 1.3–2.6). In old age, depression is also associated with acute and chronic physical illness and with self-neglect, which may contribute to any association.

There is little evidence regarding the association between delirium and other psychiatric disorders in old age, probably because the numbers of patients with conditions such as schizophrenia and mania in general medical and surgical study samples are too low for any relationship to be statistically apparent. The meta-analysis of cardiac surgery patients by Smith and Dimsdale (1989) found no association with any psychiatric disorder apart from dementia. However, factors such as self-neglect and treatment with psychotropic and anticholinergic drugs may put patients with a psychotic disorder at increased risk of developing delirium. A history of alcoholism confers a three-fold relative risk of delirium (Elie *et al.* 1998).

Physical illness factors

Within elderly in-patient populations, a number of factors related to the physical illness have been found to be associated with an increased risk of delirium, such as illness severity and instability (Rockwood 1989; Francis *et al.* 1990), burden of co-morbidity (Pompei *et al.* 1994; Marcantonio *et al.* 2000), and greater functional impairment, in terms of activities of daily living (ADL) and mobility (Williams *et al.* 1985; Marcantonio *et al.* 2000). The relative risk of functional impairments and disability is 2.5 (CI 1.4–4.2) (Elie *et al.* 1998). Marcantonio, in a large cohort of elderly undergoing elective non-cardiac surgery (Marcantonio *et al.* 1994), recorded physical function prior to surgery using a validated instrument, the Specific Activity Scale (Goldman *et al.* 1981). The most physically impaired group was 2.5 times more likely to experience delirium, even after correcting for age, alcohol abuse, cognition, metabolic abnormalities, and the type of surgery. Preoperative immobility was also found to be independently associated with delirium in a cohort presenting with hip fracture (Williams *et al.* 1985). Fracture on admission is independently associated (Schor *et al.* 1992), but a history of falls is not (Elie *et al.* 1998). Neither a history of urinary nor faecal incontinence has been causally linked to delirium.

The number of chronic medical problems appears to be associated with delirium. Pompei *et al.* (1994) found the burden of co-morbidity to be an independent predictor. Neurological co-morbidities, when identified prior to the delirium, appear to be particularly troublesome. In a cohort of elderly undergoing cardiac surgery, Rolfson *et al.* (1999) found that a previous stroke was an independent predictor of delirium and increased its risk by a factor of eight. Structural brain abnormalities, brain cancer, and cerebral metastasis are also important predisposing variables.

Laboratory investigations found to be predictive of delirium include: hypoalbuminaemia; abnormal serum sodium; hypokalaemia; hypoglycaemia; urea; and a high blood urea nitrogen (BUN)/creatinine ratio (Levkoff *et al.* 1988; Foreman 1989; Francis *et al.* 1990; Inouye *et al.* 1993; O'Keeffe and Lavan 1996). These are probably markers for the severity of the underlying illness, although some may specifically increase the risk of delirium; for example, hypoalbuminaemia may increase the levels of unbound drugs in the plasma. Mussi *et al.* (1999) found that delirious patients were more likely to have a low body mass index, and Weed *et al.* (1995) found an association between a low preoperative leukocyte count and delirium. Vitamin deficiencies, such as thiamine and cobalamin, are also believed to heighten the risk of delirium, but this has not yet been demonstrated in prospective cohort studies.

Visual impairment and hearing impairment are associated with a statistically significant risk of delirium of 1.7 and 1.9, respectively (Elie *et al.* 1998). Visual impairment has been identified as an independent risk factor in the community population (Folstein *et al.* 1991), and in medical in-patient series (Inouye *et al.* 1993; George *et al.* 1997; Martin *et al.* 2000), but not in surgical populations (Fisher and Flowerdew 1995; Weed *et al.* 1995).

Factors related to the process of care

Iatrogenesis and other extrinsic factors all too often play an initiating or perpetuating role in delirium, especially in an institutional setting. Thus, inadequate processes of care must be viewed as a potential predisposing factor. However, process of care issues, which may set the stage for delirium and its consequences, are not restricted to iatrogenesis alone. Other system-wide variables, which must also be addressed, include skills in the recognition of delirium, attitudes toward the care of the elderly, the rapid pace and technological focus of hospital care, and reductions in skilled nursing staff (Inouye *et al.* 1999b).

Other risk factors

Other factors related to the process of care that have been identified as risk factors for delirium in elderly in-patients include bladder catheterization and use of physical restraints (Werner *et al.* 1989; Inouye and Charpentier 1996). The sheer number of procedures undergone by the patient while in hospital may also be important (Martin *et al.* 2000). Environmental factors associated with hospital admission, such as sleep disturbance, sensory deprivation (and its opposite, sensory over-stimulation), and reduced mobility, may also contribute to the development of delirium in vulnerable individuals, but are difficult to identify in observational studies because most in-patients are exposed to them. Low levels of activity and social interaction were noted as risk factors by Williams *et al.* (1985), Foreman (1989) and Duppils and Wikblad (2001).

Several researchers have used their findings about risk factors to develop and validate predictive models for delirium in elderly in-patients (e.g. Schor *et al.* 1992; Inouye *et al.* 1993; Marcantonio *et al.* 1994; Fisher and Flowerdew 1995; Inouye and Charpentier 1996). Inouye and Charpentier (1996) have examined the interaction between predisposing and precipitating factors, showing that they are highly interrelated and multiplicative in their effect. Their predictive model has formed the basis for the study of interventions aimed at reducing the incidence of delirium in this population (Inouye *et al.* 1999a) (see Chapter 8).

Outcome of delirium

Cognitive recovery

Although delirium is usually regarded as a transient disorder, several studies of elderly in-patients have demonstrated its persistence in this population; for example, Rudberg *et al.* (1997) found that in about one-third of cases of delirium the episode was prolonged or recurrent. Levkoff *et al.* (1992) found that 58% of patients who developed delirium during admission were still delirious at discharge, and in only 4% was there complete recovery. Others have reported higher recovery rates by discharge, in the order of 40–70% (Rockwood 1993; O'Keeffe and Lavan 1997; Marcantonio *et al.* 2000; Brauer *et al.* 2000). Some symptoms, such as disorientation and memory impairment, appear to be particularly slow to resolve (Rockwood 1993; O'Keeffe and Lavan 1997). Longer-term follow-up studies indicate that in a minority of patients the delirium can be extremely persistent or recurrent. In a meta-analysis of eight in-patient studies (Cole and Primeau 1993), only 54.6% of patients had some degree of mental recovery at 1 month. A recent study of hip fracture patients found that delirium was still present in 32% at 1 month and 6% at 6 months following surgery (Marcantonio *et al.* 2000). Brauer *et al.* (2000) suggest that recovery rates may be better in surgical than in medical patients, because of different underlying risk factors. Conversely, delirious patients admitted to hospital from nursing homes may have a particularly poor outcome. Kelly *et al.* (2001) found that the delirium persisted until death or hospital discharge in 72%, and at 1- and 3-month follow-up in 55% and 25%, respectively. Persistence of delirium was associated with a hypoactive or mixed symptom profile. Mortality in this population was also high: 18% at 1 month and 47% at 3 months.

It is not known to what extent delirium may itself be a cause of lasting cognitive impairment. Patients who develop delirium are at increased risk of developing long-term cognitive decline over the next 2 years (Francis and Kapoor 1992). Rockwood *et al.* (1999) estimated the relative risk of dementia amongst elderly medical in-patients with no prior history of cognitive or functional impairment to be 3.23 (95% CI: 1.86–5.63), amounting to approximately 18% per year. It may be that limited cerebral reserve in the very early stages of their dementia contributed to their delirium; alternatively, the metabolic derangements during delirium may cause persistent cerebral damage in some cases (O'Keeffe and Lavan 1997).

The issue of cognitive outcome in delirium raises some of the important definitional and conceptual issues discussed in Chapter 1. If delirium as currently defined by the modern nosologies is a poor predictor of outcome, one reason for this might be that these diagnostic criteria are not efficient at excluding other disorders, notably dementia. Treloar and Macdonald (1997) have argued that, since there is no 'gold standard' for delirium, there may be merit in defining it in terms of outcome, i.e. the reversibility of the cognitive dysfunction.

Functional recovery

Given the risk factors for delirium, it is not surprising that it is associated with adverse outcomes, such as a high mortality rate, prolonged hospital admission, and a high rate of institutionalization following discharge. In the meta-analysis by Cole and Primeau (1993), at 1 month after hospital admission 14.2% of delirious patients were dead and 46.5% were in institutions, a figure that fell only slightly to 43.2% at 6 months following admission. Delirium as an in-patient is a predictor of long-term functional decline following discharge from hospital (Murray *et al.* 1993). To what extent does delirium make an independent contribution to these outcomes, separate from the underlying acute illness and associated physical and mental frailty? The evidence with regard to mortality is not consistent, at least with respect to short- to medium-term outcome. Pompei *et al.* (1994) found that delirium was independently associated with death during the hospital stay, but not at 90-day follow-up. In another series of elderly medical admissions (Ramsay *et al.* 1991), delirium was independently associated with mortality at 10-week follow-up. However, in the study by O'Keeffe and Lavan (1997), delirium was not found to be independently associated with mortality during the hospital stay, after adjustment for age, illness severity, co-morbid disease disability score, and dementia. Francis *et al.* (1990) found that delirium had no significant effect on mortality rates at 6 months following discharge; there was increased mortality associated with delirium at 2-year follow-up, but this was attributable to functional impairment (Francis and Kapoor 1992). A recent 3-year follow-up study has shown increased mortality associated with delirium (risk ratio 2.24), not accounted for by cognitive function or health status at the time of initial hospitalization (Curyto *et al.* 2001). There is a mortality rate of up to 5% specifically associated with delirium tremens, but this condition is rare in elderly patients.

Delirium does contribute to in-patient morbidity and increased length of hospital admission, independently of factors such as illness severity, cognitive impairment, and functional dependence (Thomas *et al.* 1988; Francis *et al.* 1990; Rockwood 1990; O'Keeffe and Lavan 1997). The delirious state interferes with the processes of diagnosis, treatment, and rehabilitation (Saravay and Lavin 1994), and increases the likelihood of hospital-acquired complications; patients with a hypoactive delirium are at risk of developing pressure sores and chest infections, and those with hyperactive delirium are at risk of falls (O'Keeffe and Lavan 1999). Galankis *et al.* (2001) have reported higher rates of self-destructive behaviour associated with delirium following hip surgery.

In most studies, delirium in elderly medical in-patients is independently associated with increased dependency and functional decline, both at discharge (O'Keeffe and Lavan 1997) and at long-term follow-up (Francis and Kapoor 1992; Rockwood *et al.* 1999; McCusker *et al.* 2001). In a study of hip fracture patients by Marcantonio *et al.* (2000), delirium was independently associated with poor functional outcome at 1 month after operation, but not at 6 months. There was also a 'dose-response' effect in this study, with patients whose delirium persisted at 1-month follow-up doing worse than those in whom it had resolved. Given this association with poor functional outcome, delirium is also an independent risk factor for admission into institutional care (O'Keeffe and Lavan 1997; Marcantonio *et al.* 2000). Patients with preoperative delirium appear to have worse functional outcomes than those with postoperative delirium only (Edlund *et al.* 2001).

Conclusion

A significant proportion of elderly patients are either delirious on admission to hospital, or develop delirium at some point during their hospital stay. Research has identified a number of predisposing and precipitating factors, which have the potential to identify those at risk of delirium and to prevent it occurring. Complications arising from the delirious state prolong hospital admission and contribute to adverse functional outcomes, notably increased dependency and higher rates of institutionalization. Delirium may also be a significant problem in other vulnerable elderly groups, such as nursing home residents, but research in these settings is still very limited.

References

American Psychiatric Association (1980). *Diagnostic and statistical manual of mental disorders*, 3rd edn. American Psychiatric Association, Washington.

American Psychiatric Association (1987). *Diagnostic and statistical manual of mental disorders*, 3rd edn, revised. American Psychiatric Association, Washington.

American Psychiatric Association (1994). *Diagnostic and statistical manual of mental disorders*, 4th edn. American Psychiatric Association, Washington.

Anthony, J. C., LeResche, L., Niaz, U., Von Korff, M. R. and Folstein, M. F. (1982). Limits of the 'Mini-Mental State' as a screening test for dementia and delirium among hospital patients. *Psychological Medicine*, **12**, 397–408.

Ballard, C. and McKeith, I. G. (1998). Psychiatric features in diffuse Lewy body disease. *Neurology*, **50**, 573.

Bedford, P. D. (1959). General medical aspects of confusional states in elderly people. *British Medical Journal*, **ii**, 185–188.

Berggren, D., Gustafson, Y., Eriksson, B., *et al.* (1987). Postoperative confusion after anaesthesia in elderly patients with femoral neck fractures. *Anesthesia and Analgesia*, **66**, 497–504.

Bergmann, K. and Eastham, E. J. (1974). Psychogeriatric ascertainment and assessment for treatment in an acute medical setting. *Age and Ageing*, **3**, 174–188.

Bienenfeld, D. and Wheeler, B. G. (1989). Psychiatric services to nursing homes: a liaison model. *Hospital and Community Psychiatry*, **40**, 793–794.

Bowler, C., Boyle, A., Branford, M., Cooper, S.-A., Harper, R., and Lindesay, J. (1994). Detection of psychiatric disorders in elderly medical inpatients. *Age and Ageing*, **23**, 307–311.

Brauer, C., Morrison, R. S., Silberzweig, S. B., and Siu, A. L. (2000). The cause of delirium in patients with hip fracture. *Archives of Internal Medicine*, **160**, 1856–1860.

Bucht, G., Gustafson, Y., and Sandberg, O. (1999). Epidemiology of delirium. *Dementia and Geriatric Cognitive Disorders*, **10**, 315–318.

Calabrese, J. R., Skewerer, R. G., Gulledge, A. D., *et al.* (1987). Incidence of postoperative delirium following myocardial revascularization. *Cleveland Clinical Journal of Medicine*, **54**, 29–32.

Cameron, D. J., Thomas, R. I., Mulvihill, M., and Bronheim, H. (1987). Delirium: a test of the Diagnostic and Statistical Manual III criteria on medical inpatients. *Journal of the American Geriatrics Society*, **35**, 1007–1010.

Chisholm, S. E., Deniston, O. L., Igrisan, R. M., and Barbus, A. J. (1982). Prevalence of confusion in elderly hospital patients. *Gerontological Nursing*, **8**, 87–96.

Cole, M. and Primeau, F. J. (1993). Prognosis of delirium in elderly hospital patients. *Canadian Medical Association Journal*, **149**, 41–46.

Cole, M. G., Fenton, F. R., Engelsmann, F., and Mansouri, I. (1991). Effectiveness of geriatric psychiatry consultation in an acute hospital: a randomized controlled trial. *Journal of the American Geriatrics Society*, **39**, 1183–1188.

Cole, M. G., Primeau, F. J., Bailey, R. F., *et al.* (1994). Systematic intervention for elderly inpatients with delirium: a randomized trial. *Canadian Medical Association Journal*, **151**, 965–970.

Curyto, K. J., Johnson, J., TenHave, T., Mossey, J., Knott, K., and Katz, I. R. (2001). Survival of hospitalized elderly patients with delirium: a prospective study. *American Journal of Geriatric Psychiatry*, **9**, 141–147.

Dai, Y.-T., Lou, M.-F., Yip, P.-K., and Huang, G.-S. (2000). Risk factors and incidence of postoperative delirium in elderly Chinese patients. *Gerontology*, **46**, 28–35.

Dehlin, O. and Franzen, M. (1985). Prevalence of dementia syndromes in persons living in homes for the elderly and in nursing homes in southern Sweden. *Scandinavian Journal of Primary Health Care*, **3**, 215–222.

Duppils, G. S. and Wikblad, K. (2001). Acute confusional states in patients undergoing hip surgery: a prospective observation study. *Gerontology*, **46**, 36–43.

Dyer, C. B., Ashton, C. M., and Teasdale, T. A. (1995). Postoperative delirium. A review of 80 primary data-collection studies. *Archives of Internal Medicine*, **155**, 461–465.

Edlund, A., Lundström, M., Bränström, B., Bucht, G., and Gustafson, Y. (2001). Delirium before and after operation for femoral neck fracture. *Journal of the American Geriatrics Society*, **49**, 1335–1340.

Elie, M., Cole, M. G., Primeau, F. J., and Bellevance, F. (1998). Delirium risk factors in elderly hospitalized patients. *Journal of General Internal Medicine*, **13**, 204–212.

Elie, M., Rousseau, F., Cole, M. G., Primeau, F. J., McCusker J., and Bellavance, F. (2000). Prevalence of detection of delirium in elderly emergency department patients. *Canadian Medical Association Journal*, **163**, 977–981.

Erkinjuntti, T., Wikstrom, J., Palo, J., and Autio, L. (1986). Dementia among medical inpatients. Evaluation of 2000 consecutive admissions. *Archives of Internal Medicine*, **146**, 1923–1926.

Erkinjuntti, T., Sulkava, R., Wikstrom, J., and Autio, L. (1987). Short Portable Mental Status Questionnaire as a screening test for dementia and delirium among the elderly. *Journal of the American Geriatrics Society*, **35**, 412–416.

Feldman, J., Yaretzky, A., Kaizimov, N., Alterman, P., and Vigder, C. (1999). Delirium in an acute geriatric unit: Clinical aspects. *Archives of Gerontology and Geriatrics*, **28**, 37–44.

Fisher, B. W. and Flowerdew, G. (1995). A simple model for predicting postoperative delirium in older patients undergoing elective orthopedic surgery. *Journal of the American Geriatrics Society*, **43**, 175–178.

Fisher, B. W. and Ghilchrist, D. M. (1993). Postoperative delirium in the elderly. *Annales CRMCC*, **26**, 358–362.

Flint, F. and Richards, S. (1956). Organic basis of confusional states in the elderly. *British Medical Journal*, **ii**, 1537–1539.

Folstein, M. F., Folstein, S. E., and McHugh, P. R. (1975). Mini-mental state – a practical method for grading the cognitive state of patients for the clinician. *Journal of Psychiatric Research*, **12**, 189–198.

Folstein, M. F., Bassett, S. S., Romanowski, A. J., and Nestadt, G. (1991). The epidemiology of delirium in the community: the Eastern Baltimore Mental Health Survey. *International Psychogeriatrics*, **3**, 169–179.

Foreman, M. D. (1989). Confusion in the hospitalised elderly: incidence, onset, and associated factors. *Research into Nursing and Health*, **12**, 21–29.

Francis, J. (1992). Delirium in older patients. *Journal of the American Geriatrics Society*, **40**, 829–838.

Francis, J. and Kapoor, W. N. (1990). Delirium in hospitalised elderly. *Journal of General Internal Medicine*, **5**, 65–79.

Francis, J. and Kapoor, W. N. (1992). Prognosis after hospital discharge of older medical patients with delirium. *Journal of the American Geriatrics Society*, **40**, 601–606.

Francis, J., Martin, D., and Kapoor, W. N. (1990). A prospective study of delirium in hospitalized elderly. *Journal of the American Medical Association*, **263**, 1097–1101.

Freedman, D. K., Troll, L., Mills, A. B., and Baker, P. (1965). *Acute organic disorder accompanied by mental symptoms*. California Department of Mental Hygiene, Sacramento.

Furstenberg, A. L. and Mezey, M. D. (1987). Mental impairment of elderly hospitalised hip fracture patients. *Acta Psychiatrica Scandinavica*, **62**, 13–31.

Galanakis, P., Bickel, H., Gradinger, R., Von Gumppenberg, S., and Förstl, H. (2001). Acute confusional state in the elderly following hip surgery: incidence, risk factors and complications. *International Journal of Geriatric Psychiatry*, **16**, 349–355.

Gagnon, P., Allard, P., Masse, B., and De Serres, M. (2000). Delirium in terminal cancer: a prospective study using daily screening, early diagnosis and continuous monitoring. *Journal of Pain and Symptom Management*, **19**, 412–426.

George, J., Bleasdale, S., and Singleton, S. J. (1997). Causes and prognosis of delirium in elderly patients admitted to a district general hospital. *Age and Ageing*, **26**, 423–427.

Gillick, M. R., Serrell, N. A., and Gillick, L. S. (1982). Adverse consequence of hospitalization in the elderly. *Social Science and Medicine*, **16**, 1033–1038.

Goldman, L., Hashimoto, B., Cook, E. F. and Loscalzo, A. (1981). Comparative reproducibility and validity of systems for assessing cardiovascular functional class: advantages of a new specific activity scale. *Circulation*, **64**, 1227–1233.

Golinger, R. C. (1986). Delirium in surgical patients seen at psychiatric consultation. *Surgery, Gynaecology and Obstetrics*, **163**, 104–106.

Gottlieb, G. L., Johnson, J., Wanich, C., and Sullivan, E. (1991). Delirium in the medically ill elderly: operationalizing the DSM-III criteria. *International Psychogeriatrics*, **3**, 181–196.

Gustafson, Y., Berggren, D., Brannstrom, B., *et al.* (1988). Acute confusional states in elderly patients treated for femoral neck fracture. *Journal of the American Geriatrics Society*, **36**, 525–530.

Henker, F. O. (1979). Acute brain syndromes. *Journal of Clinical Psychiatry*, **40**, 117–120.

Henon, H., Lebert, F., Durieu, I., Godefroy, O., Lucas, C., Pasquier, F., and Leys, D. (1999). Confusional state in stroke: relation to pre-existing dementia, patient characteristics and outcome. *Stroke*, **30**, 773–779.

Hole, A., Terjesen, T., and Breivik, H. (1980). Epidural versus general anaesthesia for total hip arthroplasty in elderly patients. *Acta Anaesthesiologica Scandinavica*, **24**, 279–287.

Hodkinson, H. M. (1973). Mental impairment in the elderly. *Journal of the Royal College of Physicians*, **7**, 305–317.

Hustey, F. M., Meldon, S., and Palmer, R. (2000). Prevalence and documentation of impaired mental status in elderly emergency department patients. *Academic Emergency Medicine*, **7**, 1166.

Inouye, S. K. (1999). Predisposing and precipitating factors for delirium in hospitalized older patients. *Dementia and Geriatric Cognitive Disorders*, **10**, 393–400.

Inouye, S. K. and Charpentier, P. A. (1996). Precipitating factors for delirium in hospitalized elderly persons. Predictive model and interrelationship with baseline vulnerability. *Journal of the American Medical Association*, **275**, 852–857.

Inouye, S. K., Viscoli, C. M., Horowitz, R. I., Hurst, L. D., and Tinetti, M. E. (1993). A predictive model for delirium in hospitalized elderly medical patients based on admission characteristics. *Annals of Internal Medicine*, **113**, 941–948.

Inouye, S. K., Bogardus, S. T., Charpentier, P. A., Leo-Summers, L., Acampora, D., Holford, T. R., and Cooney, L. M. (1999a). A multicomponent intervention to prevent delirium in hospitalized older patients. *New England Journal of Medicine*, **340**, 669–676.

Inouye, S. K., Schlesinger, M. J., and Lydon, T. J. (1999b). Delirium: a symptom of how hospital care is failing older persons and a window to improve quality of hospital care. *American Journal of Medicine*, **106**, 565–573.

Jacoby, R. and Bergmann, K. (1986). The psychiatry of old age. In: *Essentials of postgraduate psychiatry* (eds P. Hill, R. Murray, and A. Thorely), pp. 495–526. Sure and Shatton, London.

Jitapunkul, S., Pillay, I., and Ebrahim, S. (1992). Delirium in newly admitted elderly patients: a prospective study. *Quarterly Journal of Medicine*, **83**, 307–314.

Johnson, J. C., Gottlieb, G. L., Sullivan, E., *et al.* (1990). Using DSM-III criteria to diagnose delirium in elderly general medical patients. *Journal of Gerontology*, **45**, M113–M119.

Kaneko, T., Takahashi, S., Naka, T., Hirooka, Y., Inoue, Y., and Kaibara, N. (1997). Postoperative delirium following gastrointestinal surgery in elderly patients. *Surgery Today*, **27**, 107–111.

Kelly, K. G., Zisselman, M., Cutillo-Schmitter, T., Reichard, R., and Payne, D. (2001). Severity and course of delirium in medically hospitalized nursing facility patients. *American Journal of Geriatric Psychiatry*, **9**, 72–77.

Kobayashi, K., Takeuchi, O., Suzuki, M., and Yamaguchi, N. (1992). A retrospective study on delirium type. *Japanese Journal of Psychiatry and Neurology*, **46**, 911–917.

Kolbeinsson, H. and Jonsson, A. (1993). Delirium and dementia in acute medical admissions of elderly patients in Iceland. *Acta Psychiatrica Scandinavica*, **87**, 123–127.

Koponen, H., Stenbäck, U., Mattila, E., *et al.* (1989). Delirium in elderly persons admitted to a psychiatric hospital: clinical course during the acute stage and one-year follow-up. *Acta Psychiatrica Scandinavica*, **79**, 579–585.

Lawlor, P. G., Gagnon, B., Mancini, I. L., *et al.* (2000). Occurrence, causes and outcome of delirium in patients with advanced cancer: a prospective study. *Archives of Internal Medicine*, **160**, 786–794.

Lerner, A. J., Hedera, P., Koss, E., Stuckey, J., and Friedland, R. P. (1997). Delirium in Alzheimer's disease. *Alzheimer's Disease and Associated Disorders*, **11**, 16–20.

Levkoff, S. E., Safran, C., Cleary, P. D., *et al.* (1988). Identification of factors associated with the diagnosis of delirium in elderly hospitalized patients. *Journal of the American Geriatrics Society*, **36**, 1099–1104.

Levkoff, S. E., Safran, C., Cleary, P. D., Gallop, J., and Phillips, R. S. (1991). Identification of factors associated with the diagnosis of delirium in elderly hospitalized patients. *Journal of the American Geriatrics Society*, **36**, 1099–1104.

Levkoff, S. E., Evans, D. A., Liptzin, B., *et al.* (1992). Delirium. The occurrence and persistence of symptoms among elderly hospitalised patients. *Archives of Internal Medicine*, **152**, 334–340.

Lipowski, Z. J. (1989). Delirium in the elderly patient. *New England Journal of Medicine*, **320**, 578–582.

Lipsitz, B., Levkoff, S. E., Cleary, P. D., *et al.* (1991). An empirical study of diagnostic criteria for delirium. *American Journal of Psychiatry*, **148**, 451–457.

Liptzin, B. and Levkoff, S. E. (1992). An empirical study of delirium subtypes. *British Journal of Psychiatry*, **161**, 843–845.

Magaziner, J., Simonsick, E. M.,Kashner, T. M., Hebel, J. R., and Kenzora, J. E. (1990). Predictors of functional recovery one year following hospital discharge for hip fracture: a prospective study. *Journal of Gerontology*, **45**, M101–M107.

Marcantonio, E. R., Goldman, L., Mangione, C. M., *et al.* (1994). A clinical prediction rule for delirium after elective noncardiac surgery. *Journal of the American Medical Association*, **271**, 134–139.

Marcantonio, E. R., Flacker, J. M., Michaels, M., and Resnick, N. M. (2000). Delirium is independently associated with poor functional recovery after hip fracture. *Journal of the American Geriatrics Society*, **48**, 618–624.

Martin, N. J., Stones, M. J., Young, J. E., and Bedard, M. (2000). Development of delirium: A prospective cohort study in a community hospital. *International Psychogeriatrics*, **12**, 117–127.

McCusker, J., Cole, M., Dendukuri, N., Belzile, E., and Primeau, F. (2001). Delirium in older medical inpatients and subsequent cognitive function status: a prospective study. *Canadian Medical Association Journal*, **165**, 575–583.

McKeith, I. G., Galasko, D., and Kosaka, K. (1996). Consensus guidelines for the clinical and pathologic diagnosis of dementia with Lewy bodies (DLB): report of the consortium on DLB international workshop. *Neurology*, **47**, 1113–1124.

Millar, H. R. (1981). Psychiatric morbidity in elderly surgical patients. *British Journal of Psychiatry*, **138**, 17–20.

Milstein, A., Barak, Y., Kleinman, G., and Pollack, A. (2000). The incidence of delirium immediately following cataract removal surgery: a prospective study in the elderly. *Aging and Mental Health*, **4**, 178–181.

Murray, A. M., Levkoff, S. E., Wetle, T. T., *et al.* (1993). Acute delirium and functional decline in the hospitalized elderly patient. *Journal of Gerontology*, **48**, M181–M186.

Mussi, C., Ferrari, R., Ascari, S., and Salvioli, G. (1999). Importance of serum anticholinergic activity in the assessment of elderly patients with delirium. *Journal of Geriatric Psychiatry and Neurology*, **12**, 82–86.

Myers, J. K., Weissman, M. M., Tischler, G. L., *et al.* (1984). Six month prevalence of psychiatric disorders in three communities. *Archives of General Psychiatry*, **41**, 959–967.

Naughton, B. J., Moran, M. B., Kadah, H., Heman-Ackah, Y., and Longano, J. (1995). Delirium and other cognitive impairment in older adults in an emergency department. *Annals of Emergency Medicine*, **25**, 751–755.

O'Keeffe, S. T. (1999). Clinical subtypes of delirium in the elderly. *Dementia and Geriatric Cognitive Disorders*, **10**, 380–385.

O'Keeffe, S. T. and Lavan, J. N. (1996). Subcutaneous fluids in elderly hospital patients with cognitive impairment. *Gerontology*, **42**, 36–39.

O'Keeffe, S. T. and Lavan, J. N. (1997). The prognostic significance of delirium subtypes in older people. *Journal of the American Geriatrics Society*, **45**, 174–178.

O'Keeffe, S. T. and Lavan, J. N. (1999). Clinical significance of dementia subtypes in older people. *Age and Ageing*, **28**, 115–119.

O'Keeffe, S. T. and Ni Chonchubhair, A. (1994). Postoperative delirium in the elderly. *British Journal of Anaesthesia*, **73**, 673–687.

Okita, Y., Takamoto, S., Ando, M., *et al.* (1998). Mortality and cerebral outcome in patients who underwent aortic arch operations using deep hypothermic circulatory arrest with retrograde cerebral perfusion: no relation of early death, stroke and delirium to the duration of circulatory arrest. *Journal of Thoracic and Cardiovascular Surgery*, **115**, 129–138.

Platzer, H. (1989). Post-operative confusion in the elderly – a literature review. *International Journal of Nursing Studies*, **26**, 369–379.

Pochard, F., Lanore, J. J., Bellevir, F., *et al.* (1995). Subjective psychological status of severely ill patients discharged from mechanical ventilation. *Clinical Intensive Care*, **6**, 57–61.

Pompei, P., Foreman, M., Rudberg, M. A., Inouye, S. K., Braund, V., and Cassel, C. (1994). Delirium in hospitalized older persons: Outcomes and predictors. *Journal of the American Geriatrics Society*, **42**, 809–815.

Rahkonen, T., Eloniemi-Sulkava, U., Halonen, P., *et al.* (2001) Delirium in the non-demented oldest old in the general population: risk factors and prognosis. *International Journal of Geriatric Psychiatry*, **16**, 415–421.

Ramsay, R., Wright, P., Katz, A., Bielawska, C., and Katona, C. (1991). The detection of psychiatric morbidity and its effects on outcome in acute elderly medical admissions. *International Journal of Geriatric Psychiatry*, **6**, 861–866.

Robertsson, B., Blennow, K., Gottfries, C. G., and Wallin, A. (1998). Delirium in dementia. *International Journal of Geriatric Psychiatry*, **13**, 49–56.

Robinson, G. W. (1956). The toxic delirious reactions of old age. In: *Mental disorder in later life* (ed. D. J. Kaplan), pp. 332–51. Stanford University Press, Stanford.

Rockwood, K. (1989). Acute confusion in elderly medical patients. *Journal of the American Geriatrics Society*, **37**, 150–154.

Rockwood, K. (1990). Delays in the discharge of elderly patients. *Journal of Clinical Epidemiology*, **43**, 971–975.

Rockwood, K. (1993). The occurrence and duration of symptoms in elderly patients with delirium. *Journal of Gerontology*, **48**, M162–M166.

Rockwood, K., Stolee, P., and Brahim, A. (1991). Outcomes of admissions to a psychogeriatric service. *Canadian Journal of Psychiatry*, **36**, 275–279.

Rockwood, K., Cosway, S., Stolee, P., *et al.* (1994). Increasing the recognition of delirium in elderly patients. *Journal of the American Geriatrics Society*, **42**, 252–256.

Rockwood, K., Cosway, S., Carver, D., *et al.* (1999). The risk of dementia and death following delirium. *Age and Ageing*, **28**, 551–556.

Rogers, M. P., Liang, M. H., Daltroy, L. H., *et al.* (1989). Delirium after elective orthopedic surgery: Risk factors and natural history. *International Journal of Psychiatry in Medicine*, **19**, 109–121.

Rolfson, D. B., McElhaney, J. E., Rockwood, K., *et al.* (1999). Incidence and risk factors for delirium and other adverse outcomes in older adults after coronary artery bypass graft surgery. *Canadian Journal of Cardiology*, **15**, 771–776.

Rolfson, D., Majumdar, S. R., Taher, A., and Tsuyuki, R. T. (2000). Development and validation of a new instrument for frailty. *Clinical and Investigative Medicine*, **23**, 336.

Rovner, B. W., Kafonek, S., Filipp, L., Lucas, M. J., and Folstein, M. F. (1986). Prevalence of mental illness in a Community Nursing Home. *American Journal of Psychiatry*, **143**, 1446–1449.

Rubinstein, D. and Thomas, J. K. (1970). Psychiatric findings in cardiotomy patients. *AORN Journal*, **11**, 71–82.

Rudberg, M. A., Pompei, P., Foreman, M. D., Ross, R. E., and Cassel, C. K. (1997). The natural history of delirium in hospitalised older people: a syndrome of heterogeneity. *Age and Ageing*, **26**, 169–174.

Sabin, T. D., Vitug, A. J., and Mark, V. H. (1982). Are nursing-home diagnosis and treatment adequate? *Journal of the American Medical Association*, **248**, 321–322.

Sandberg, O., Gustafson, Y., Brännström, B., *et al.* (1998). Prevalence of dementia, delirium, and psychiatric symptoms in various care settings for the elderly. *Scandinavian Journal of Social Medicine*, **26**, 56–62.

Saravay, S. M. and Lavin, M. (1994). Psychiatric comorbidity and length of stay in the general hospital. A critical review of outcome studies. *Psychosomatics*, **35**, 233–252.

Schor, J. D., Levkoff, S. E., Lipsitz, L. A., *et al.* (1992). Risk factors for delirium in hospitalized elderly. *Journal of the American Medical Association*, **267**, 827–831.

Seymour, D. G. and Pringle, R. (1983). Post-operative complications in the elderly surgical patient. *Gerontology*, **29**, 262–270.

Seymour, D. G., Henschke, P. J., Cape, R. D. T., *et al.* (1980). Acute confusional states and dementia in the elderly: the role of dehydration/volume depletion, physical illness and age. *Age and Ageing*, **9**, 137–146.

Shaw, P. J., Bates, D., Cartilidge, N. E. F., *et al.* (1986). Early intellectual dysfunction following coronary bypass surgery. *Quarterly Journal of Medicine*, **225**, 59–68.

Simon, A. and Cahan, R. B. (1963). The acute brain syndrome in geriatric patients. *Psychiatric Research Reports*, **16**, 8–21.

Simpson, C. J. and Kellett, J. M. (1987). The relationship between pre-operative anxiety and post-operative delirium. *Journal of Psychosomatic Research*, **31**, 491–497.

Sirois, F. (1988). Delirium: 100 cases. *Canadian Journal of Psychiatry*, **33**, 375–378.

Smith, L. W. and Dimsdale, J. E. (1989). Postcardiotomy delirium: conclusions after 25 years? *American Journal of Psychiatry*, **146**, 452–458.

Summers, W. K. and Reich, T. C. (1979). Delirium after cataract surgery: review and two cases. *American Journal of Psychiatry*, **136**, 386–391.

Thomas, R. I., Cameron, D. J., and Fahs, M. C. (1988). A prospective study of delirium and prolonged hospital stay. *Archives of General Psychiatry*, **45**, 937–940.

Treloar, A. J. and Macdonald, A. J. D. (1997). Outcome of delirium: Part 1. Outcome of delirium diagnosed by DSM-III-R, ICD-10 and CAMDEX and derivation of the Reversible Cognitive Dysfunction Scale among acute geriatric inpatients. *International Journal of Geriatric Psychiatry*, **12**, 609–613.

Tune, L. E., Holland, A., Folstein, M. F., Damlouji, N. F., Gardner, T. J., and Coyle, J. T. (1981). Association of postoperative delirium with raised serum levels of anticholinergic drugs. *Lancet*, **ii**, 651–653.

Uwakwe, R. (2000). Psychiatric morbidity in elderly patients admitted to non-psychiatric wards in a general/teaching hospital in Nigeria. *International Journal of Geriatric Psychiatry*, **15**, 346–354.

Van der Mast, R. C. and Roest, F. H. (1996). Delirium after cardiac surgery: a critical review. *Journal of Psychosomatic Research*, **41**, 13–30.

Vetter, N. J. and Ford, D. (1989). Anxiety and depression scores in elderly fallers. *International Journal of Geriatric Psychiatry*, **4**, 159–164.

Weed, H. G. Lutman, C. V., Young, D. C., and Schuller, D. E. (1995). Preoperative identification of patients at risk for delirium after major head and neck cancer surgery. *Laryngoscope*, **105**, 1066–1068.

Werner, P., Cohen-Mansfield, J., Braun, J., and Marx, M. S. (1989). Physical restraints and agitation in nursing home residents. *Journal of the American Geriatrics Society*, **37**, 1122–1126.

Williams, M. A., Campbell, E. B., Raynor, W. J., Musholt, M. A., Mlynarczyk, S. M., and Crane, L. F. (1985). Predictors of acute confusional states in hospitalised elderly patients. *Research in Nursing and Health*, **8**, 31–40.

Williams-Russo, P., Urquhart, B. L., Sharrock, N. E., and Chisholm, M. E. (1992). Post-operative delirium: predictors and prognosis in elderly orthopedic patients. *Journal of the American Geriatrics Society*, **40**, 759–767.

World Health Organization (1992). *International classification of diseases*, 10th revision. World Health Organization, Geneva.

Chapter 4

The neuropathophysiology of delirium

Paula Trzepacz and Roos van der Mast

Introduction

Multiple higher cortical functions and neural circuits are affected in delirium, hence Lipowski's description of the disorder as 'acute brain failure'. With its characteristic abrupt onset and fluctuating symptom severity, delirium is a severe neuropsychiatric disorder. It is usually associated with generalized EEG slowing, consistent with widespread cortical dysfunction causing a range of symptoms arising from different functional brain regions. Additionally, evoked potential abnormalities suggest involvement of subcortical areas including the brainstem and thalamus (Trzepacz 1994). Lack of primary motor and sensory signs (unless related to specific aetiologies, like asterixis) suggests that association cortices (secondary and tertiary), limbic structures and ascending neurotransmitter systems are principally affected in delirium. Neuroimaging and lesion reports suggest that prefrontal cortex, anterior thalamus, non-dominant parietal and fusiform cortex are also involved (Trzepacz 1999).

Though a number of neurotransmitters have been implicated in delirium, particularly important roles for acetylcholine and dopamine systems have been hypothesized (Trzepacz 2000). A state of cholinergic deficiency and dopaminergic excess, either absolute and/or relative to each other, is the dominant theory of neurotransmission abnormality that may underlie the final common pathway of delirium (Trzepacz 1999, 2000). In addition, serotonin, which interacts with and may regulate cholinergic and dopaminergic systems, is associated with delirium either when it is increased or decreased. Perturbations of other neurotransmitters such as noradrenaline (norepinephrine), gamma-aminobutyric acid (GABA), and glutamate may also play a role in delirium neuropathophysiology, though there is much less literature implicating them, and they may interact with the above-mentioned systems in causing delirium (Trzepacz 2000; Van der Mast 1998). Evidence for this as well as for interaction between these neurotransmitters in the brain is discussed in this article.

Delirium is commonly associated with severe medical illness, trauma, and postoperative states, in addition to pharmacological causes. Because illness and tissue injury lead to a physiological stress response, their accompanying metabolic changes contribute significantly to the pathophysiology of delirium. The brain's metabolism is dependent on delivery of glucose and oxygen from the bloodstream, without which it cannot function. The stress response differs depending on the level of acuteness of the stage of illness. Acute stress is accompanied by neuroendocrine adaptation, while chronic stress seems to provoke neuroendocrine exhaustion with enduring hypercortisolism. Stress affects the cortisol axis, thyroid hormone metabolism, and cytokine production. Since these stress-induced metabolic changes may alter amino acid availability from plasma for the brain, cerebral neurotransmission, and secretion of cytokines, immune and brain function may be influenced in a maladaptive way (Flacker and Lipsitz 2000; Van der Mast 2000; Van der Mast and Fekkes 2000; Van der Mast *et al.* 2000). Certain neuroanatomical and neurotransmitter systems may represent final common pathways for the otherwise diverse aetiologies of delirium (Trzepacz 1999, 2000), or delirium may be the final common symptom of multiple neurotransmitter abnormalities (Flacker and Lipsitz 1999).

Severe illness, stress response, and the brain

The initial metabolic response to illness, trauma, and starvation involves an increased availability of glucose, amino acids and free fatty acids. However, the body's overall utilization of these substrates is reduced in favour of diversion to vital organs like the immune system and the brain. These metabolic changes are evoked by, among other things, an activation of the sympathetic nervous system and the hypothalamic-pituitary-adrenocortical (HPA) axis, hypersecretion of prolactin and growth hormone (GH), and reduced activity of the thyroid axis (Van den Berghe *et al.* 1998; Van den Berghe 2000) (see Fig. 4.1). The greater the severity of the stressor, the higher the levels of catecholamines and cortisol.

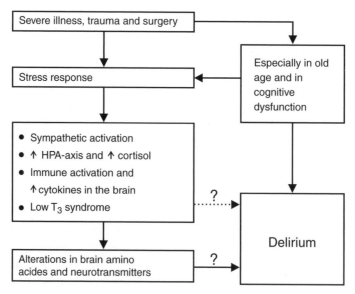

Fig. 4.1 Illness, stress response, and delirium.

This acute stress response is considered adaptive and beneficial, as it reduces and redirects energy consumption, postpones anabolism, and activates the immune response. Simultaneously, hypercortisolism constrains this sympathetic activation and protects against the deleterious effects of the immune response by muting its inflammatory cascade and preventing over-responses. Increased adrenocorticotrophin hormone (ACTH) release, presumably driven by corticotrophin releasing hormone (CRH), cytokines, and the noradrenergic system, causes elevated cortisol levels soon after surgery, trauma, or critical illness (Van den Berghe *et al.* 1998; Van den Berghe 2000).

By contrast, during prolonged illness inappropriate neuroendocrine function develops with reduced secretion of the anterior pituitary hormones and decreased activity of its target organs, while cortisol concentrations usually remain elevated. At the same time, levels of the adrenocortical hormone dehydroepiandrosterone sulphate (DHEAS), which has immunostimulatory properties, are low (Van den Berghe *et al.* 1998; Van den Berghe 2000).

Stress, the limbic system, and the hypothalamic-pituitary-adrenocortical (HPA) axis

Exposure to severe illness and trauma results in biological responses that help the body to deal with the physical stress and to restore homeostasis. The amygdala is the brain centre that mediates between cortical somatic sensory and emotional input, and autonomic and endocrine responses through the sympathetic nervous system and the HPA axis. In the hippocampus, which is involved in learning and memory, projections of the suprachiasmatic nucleus ensure circadian rhythmicity of the HPA axis. The amygdala and hippocampus interact in controlling the HPA axis under daily basal conditions and in reaction to stress (De Kloet *et al.* 1998; Kandel 2000). Stress results in an increase in catecholamines and induces activation of the HPA axis, leading to elevated levels of CRH, ACTH, and cortisol. Under normal circumstances, the stress response is of short duration. Through negative-feedback inhibition, cortisol acts at the pituitary, hypothalamus, hippocampus, and amygdala to keep its levels within physiological limits (De Kloet *et al.* 1998; Kandel 2000). Furthermore, DHEAS may protect limbic structures against the deleterious effects of cortisol. For example, in healthy elderly individuals the cortisol/DHEAS ratio, more than cortisol levels alone, is associated with cognitive decline (Kalmijn *et al.* 1998). However, chronic physical stress produces tolerance to elevated glucocorticoid levels and leads to further dysregulation of the HPA axis. The brain suffers from this increased activity of the HPA axis and cortisol overexposure (De Kloet *et al.* 1998). In the end, neuroendocrine stimulation may become reduced with low ACTH and DHEAS levels and ongoing hypersecretion of cortisol, possibly driven through an alternative peripheral pathway.

The vulnerability for stress-related psychopathology differs among individuals (De Kloet *et al.* 1998). Changes in corticosteroid levels may account for a variety of disturbances in behaviour and cognition, including delirium (Ismail and Wessely 1995;

Vincent 1995; Van der Mast and Fekkes 2000). This may be due to the direct influence of corticosteroids on metabolism and function of various cerebral neurotransmitters as well as the deleterious effects of chronic hypercortisolism on hippocampal 5-HT$_{1A}$ receptors (Fogel *et al.* 1996; Meijer and de Kloet 1998). At the same time, hypercortisolism inhibits the release of thyroid stimulating hormone (TSH), thus maintaining a low activity of the thyroid axis, which may also influence cerebral neurotransmitter balance.

Stress and thyroid hormone metabolism

A low activity state of the thyroid axis is part of the stress response to severe illness, starvation, and major accidental and surgical trauma (McIver and Gorman 1997; Van den Berghe *et al.* 1998; Van den Berghe 2000). This 'low T3 syndrome' is characterized by abnormal thyroid hormone concentrations in the absence of clinically evident thyroid illness. Triiodothyronine (T3) levels are low, often accompanied by elevated levels of the inactive metabolite of thyroxine (reverse T3), as well as normal or decreased total thyroxine (T4) and thyroid stimulating hormone (TSH) levels. The degree of thyroid hormone change is dependent on the severity of disease. Low levels of thyroid hormones predict poor prognosis in several illnesses and, in critically ill patients, low serum T4 correlates with the probability that the patient will die (Felicetta 1989; Cherem *et al.* 1992; McIver and Gorman 1997; Reinhardt *et al.* 1997). The absence of a TSH elevation in the face of low circulating T3 levels suggests that there is also an altered feedback setting at the HP axis (Van den Berghe *et al.* 1998; Van den Berghe 2000). Diminished availability of active thyroid hormone leads to reduced tissue energy expenditure, which may be seen as part of an adaptive stress response (Felicetta 1989; McIver and Gorman 1997; Van den Berghe *et al.* 1998; Camacho and Dwarkanathan 1999; Van den Berghe 2000). However, during the prolonged phase of critical illness, a low T3 syndrome may also be considered as a maladaptive response inducing hypothyroidism and further catabolism (Van den Berghe *et al.* 1998).

The clinical consequences of low serum and tissue concentrations of T3 are not clear, and it remains speculative whether a low T3 syndrome affects arousal, cognition, emotion or behaviour. However, one may hypothesize that the resulting reduced transport of amino acids and sugars into the cell, diminished protein synthesis, and decreased production of ATP lead to widespread reduction of cerebral oxidative metabolism and alterations in neurotransmission, especially in prolonged critical illness.

Stress and cytokines

Physical stress activates the immune system and cytokine production. Cytokines play a key role in mediating inflammatory and immune responses. In addition to providing communication between immune cells, specific cytokines may also signal the brain to produce neurochemical, neuroendocrine, neuroimmune, and behavioural changes.

Thus, cytokines may act as neuromodulators affecting important brain activities such as sleep, appetite, and neuroendocrine regulation (Kronfol and Remick 2000). Cytokines are small polypeptides that can be secreted by various cells regulating the immune response being part of the response to stress. The activity of cytokines is regulated in cascades, where the induction of early cytokines [such as interleukin-1 (IL-1)] serves to increase the production of later cytokines (such as IL-2, IL-6, etc.). The response to cytokines is provided by unique cytokine receptors. There are cytokine receptors in the brain, and astrocytes and/or microglia, in turn, may secrete various cytokines in response to brain insult (Kronfol and Remick 2000; Broadhurst and Wilson 2001).

According to the inflammatory hypothesis, cytokines may directly or indirectly play a role in the pathophysiology of delirium. For example, IL-1 released in the brain stimulates the production of other cytokines such as TNF-α, IL-2 and IL-6. Furthermore, IL-1 cytokines, such as IL-2, IL-6, TNF and interferon, are associated with activation of the HPA axis, resulting in increases of CRH, ACTH, and cortisol, while feedback mechanisms include negative feedback exerted by cortisol (Kronfol and Remick 2000). Cytokines can also modulate the hypothalamic-pituitary-thyroid (HPT) axis, contributing to the occurrence of a low T3 syndrome, and cytokines seem to play a role in the suppression of the hypothalamic-pituitary-gonadal (HPG) axis (Van den Berghe et al. 1998; Kronfol and Remick 2000). Thus, immune activation can interface with neuroendocrine systems that become perturbed during the stress associated with severe illness.

In addition, cytokines are directly linked with certain brain functions. They may change the permeability of the blood–brain barrier and cerebral neurotransmission (Müller 1997; Kronfol and Remick 2000). They can alter activity of dopaminergic, noradrenergic, serotonergic, and cholinergic neurotransmitter systems. Certain cytokines cause increased activity of the dopaminergic and noradrenergic systems, reduced acetylcholine release, and elevated cerebral tryptophan (Trp) and serotonin turnover, all of which have been hypothesized as underlying delirium (Stefano et al. 1994; Hopkins and Rothwell 1995; Müller 1997; Kronfol and Remick 2000). In depressed patients, a relationship between immune activation and decreased plasma Trp availability has been found (Maes et al. 1994, 1997).

On the other hand, cytokine production is related to the activity of the peptides insulin-like growth factor (IGF-I) and somatostatin that have important neurotrophic properties (for an overview see Broadhurst and Wilson 2001). Delirium has been associated with reversible somatostatin reduction, and elevated levels of IGF-I and somatostatin may represent a neuroprotective response suggesting a potential role in the treatment or prevention of delirium (Broadhurst and Wilson 2001).

In summary, the release of cerebral cytokines, such as IL-1, in response to significant illness or trauma lead to activation of the HPA axis and hypercortisolism, decreased activity of the HPT and HPG axes, altered permeability of the blood–brain barrier, and interference with neurotransmission. Thus, cytokines may play an intriguing and complex role in psychiatric disturbances such as delirium (Stefano *et al.* 1994; Hopkins and Rothwell 1995; Müller 1997; Kronfol and Remick 2000). This is consistent with dose-dependent psychiatric adverse events associated with cytokine levels of patients (e.g. interferon-alpha, IL-2, and lymphokine-activated killer cells) (Denicoff *et al.* 1987; Renault and Hoofnagle 1989; Müller 1997; Kronfol and Remick 2000; Broadhurst and Wilson 2001). Also, reduction of the neuroprotective peptides IGF-I and somatostatin may have a role in the pathogenesis of delirium (Broadhurst and Wilson 2001).

The final common neural pathway in delirium

Delirium involves a generalized disturbance of higher cerebral cortical processes, as reflected by diffuse slowing on EEG and a wide range of symptoms (cognition, perception, sleep, motor, language, and thought). However, not all brain regions are equally affected in delirium. Certain regions, circuits, and neurochemistry may be integral in the neuropathogenesis of delirium (Trzepacz 1994, 1999, 2000). Supporting this hypothesis, Henon *et al.* (1999) found that laterality of lesion location and not metabolic factors accounted for the differences in delirium incidence for superficial cortical lesions in a series of stroke patients.

Delirium is caused by many different aetiologies, each with its own physiological effects on the body. Somehow, this diversity of physiological perturbations produces a common clinical expression – 'core symptoms' – that are at times acompanied by 'associated symptoms' (Trzepacz 1999). A final common neural pathway (Trzepacz 1994, 1999, 2000; Trzepacz *et al.* 2001) (see Figure 4.2) may underlie these symptoms. This common neural circuitry may comprise bilateral or right prefrontal cortex, superficial right posterior parietal cortex, basal ganglia, fusiform (ventromesial temporoparietal) and

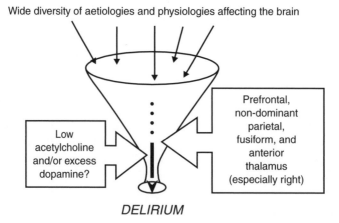

Fig. 4.2 Delirium final common pathway. Reproduced with permission from Trzepacz *et al.* 2001.

lingual gyrus on either side, and right anterior thalamus. Pathways linking these areas (thalamic-frontal-subcortical and temporolimbic-frontal/subcortical) are also probably involved. These brain regions are suggested by structural neuroimaging case reports (see Table 4.1) and several consecutive, prospective studies that are largely consistent with functional neuroimaging studies.

Lateralization to right-sided circuitry involvement in delirium – in contrast to left anterior in major depression – has been suggested (Trzepacz 1994, 2000; Trzepacz *et al.* 2001). Because right prefrontal cortex processes novel situations cognitively while the left processes familiar ones (Goldberg 1998), this may account for difficulties comprehending new environments. Right (non-dominant) posterior parietal cortex is a region associated with severe delirium after stroke; it subserves sustained attention and attention to the environment, and attentional difficulties are a key criterion for delirium diagnosis (Posner and Bois 1971). Bipolar patients had the highest incidence of delirium (35.5%) among 199 psychiatric inpatients (Ritchie *et al.* 1996). Their greater

Table 4.1 Lesions associated with delirium in structural neuroimaging studies

Authors	Lesions associated with delirium
Mesulam (1979); Price and Mesulam (1985)	CVA in R posterior parietal, R prefrontal, ventromedial temporal or occipital cortex
Horenstein *et al.* (1967)	CVAs in fusiform and calcarine cortex
Medina *et al.* (1977)	L or bilateral mesial temporal-occipital CVA
Medina *et al.* (1974)	L hippocampal or fusiform CVA
Valphiades *et al.* (1996)	R mesial occipital, parahippocampal and hippocampus (with visual hallucinations)
Nighoghossian *et al* (1992)	R subcortical CVA (with frontal deactivation)
Bogousslavsky *et al.* (1988)	R anterior thalamus CVA on preexisting L caudate lesion (with ↓ frontal perfusion on SPECT)
Figiel *et al.* (1989); Martin *et al.* (1992)	Lesions in caudate (in depressed patients treated with ECT or meds)
Figiel *et al.* (1991)	Parkinson's patients (depressed and treated with ECT or meds)
Koponen *et al.* (1989)	R prefrontal or posterior parietal cortex CVA (many with co-morbid dementia)
Dunne *et al.* (1986)	R temporoparietal CVA
Mullally *et al.* (1982)	R temporal or parietal CVA
Boiten and Lodder (1989)	R inferior parietal lobule CVA
Santamaria *et al.* (1984); Friedman (1985)	R anteromedial thalamus CVA
Henon *et al.* (1999)	R superficial CVA (prospective sample)

Note: R, right; L, left; CVA, stroke.

Reproduced with permission from Trzepacz (2000).

predisposition for delirium may be related to dysfunction of right-sided anterior and subcortical pathways implicated in mania (Blumberg *et al.* 1999). 'Bell's mania' is a severe confusional state of acute mania that mimics delirium. Visual attention and memory tests were able to distinguish delirious from non-delirious patients, supporting the importance of non-dominant hemisphere dysfuction in delirium (Hart *et al.* 1997). Even dopamine neurotransmission is lateralized such that activity is normally higher in the left prefrontal cortex (Glick *et al.* 1982), which may become relevant in delirium.

Severe and persistent delirium can result from right posterior parietal cortex lesions (Mesulam *et al.* 1976; Price and Mesulam 1985; Boiten and Lodder 1989; Koponen *et al.* 1989), whereas agitated delirium can result from infarctions of the right middle cerebral artery distribution (Schmidley and Messing 1984). Fusiform cortex (inferior, mesial temporal-occipital cortex) may be associated with an acute, agitated delirium that is accompanied by visual impairment (Horenstein *et al.* 1967; Medina *et al.* 1974, 1977). There are only a small number of studies examining the relationship between delirium and stroke. In a retrospective study of 661 stroke patients, nearly all 19 cases diagnosed with delirium had right-sided temporoparietal cortex lesions (Dunne *et al.* 1986). Another 26 cases with similar lesions were not diagnosed with delirium because they lacked 'clouded consciousness', probably resulting in an underestimate of the association of delirium with such lesions. In a retrospective study where 60 of 309 neurology consultations had an acute confusional state, cases with focal lesions were dominated by right temporal or parietal locations (Mullaly *et al.* 1982).

Prospective studies of stroke location and delirium incidence largely support findings from retrospective studies and case reports. Using DSM-IV criteria and a DRS score ≥ 10 points to define cases, Henon *et al.* (1999) found a 25% incidence of delirium among 202 consecutive stroke patients. Right-sided superficial cortical lesions were more associated with delirium than left ($P = 0.009$), although a comparison of cases with deep lesions did not reveal laterality. Using DSM-III–R criteria, 69 consecutively admitted delirious elderly patients (most with co-morbid dementia) had more generalized atrophy and focal changes on CT scan, in particular right hemisphere lesions in the parieto-occipital association area, when compared to 31 age-matched controls with other neurological disorders (Koponen *et al.* 1989). By contrast, a study not designed to assess effects of laterality found that 58% of 155 consecutive stroke patients with left-sided lesions were acutely confused (DSM-III–R criteria) versus 38% with right-sided lesions (Gustafson *et al.* 1991).

Frontal, thalamic and subcortical regions have also been implicated in delirium. Anterior, medial, and dorsal thalamic nuclei interconnect with prefrontal, subcortical, and limbic areas that are involved in cognitive and behavioural functions. The thalamus is involved in sensory gating, maintenance of waking EEG activity, reciprocal interactions with all brain regions. Its position in the frontal-striatal-thalamic circuits means that a relatively small thalamic lesion can cause delirium, including a stroke in the right paramedian and anteromedial thalamus (Santamaria *et al.* 1984; Friedman 1985; Bogousslavsky *et al.* 1988). The thalamus is rich in GABAergic interneurons and glutamatergic neurons (Sherman and Kock 1990) and receives cholinergic, noradrenergic, and serotonergic afferents from brainstem nuclei. Muscarinic activity at the thalamus helps maintain EEG rhythm. Basal ganglia lesions disrupt fronto-striatal-thalamic circuits.

Pre-existing lesions of the caudate (Figiel *et al.* 1989; Martin *et al.* 1992) and Parkinson's disease (Figiel *et al.* 1991) both increase the risk of delirium during ECT or with tricyclic antidepressants. Robertsson *et al.* (1998) found that subcortical damage increased delirium risk among 175 consecutive dementia patients, where vascular dementia carried more risk than early Alzheimer's or frontal types.

Thus, though many patients with strokes can become delirious through a variety of chemical or structural mechanisms (including glutamatergic surges and cholinergic deficiency), the majority of evidence from stroke reports supports the importance of right-sided laterality for cortical and thalamic lesions. Findings from single photon emission computed tomography (SPECT) and positron emission tomography (PET) scans also support the relevance of the prefrontal cortex and subcortical regions in patients with delirium (Trzepacz 1994). These usually show reduced flow or metabolism in the frontal cortex and either increased or decreased flow in subcortical regions. Dysfunction in both cortical and subcortical regions in delirium is also supported by slowing of EEG and evoked potentials.

Neurotransmission in delirium

A final common neural pathway for delirium would involve certain neurotransmitters as well as neuroanatomical circuitry. The predominance of evidence in the literature supports a low cholinergic-excess dopaminergic state. This does not preclude involvement of other neurotransmitter systems that can alter the activity of cholinergic and dopaminergic pathways, including serotonin, endogenous opiates, GABA, and glutamate. Neuroendocrine and inflammatory perturbations during stress or severe illness can also alter neurotransmission (see *Stress and cytokines* above). Neurotransmission also can be altered through widespread effects on oxidative metabolism. Metabolic pathways for the oxidation of glucose that produces ATP utilize glucose, oxygen, and vitamins as cofactors for enzymes, such that deficiency in any of these could result in less ATP and fewer substrates for optimal neurotransmission (e.g. amino acids and acetyl coenzyme A). Even ratios of plasma amino acids affect neurotransmitter synthesis during severe illness, surgery and trauma when associated with immune activation and adaptive metabolic changes that redirect energy consumption (Van der Mast and Fekkes 2000).

There is evidence for both widespread effects on neurotransmission (general metabolism) and interference with specific receptors and neurotransmitters in delirium. Neurotoxic metabolites, such as quinolinic acid from tryptophan metabolism

(Basile *et al.* 1995), and false neurotransmitters (octopamine in hepatic insufficiency), can alter neurotransmission as a mechanism in the neuropathogenesis of delirium. Glial dysfunction might also play a role, as glia can regulate synaptic neurotransmitter levels.

Acetylcholine and delirium

A deficiency of muscarinic cholinergic activity has received the most study in delirium. Acetylcholine (Ach) in the brain is a good candidate because of its role in attention, memory, visuospatial ability, executive functions, delusions, visual hallucinations, sensory gating, REM sleep, motor activity, and thalamic EEG rhythm (see Table 4.2). These different functions and behaviours may be mediated by different receptor subtypes (Reiner and Fibiger 1995). Cholinergic neurons project from lateral tegmentum and basal forebrain to cortical targets across the cortex (Selden *et al.* 1998).

The five muscarinic cholinergic receptor subtypes are designated as m1–m5 by gene cloning techniques, or M1–M3 by pharmacological probes. Subtype distribution in human CNS as determined by autoradiography (Ehlert *et al.* 1995) reveals that m1 receptors are the most prevalent subtype post-synaptically, and distributed reciprocally from nicotinic receptors. M1, m3 and m4 receptors are most abundant in forebrain, decreasing in density along a rostral–caudal gradient (Cortes *et al.* 1986; Lin *et al.* 1986). By contrast, m2 receptors are less prevalent than m1 receptors, presynaptic, distributed similarly to nicotinic receptors, and increasing in density going caudally (greatest density in brainstem, cerebellum, and thalamus).

Evidence for cholinergic deficiency in delirium is supported by a number of different lines of evidence (see Table 4.3) ranging from anticholinergic drug-induced delirium to serum anticholinergic assays to EEG slowing. Metabolic (e.g., hypoxia, hyperglycemia) or structural perturbations (e.g. stroke, traumatic brain injury) that reduce Ach synthesis or release are considered 'anticholinergic' as part of their mechanism in causing delirium. Even at low doses, anticholinergic medications cause cognitive impairment without causing full-blown delirium (Miller *et al.* 1988), and are often identified as risk factors for delirium in epidemiological studies (Gustafson *et al.* 1988). Centrally active anticholinergic drugs can cause EEG slowing and reduced verbal memory (Sloan *et al.* 1992).

Table 4.2 Acetylcholine (Ach) and brain functions

Cortical arousal

Induction of REM sleep

EEG fast wave activity

Learning and memory

Attentional processes

Mood

Motor components of behaviour

Sensory gating

Table 4.3 Evidence for cholinergic deficiency in delirium

- Acetylcholine maintains thalamic EEG fast wave activity
- Anticholinergic drugs cause delirium
- Cholinergic agonists reverse anticholinergic drug-induced delirium
- Higher serum anticholinergic activity correlates with delirium severity and incidence
- Lewy body dementia mimics delirium
- Atropine animal delirium model shows EEG slowing, maze impairment and hyperactivity
- Hypoxia, hyperglycaemia, thiamine deficiency associated with decreased Ach release
- Stroke and traumatic brain injury associated with decreased Ach activity
- Alzheimer's and vascular dementias that disrupt Ach pathways have increased risk for delirium
- Age-associated decreased acetylcholine system activity has increased risk for delirium

Adapted from Trzepacz (2000).
Ach = acetylcholine

Many drugs exert their anticholinergic effects by antagonizing post-synaptic muscarinic receptors (e.g. m1). Muscarinic blockade from atropinic drugs is receptor subtype non-specific. Reports of anticholinergic drugs causing delirium include homatropine eye drops, mefloquine, pheniramine aminosalicylate, meperidine, diphenhydramine, benztropine, atropine, Ditran, clozaril, tricyclic antidepressants, belladonna alkaloids, lorazepam, H2 blockers, anesthetics, and ingestion of Angels' trumpet flowers (Trzepacz 2000). In addition, normeperidine and norfentanyl are highly anticholinergic metabolites of their parent opiate compounds (Coffman and Dilsaver 1988). Other drugs are anticholinergic by affecting presynaptic sites or other neurotransmitters that regulate the cholinergic activity to cause anticholinergic delirium, including barbiturates, opiate agonists, cannibinoids, β-adrenergic agonists, dopaminergic agonists, and ethanol (Coffman and Dilsaver 1988).

Efforts to measure anticholinergicity and to correlate it with delirium include a drug scoring system and a serum anticholinergic activity assay. A drug risk ranking system was assigned to drugs with anticholinergic effects; post-cardiotomy, post-cataractectomy and post-ECT patients with delirium had significantly higher total risk scores than those without delirium (Summers 1978). Delirium severity in 278 elderly medical in-patients was assessed longitudinally using the Delirium Index and Summers' drug risk rankings (Han *et al.* 2001). An increase in delirium severity was significantly and independently associated with exposure to anticholinergic medications given the prior day – even after adjusting for dementia, baseline delirium severity, length of follow-up, and number of non-anticholinergic drugs taken.

Tune *et al.*'s (1981) technique measures serum anticholinergic activity (SAA) in atropine equivalents using a radioimmunoassay (see review by Tune 2000). Tune *et al.* (1992) measured 10^{-8} molar amounts of 25 drugs commonly prescribed to the elderly using this radioimmunoassay and found that 14 drugs had detectable anticholinergic activity. A study of healthy elderly subjects given low dose scopolamine prior to surgery found a high correlation ($r = 0.69$) between SAA and CSF anticholinergic activity levels, suggesting a relationship between peripheral and central levels (Miller *et al.* 1988). SAA levels exceeding 0.83 ng/ml of atropine equivalents predicted a significant deleterious effect on self-care ability of demented nursing home patients, likely related to cognitive impairments (Rovner *et al.* 1988). Using a SAA assay cut-off value of 1.5 pmol/ml atropine equivalents, Tune *et al.* (1981) distinguished delirious and non-delirious post-cardiotomy patients. Their MMSE scores correlated inversely ($r = -0.83$) with SAA levels supporting a relationship between anticholinergicity and cognitive impairment. Similarly, Mondimore *et al.* (1983) found a correlation between SAA levels and MMSE scores in 20 post-ECT patients. SAA levels were significantly higher in nine delirious than in 16 non-delirious surgical ICU patients (Golinger *et al.* 1987). A double-blind intervention study by Tollefson *et al.* (1991) in nursing home residents with elevated SAA levels found that cognitive status improved in patients whose anticholinergic medications were reduced. SAA levels correlated with more delirium symptoms as measured on the Delirium Symptom Interview and these elevated SAA levels were independently associated with delirium (Flacker *et al.* 1998). In delirious hospitalized medically ill elderly patients SAA levels were significantly higher than in non-delirious patients and declined when the delirium resolved (Mach *et al.* 1995). When an anticholinergic activity score for medications given to ICU patients the day before surgery was calculated based on individual drug SAA potencies, these sums distinguished patients with post-operative delirium (Tune *et al.* 1993). Mussi *et al.* (1999) found higher SAA (23 versus 3.9 pmol/ml atropine equivalents, $P < 0.004$) in elderly medically ill patients who were delirious ($n = 12$) than those without delirium ($n = 49$). The majority of these studies link higher serum anticholinergicity with central nervous system impairment, consequences of delirium, poor self-care, and/or worse cognitive deficits. However, in contrast to these studies, Flacker *et al.* (1998) found no difference in SAA levels between eight delirious and 14 non-delirious elderly nursing home residents who became febrile due to acute medical illnesses. Rather, levels were higher in both groups during febrile illness and lower after recovery. The authors proposed that peptides released during fever, such as dynorphin A, could have acted at the muscarinic receptors and may have masked differences between these groups.

Methodological issues surrounding the SAA technique include not differentiating between muscarinic receptor subtypes. Therefore, the SAA could be detecting opposite effects – for example, M1 blockade activity that would be deliriogenic as well as procholinergic M2 blockade that would be delirium protective. Not only does this method not have specificity for muscarinic receptor subtypes, it also may be affected by non-muscarinic drugs such as peptides released during febrile illness or inflammatory responses such as dynorphin A. In addition, wide interindividual variation in SAA levels makes it difficult to determine meaningful cut-off values that indicate increased delirium risk.

There is other evidence that delirium involves cholinergic dysfunction. A human experimental model of delirium was induced using anticholinergic drugs and resulted in EEG slowing, hyperactivity, psychosis, and cognitive impairment (Itil 1966; Itil and Fink 1966). These symptoms and EEG changes reversed after treatment with either tacrine, physostigmine, or chlorpromazine – that is, either enhancing Ach or blocking dopamine. Lewy body dementia bears similarities to delirium – diffuse cognitive impairment, fluctuating symptom severity, visual hallucinations, and EEG slowing (Perry and Perry 1995). It is associated with severe degeneration of basal forebrain cholinergic neurons and some of its symptoms may be responsive to treatment with donepezil, a cholinergic enhancer (Kaufer *et al.* 1998).

If delirium can be caused by anticholinergic drugs, then it follows that treatment with acetylcholinesterase inhibitor drugs, which raise levels of Ach by inhibiting its breakdown in the synapse, should reverse anticholinergic drug-induced delirium. In fact, physostigmine has been reported to reverse cases of delirium associated with the use of ranitidine, meperidine, cimetidine, homatropine eyedrops, belladonna alkaloids, mefloquine, anaesthetics, clozaril, amitriptyline, and lorazepam (Trzepacz 2000). In addition, tacrine resolved pheniramine delirium (Mendelson 1977) and galanthamine reversed scopolamine delirium (Baraka and Harik 1977). More recently, cholinesterase inhibitors have been used for non-drug-induced delirium cases, supporting a broader role for cholinergic deficiency in delirium. Physostigmine has been reported to treat delirium tremens (Powers *et al.* 1981; Daunderer 1983). A retrospective study of 52 consecutive consultations to a toxicology service showed that delirium and anticholinergic agitation were better controlled by physostigmine than benzodiazepines (Burns *et al.* 2000). Physostigmine-treated patients had a lower incidence of clinical complications (7% versus 46%, $P < 0.002$) and shorter median time to recovery (12 versus 24 hours, $P = 0.004$). Donepezil improved delirium in a mildly demented alcoholic patient (Wengel *et al.* 1998), perhaps because he may have had thiamine deficiency-related degeneration of the cholinergic nucleus basalis (Cullen and Halliday 1995). Visual hallucinations in a postoperative patient who had EEG slowing and mild cognitive impairment improved using donepezil, though he may have had early Lewy body dementia (Burke *et al.* 1999). Donepezil also improved a mildly demented Alzheimer's patient who had a prolonged postoperative delirium episode (Wengel *et al.* 1999). Rivastigmine was reported to treat a 17-day delirium episode secondary to lithium intoxication within 48 hours and the Delirium Rating Scale score decreased from 29 to 8 (Fischer 2001). However, these case reports remain unsupported by double-blind studies.

In addition to medications, several medical conditions can reduce cholinergic neurotransmission, including thiamine deficiency, hypoxia, and hypoglycemia. The rate-limiting step in synthesis of Ach combines choline and acetyl coenzyme A (CoA). Choline is derived from dietary sources. Because acetyl CoA is produced from glucose oxidation in the citric acid cycle, hypoglycaemia or niacin deficiency can reduce

Ach synthesis (Ghajar *et al.* 1985). Thus, cholinergic neurotransmission is vulnerable to impairments of cerebral metabolism (Blass and Gibson 1999). In animal models, hypoxia reduces Ach release and synthesis, which is accompanied by increased dopamine release (Gibson *et al.* 1975). Because thiamine is necessary for cholinergic neuron function, its deficiency reduces cholinergic neurotransmission (Gibson *et al.* 1982), as can occur in alcoholic dependence or nutritional deficiency. Consistent with these findings, glucose has been shown to enhance memory performance via a CNS muscarinic mechanism (Kopf and Baratti 1994). Parietal cortex levels of choline are reduced in chronic hepatic encephalopathy, as measured by magnetic resonance imaging (MRI) spectroscopy (Kreis *et al.* 1991).

Stroke and traumatic brain injury are associated with decreased cholinergic activity, especially in the thalamus, amygdala, frontal cortex, hippocampus, and basal forebrain (Yamamoto *et al.* 1988). These patients are vulnerable to side effects from anti-muscarinic drugs (Dixon *et al.* 1994). Both traumatic brain injury (Dixon *et al.* 1994) and stroke (Scremin and Jenden 1989; Bertrand *et al.* 1993) result acutely in surges of glutamate and Ach at the time of injury, followed by a decline in cholinergic activity that can persist for weeks (Lyeth *et al.* 1988; Saija *et al.* 1988). The low cholinergic state seems to temporally coincide with the emergence of delirium after the initial neurolog-ical damage. In stroke patients, cholinergic agonists result in increased Ach synthesis as well as membrane regeneration (D'Orlando and Sandage 1995). Ischaemia reduces hippocampal Ach neurotransmission (Ishimaru *et al.* 1995), even in the presence of intact neurons.

Elderly people are more vulnerable to delirium. Neuroanatomical changes with ageing or damage, multiple medical problems, and more complex pharmacological needs combine to increase their delirium risk. An index delirium episode in an elderly person may indicate an undiagnosed or subclinical dementia and therefore explain so-called 'persistent cognitive deficits' noticed during the year after hospital discharge. Koponen *et al.*'s work supports this hypothesis. They found a correlation between CSF acetylcholinesterase levels and survival duration during a 4-year follow-up period for delirious patients, in whom serial CSF levels decreased with the progression of underlying Alzheimer's or vascular dementia (Koponen *et al.* 1991, 1994). Cholinergic neuronal degeneration (e.g. nucleus basalis) in the early stages of Alzheimer's dementia increases susceptibility to delirium. Vascular lesions that disrupt cholinergic projection pathways and receptor density can also increase vulnerability to delirium (Nagasawa *et al.* 1994; Kondo *et al.* 1995). Age-associated changes of the cholinergic system differ from Alzheimer's disease (Muller *et al.* 1991). These include reductions of muscarinic receptor plasticity, quantal release of Ach, second messenger responsivity, and m1 and m2 receptor density in cerebral cortex, hippocampus, and striatum. Advanced age is identified as a risk factor for delirium, suggesting that age-associated cholinergic changes alone may increase delirium vulnerability though comparisons of delirium incidence between non-demented elderly and younger adults are needed. There is also an increased sensitivity with ageing to adverse events associated with anticholinergic medications (Molchan 1992; Ray *et al.* 1992).

In contrast to the plethora of support for a cholinergic deficiency state in delirium, there is only scant evidence that cholinergic intoxication can result in delirium, because therapeutic agents are more often anticholinergic than cholinergic-enhancing. Delirium has been associated with the use of organophosphate insecticides, nerve poisons, and tacrine (Trzepacz 1996). Perhaps delirium results from extreme imbalances of cholinergic neurotransmitter activity levels.

Dopamine and Ach systems interact with each other. Increased dopamine activity can result from reduced cholinergic activity, conceptualized as an imbalance of their activities relative to each other. Hypoxia results in increased release of dopamine and decreased release of acetylcholine (Broderick and Gibson 1989). In the striatum, D2 receptor stimulation reduces acetylcholine release whereas D1 stimulation increases it (Ikarashi *et al.* 1997) (see Figure 4.3). D2 blockade, therefore, would be expected to be associated with enhanced Ach release.

Serotonin can also affect Ach activity. The serotonin system involves many receptor subtypes. Serotonergic neurons of the median raphe nuclei innervate the basal forebrain – a cholinergic-rich region – where they may interact. Figure 4.4 depicts the relationship between presynaptic serotonergic receptor subtypes on a cholinergic neuron and Ach release into the synapse. *In vivo* microdialysis rat studies suggest synergism between serotonin and Ach for learning, memory, and regulating cortical EEG activity (Hirano *et al.* 1995).

Low voltage fast-wave activity on EEG can be abolished by serotonin antagonists when combined with scopolamine, suggesting a role for serotonin maintaining EEG activation at the thalamus in addition to Ach (Dringenberg and Vanderwolf 1995). Serotonin deficiency, which occurs in some cases of delirium, may cause EEG slowing.

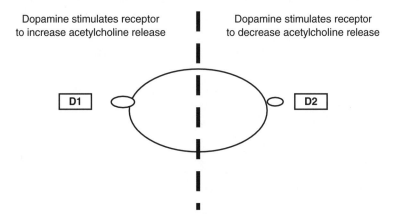

Fig. 4.3 Dopamine receptor subtype effects on acetylcholine release. Reproduced with permission from Trzepacz (2000).

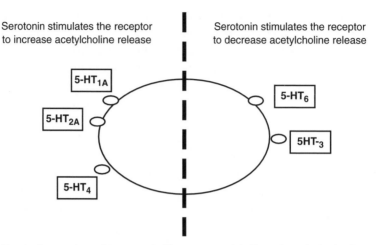

Fig. 4.4 Serotonin receptor subtypes and effects on acetylcholine release in brain. Reproduced with permission from Trzepacz (2000).

In rat frontal cortex, serotonin regulation of acetylcholine neurons occurs when stimulation of 5-HT$_2$ receptors results in increased Ach release (Hirano *et al.* 1995). Terminals of basal forebrain cholinergic neurons also have 5-HT$_2$ receptors (Quirion *et al.* 1985). 5-HT$_4$ receptors also mediate increased Ach release in rat frontal cortex (Yamaguchi *et al.* 1997). In addition, stimulation of 5-HT$_3$ and 5-HT$_6$ receptors, as well as presynaptic m2 receptors, inhibit Ach release and enhance release when blocked (Kennedy *et al.* 2001) (see Figure 4.4). 5-HT$_6$ receptors localize only in the brain (Monsoma *et al.* 1993) and its antagonists raise Ach activity (Sleight *et al.* 1998). Ach release in rat hippocampus is inhibited by serotonin stimulation of hippocampal 5-HT$_3$ receptors whilst their blockade enhances Ach release (Ramirez *et al.* 1996). Thus, findings from these *in vivo* microdialysis studies of synaptic activity in freely moving rats suggest that serotonin can enhance cholinergic activity in the forebrain depending on how and which combination of 5-HT receptor subtypes are affected. Such *in vivo* microdialysis studies probably more accurately reflect neurotransmission because the whole synaptic system is assessed in live animals in contrast to *in vitro* receptor studies.

In summary, there is evidence from a variety of reports in humans and animals suggesting that cholinergic deficiency may be neurochemically responsible for the final common neural pathway for delirium. Interrelationships between dopamine excess or serotonin deficiency with reduced cholinergic function also may be important.

Dopamine and delirium

Dopamine (DA) neurotransmission, which may be largely regulatory, plays a role in motor activity, stereotypies, attention, mood, motivation, memory, thought, language, and perceptions. Dopamine excess, either absolute or relative to acetylcholine activity,

Table 4.4 Evidence for dopaminergic excess in delirium

- DA agonists cause delirium (e.g. levodopa, bupropion)
- DA blockers treat delirium
- ECT increases dopamine
- Cocaine overdose causes delirium
- D2 density declines with ageing and correlates with frontal cognitive test scores
- DA transporter gene allele A-9 is more prevalent in alcoholics with withdrawal delirium and seizures
- DA agonists cause EEG slowing
- DA release ↑ in hypoxia (when Ach ↓)
- DA is important in prefrontal and temporo-limbic areas

Adapted from Trzepacz (2000).

has been hypothesized as underlying delirium based on a variety of observations (see Table 4.4). Delirium is associated with intoxication from dopaminergic drugs, including levodopa, dopamine, and bupropion (Dager and Heritch 1990; Rudrofer *et al.* 1991; Ames *et al.* 1992), as well as from cocaine binges (Wetli *et al.* 1996). Parkinson's patients are vulnerable to delirium related to dopaminergic medications. Opiates commonly cause delirium, especially via their anticholinergic metabolites, but they also increase brain DA and glutamate activity. During hepatic encephalopathy excess dopamine levels occur, likely related to increased CSF levels of tyrosine and phenylalanine (Knell *et al.* 1974) or to changes in dopamine regulation by altered serotonin activity. Increased availability of tyrosine increases mesoprefrontal DA synthesis and release (Tam and Roth 1997). Hypoxia increases the release of dopamine (Broderick and Gibson 1989), in addition to decreasing acetylcholine (Gibson *et al.* 1975).

Patients with alcohol withdrawal delirium are more likely to have the A-9 allele of the dopamine transporter gene compared to matched controls without delirium (Sander *et al.* 1997), suggesting a role for abnormal dopamine neurotransmission in delirium. Dopamine agonists that are active at D1 and D2 receptors cause EEG slowing and behavioural arousal in rats (Ongini *et al.* 1985), findings similar to those seen in atropine-treated rats (Leavitt *et al.* 1994; Trzepacz *et al.* 1992).

Delirium during ECT may be related to excess DA, the seizure itself, or anticholinergic effects of drugs given. Patients with higher SAA levels were at greater risk for post-ECT delirium (Mondimore *et al.* 1983). ECT causes EEG slowing (Ishikara and Sasa 1999). ECT may be efficacious in part by increasing dopamine release, which can cause delirium. ECT causes an increased release of dopamine (Ishikara and Sasa 1999) including in the frontal cortex (Yoshida *et al.* 1998), and increased D1 and D2 receptor mRNA levels in the nucleus accumbens (Smith *et al.* 1995). Parkinson's patients undergoing ECT while still receiving levodopa are particularly susceptible to interictal delirium (Nymeyer and Grossberg 1997). The same dopamine release responsible for causing delirium and EEG slowing may be necessary for improvement from depression.

Cocaine binges can cause agitated delirium and hyperthermia that does not occur with chronic cocaine abuse (Wetli *et al.* 1996), probably because bingers lack the adaptive compensatory mechanisms found in chronic abusers. Compensatory decreased D1 and D2 receptor density and increased DA transporter density does not occur in bingers, which culminates in excessive DA activity and delirium (Wetli *et al.* 1996).

In the brain there are three main groups of dopaminergic neurons: nigrostriatal, hypothalamic-pituitary, and ventral tegmental. These pathways serve anterior cerebral cortex and limbic structures where neuropsychiatric symptoms may result, and frontal and striatal regions where motor functions occur. For neuropsychiatric symptoms, ventral tegmental DA neurons are important. Neurons from this midbrain nucleus project *via* the mesocortical pathway up to prefrontal, anterior cingulate, and entorhinal cortices, and *via* mesolimbic pathway project over to nucleus accumbens, septum, and amygdala. There are two families of DA receptors: D1 and D2. D1 and D5 receptor subtypes comprise the D1 family and activate adenylate cyclase, whilst D2, D3, and D4 receptor subtypes constitute the D2 family and inhibit adenylate cyclase, in addition to activating other pathways (Wilson *et al.* 1998). D3 density is highest in the nucleus accumbens while D4 is highest in frontal cortex, amygdala, thalamus, hypothalamus, pituitary, and hippocampus (Wilson *et al.* 1998). D1, D3, D4, and D5 receptor proteins are abundant in the prefrontal cortex where DA neurons interface with glutamate and GABA neurons to modulate pyramidal cell firing (Goldman-Rakic 1998). In the striatum, D4 receptors modulate DA turnover; D4 antagonists increase DA release. Though the highest density of D2 receptors is in striatum, nucleus accumbens, olfactory tubercle, and substantia nigra, they are prominent elsewhere also (Wilson *et al.* 1998). D1 receptors are mainly post-synaptic, while D2 receptors occur both pre- and post-synaptically (Jaber *et al.* 1996).

Though it is not known which DA receptor subtypes are involved in delirium, evidence suggests they could play a role in many delirium symptoms, including motor behaviour, learning and memory. In addition, they are widely distributed in brain regions relevant to delirium, based on neuroanatomical reports (see above section). D1 and D2 agonists cause EEG slowing accompanied by behavioural arousal in rats (Ongini *et al.* 1985; Keane and Neal 1981), similar to the effects on EEG and motor behaviour with anticholinergic drugs – a pattern often seen in delirium. Regional differences in DA synapses may play a role in determining delirium's constellation of symptoms. Regulation of DA neurotransmission in the mesoprefrontal cortex is unique compared to other DA neurons. Compared to striatum and nucleus accumbens, the mesial prefrontal cortex has an enhanced rate of DA synthesis and turnover, less efficient DA reuptake, and fewer DA transporters (Cass and Gerhardt 1995). This slower clearance of DA may result in more widespread effects for DA diffusing in the prefrontal cortex.

That DA plays a major role in motor learning was substantiated when CSF levels of DA metabolite were shown to correlate with cognitive measures – while serotonin and noradrenaline metabolites did not (McEntee *et al.* 1987). Novel learning involves DA release in the mesial prefrontal cortex (Wilkinson 1997). D1 receptors in the PFC modulate visuospatial working memory in humans (Sawaguchi and Goldman-Rakic 1991; Muller *et al.* 1998). D1 receptors also modulate hippocampal-prefrontal circuits needed for delayed responses – in addition to their role in short-term retention – suggesting DA is even involved in long-term memory (Seamans *et al.* 1998).

Opposite psychomotor presentations of delirium (hypoactive and hyperactive) are difficult to reconcile on a neurochemical basis if a single DA-Ach hypothesis is presumed. DA controls spontaneous and voluntary movements, and associative learning, through activity in both the nigrostriatal and mesocorticolimbic pathways (Seamans *et al.* 1998). DA activity in the ventral striatum is involved with locomotor behaviour (Wilkinson 1997). D1 receptors in the nucleus accumbens (part of the ventral striatum) are mainly involved with locomotor activity and reward mechanisms (Nakamura *et al.* 1998). Increased DA, like decreased Ach activity, is associated with hyperactivity. Both D3 and D1 receptors are involved in regulation of motor function in the nucleus accumbens, where they can interact to enhance or oppose each other's effects (Schwartz *et al.* 1998). D3 receptor stimulation has an inhibitory role on motor activity (Accili *et al.* 1996), whereas D1 agonists increase motor activity. DA activity in dorsal striatum can lead to stereotypies and D2 agonists increase stereotypies. Thus, individual differences in regional DA receptor subtype responsivity or differential effects on certain DA systems of the brain from physiologies of different delirium aetiologies might explain why some patients' delirium episodes are hyperactive, hypoactive, or mixed – even though DA effects related to other delirium symptoms, such as cognition, consistently result in deficits.

Changes in DA receptors throughout the life cycle, including during ageing, may play a role in susceptibility to delirium. In humans, D1 receptor density in the caudate and putamen declines during the transition between infancy and adulthood (Montague *et al.* 1999). Caudate and putamen D2 receptor density declines during the transition from adult to old age, correlating with frontal lobe motor and cognitive performances (Volkow *et al.* 1998).

The laminar distribution of DA receptors in the cerebral cortex varies regionally. D2 receptor binding is greatest in the striatum compared to all other regions. In frontal and parietal cortices, D2 receptors are most dense in layers V and VI. In human and primate prefrontal cortex, D2 receptors are in highest density in layer V, while D1 receptors are densest in layers I, II and IIIa (Goldman-Rakic *et al.* 1992). However, D2 receptor density is greatest in layers I, II, V, and VI in temporal cortex where, regionally, they are highest in subiculum, CA3 and dentate gyrus of the hippocampal complex, and almost nonexistent in entorhinal cortex (Joyce *et al.* 1991). Such differential geographical distribution may relate to their role in memory and other aspects of cognition. In addition, D2 receptors are dense in auditory-visual association, auditory and speech areas (Goldsmith *et al.* 1997) – regions related to hallucinations, language and thought disturbances.

The hypothesis that Ach and DA neurotransmitter activities are inversely involved in causing delirium symptoms can be supported by neuroanatomical and pharmacological evidence that these systems interface. Cholinergic fibres show bilaminar distribution in the prefrontal cortex, with highest density in layers IIIb and V, as well as layer I (Mrzljak and Goldman-Rakic 1992). D2 receptors block the release of Ach, while D1 receptors stimulate Ach release (Ikarashi *et al.* 1997). Thus, D2 antagonism by neuroleptic drugs not only blocks DA effects, but also enhances Ach release, thereby 'rebalancing' Ach and DA neurotransmitter activites. In another cholinergic deficiency disorder, Alzheimer's disease, both haloperidol and physostigmine ameliorate delusions and hallucinations (Cummings *et al.* 1993). Dopamine antagonists, particularly neuroleptics, appear to treat delirium, including that arising from anticholinergic causes (Itil and Fink 1966; Platt *et al.* 1994). Chlorpromazine reverses anticholinergic drug-induced delirium in humans, as does tacrine (Itil and Fink 1966). Haloperidol partially reverses scopolamine-induced verbal short-term memory deficits in humans (Vitiello *et al.* 1997).

Serotonin may regulate DA activity in various brain regions, including striatum and limbic structures (Meltzer 1993). Serotonergic agents can enhance DA release in PFC (Tanda *et al.* 1994). In addition, noradrenaline exhibits tonic excitatory control over mesocortical DA neurons with effects on the PFC but not nucleus accumbens (Tassin 1998). Thus, other neurotransmitters can interface with DA to cause delirium.

Recent reports of delirium occurring after withdrawal of amantadine in Parkinson's patients suggests the possibility that an extreme deficiency of DA may also result in delirium (Factor *et al.* 1998; Miyasaki *et al.* 1999). Thus, DA may have an inverted U-shaped dose–response relationship to symptoms such that delirium results at either extreme. When delirium occurs in the context of neuroleptic malignant syndrome, it may be related to excessive DA blockade.

Serotonin and delirium

Changes in brain serotonin functioning have been associated with a variety of psychiatric disturbances. In humans, low serotonin functioning has been related to symptoms such as aggression, impulsivity, and suicidal behaviour. Furthermore, serotonin has been implicated to play a role in anxiety and affective disorders, and psychosis. Increased as well as decreased serotonergic activity in the brain has been associated with delirium under various clinical conditions (Fogel *et al.* 1996; Van der Mast 1998; Van der Mast and Fekkes 2000). Increased tryptophan uptake may result in increased brain serotonin activity in hepatic encephalopathy (Mousseau and Butterworth 1994; Van der Mast and Fekkes 2000). Sepsis (Mizock *et al.* 1990) and serotonergic syndromes (Goldberg and Huk 1992) may also involve increased serotonin activity.

Increased free tryptophan plasma levels correlate with reductions in cerebral blood flow on xenon computed tomography (CT) scans in patients with subclinical hepatic encephalopathy (Rodriguez *et al.* 1987), and l,5-hydroxytryptophan can induce delirium (Irwin *et al.* 1986). By contrast, in patients with post-cardiotomy delirium tryptophan was found to be decreased (Van der Mast *et al.* 1994).

All serotonin pathways in the brain have their origin in the raphe nuclei that are located in the midline of the brainstem nuclei. Within the brainstem, serotonergic neurons play a role in arousal and sleep, while ascending pathways distributed to the basal ganglia, thalamus, hypothalamus, amygdala, hippocampus, and cortex regulate functions such as motor activity, aggressive and impulsive behaviour, mood, anxiety, and memory – functions that may all be disturbed in delirium. Descending serotonergic pathways from the raphe nuclei project to the motor and autonomic systems in the spinal cord (Ross 1991; Fogel *et al.* 1996; Kandel 2000).

Serotonin is synthesized within the nerve ending from its precursor, the essential amino acid tryptophan (Trp). On entering the nerve terminal, Trp is hydroxylated into 5-hydroxytryptophan by Trp hydroxylase, which is the rate-limiting step in serotonin synthesis. The enzyme Trp-hydroxylase needs oxygen and the cofactor tetrahydrobiopterin for its activity. 5-Hydroxytryptophan is decarboxylated to serotonin, which is metabolized by monoamine oxidase to 5-hydroxyindoleacetic acid. In the pineal gland, serotonin is O-methylated to form melatonin, which plays an important role in regulating the circadian rhythm (Leonard 1992).

Brain serotonin levels are dependent on the concentration of brain tryptophan. Tryptophan is transported into the brain and nerve terminal by an active carrier transport system which it shares with the other large neutral amino acids (LNAA) tyrosine, phenylalanine, valine, leucine, and isoleucine. The production rate of brain serotonin is dependent on the plasma availability of Trp (Wurtman *et al.* 1980), which competes with these other LNAAs for uptake from blood across the blood–brain barrier into the brain. This competition is best represented by the ratio of the plasma level of Trp to the sum of the plasma levels of the other LNAAs. Thus, the plasma ratio of Trp/LNAA determines the amount of Trp that reaches the brain (Fernström and Wurtman 1972). Trp is mostly obtained from dietary sources and unique among the LNAAs in that it is about 85% bound to the plasma protein albumin inhibiting storage into muscle tissue. Changes in liver Trp-pyrrolase activity that may be brought about by steroids, insulin, changes in diet, and by the circadian rhythm, may play a secondary role in regulating serotonin synthesis.

The carrier transport system at the blood–brain barrier has a high affinity for the LNAAs, with the highest affinity for phenylalanine. Phenylalanine is also an inhibitor of the monoamine-synthesizing enzymes such as tyrosine hydroxylase and tryptophan hydroxylase, thus interfering with dopamine, noradrenaline, adrenaline (epinephrine), and serotonin synthesis, respectively (Richardson 1990).

In illness and trauma, both psychological and physical chronic stress is of major importance. Data on the effects of 'psychological' stress on serotonin systems are somewhat contradictory. Animal research has shown an increase in serotonin turnover in acute stress, while chronic 'inescapable' stress has been associated with reduced *in vivo* release of serotonin in the cerebral cortex. Moreover, chronic stress leads to an increase of cortical 5-HT_2 receptors and a reduction of hippocampal 5-HT_{1A} receptors (Fogel *et al.* 1996). Transiently increased concentrations of corticosteroids, as induced by stress, lead to increases in brain Trp and serotonin and result in increased activity of the raphe-hippocampal serotonergic system. The serotonergic stress response depends on sympathetic nervous system activity and the elevation of cortical 5-HT_2 receptors by stress on the integrity of brain noradrenergic neurons. In addition, there is considerable preclinical evidence that serotonin has inhibitory effects on noradrenergic function in the locus ceruleus and the cortex (Fogel *et al.* 1996). Under (pathological) conditions of chronically elevated corticosteroid concentrations, however, serotonergic neurotransmission is impaired. Human depression is an important example of a condition of combined hypercortisolism and an apparent hypoactivity of serotonergic transmission (De Kloet *et al.* 1998). Thus, it may be that acute stress causes neuroendocrine adaptation with initially increased plasma Trp availability and brain serotonin function, whilst chronic stress leads to neuroendocrine exhaustion, depletion of plasma Trp and consequently decreased serotonergic activity. Moreover, persistent hypercortisolism during chronic stress is associated with hippocampal damage, hippocampal receptor insensitivity, cognitive disturbances, and a decreased negative feedback mechanism maintaining hypercortisolism (Fogel *et al.* 1996; Van den Berghe *et al.* 1998).

Postoperatively, delirium has been associated with reduced cerebral availability of tryptophan from plasma, suggesting diminished serotonergic function in the brain – possibly due to poor physical condition and a sustained stress response (Skaug 1984; Caston *et al.* 1989; Van der Mast *et al.* 1991, 1999, 2000). During chronic physical stress, transport of Trp across the blood–brain barrier may be reduced by two important mechanisms. First, the plasma concentrations of the LNAAs, except Trp, rise due to degradation of muscle proteins, leading to increased competition for transport across the blood–brain barrier. Second, plasma Trp decreases because of induction of Trp pyrrolase in the liver through lasting hypercortisolism, leading to increased catabolism and depletion of plasma Trp (Lehman 1982). Furthermore, immune activation, common in tissue injury, has been associated with lower Trp availability for the brain in depressed patients (Maes *et al.* 1997). In addition, poor physical state may be accompanied by a low T3 syndrome, during which cell metabolism is generally decreased through reduced synthesis of adenosine triphosphate (ATP). The consequently deficient synthesis of tetrahydrobiopterin, a cofactor for Trp hydroxylase, may also endanger the production of serotonin in the brain.

Drug-induced excess serotonergic activity in the brain due to the concomitant use of selective serotonin reuptake inhibitors (SSRI) or tryptophan as well as monoamine oxidase inhibitors (MAOI) has been related to the development of the 'serotonin syndrome', of which delirium is a main symptom (Sternbach 1991). Illness severity is strongly associated with the degree of elevation of intrasynaptic serotonin, which is greatest following combinations of irreversible MAOI-A and MAOI-B with potent SSRIs. The serotonin syndrome can be fatal and no effective drug treatment has been established (Gillman 1998, 1999).

In hepatic encephalopathy (HE) levels of tyrosine, phenylalanine, and Trp are increased as a consequence of impaired hepatic oxidative deamination which may give rise to altered synthesis in the brain of, respectively, dopamine and serotonin. The excess of cerebral glutamine due to increased ammonia levels may also stimulate Trp uptake in the brain, and thereby enhance the synthesis of serotonin (James *et al.* 1979). Thus, altered neurotransmitter balance due to, among other things, increased activity of serotonin may be partly responsible for the clinical picture of HE, which resembles the serotonin syndrome (Van der Mast 1998).

Alcohol withdrawal delirium has been associated with monoaminergic dysfunction, in particular of noradrenaline and serotonin (Van der Mast 1998). Chronic alcoholism may lead to reduced cerebral availability of Trp from plasma due to nutritional deficiencies and metabolic derangement, since alcohol itself enhances the metabolism of liver Trp, thereby decreasing its availability for the brain (Badawy 1988; Buydens-Branchey *et al.* 1988). This process may be further stimulated by the elevated levels of corticosteroids that can occur under stressful circumstances such as withdrawal. Thus, alcohol withdrawal delirium may be partly the result of decreased function of the serotonergic system.

In chronic levodopa-treated Parkinson patients, altered serotonergic function may contribute to delirium, as levodopa reduces plasma and brain levels of tryptophan by competing with tryptophan for uptake from the gut and at the blood–brain barrier. The initially reduced serotonergic activity would, at a later stage of the disease and duration of treatment with levodopa, be followed by sensitization and increased activity of the serotonin receptors (Nausieda *et al.* 1982). The inconclusive results of Trp and 5-hydroxytryptophan supplementation in Parkinson's patients may be explained by implicating variable disease stages and durations of treatment with levodopa (Beasley *et al.* 1980).

Rat models of human delirium

Rat models for delirium exist but have not yet been used to test treatments or neuro-chemical hypotheses. Anticholinergic and dopaminergic models have been described. Because rats cannot be interviewed, models that incorporate EEGs to measure degree of slowing are more likely to parallel human delirium. Rat EEGs are comparable to human EEGs, with a similar normal frequency distribution (Benigmus 1984). One anticholinergic rat model of delirium assessed a range of atropine doses from 3.44 to 55 mg/kg intravenously, and rats were compared to themselves as saline controls (Trzepacz *et al.* 1992; Leavitt *et al.* 1994). This model demonstrated similarities to human delirium across several dimensions: EEG slowing (frequency and amplitude), cognitive impairment as measured by a maze, and objectively monitored hyperactivity. A different rat model used lower atropine doses from 0.1 to 3 mg/kg intraperitoneally (O'Hare et al. 1997). O'Hare et al. (1997) demonstrated cognitive impairment during an operant response procedure, but because EEGs were not included in this putative model, only cognitive impairment was demonstrated and not delirium. These investigators measured SAA levels as a surrogate for EEGs; however, rat SAA levels may not be comparable to those found in delirious humans. In fact, human SAA levels show very wide interindividual variability, so cut-off levels for human delirium occurrence are also not determinable.

There is a rat DA delirium model using apomorphine (a direct D1 and D2 agonist) in a choice reaction performance task (Nakamura et al. 1998). Rats had attentional deficits, but the lowest apomorphine dose resulted in hypoactivity attributed to preferential stimulation of DA autoreceptors in the mesolimbic system. The highest apomorphine doses resulted in hyperactivity attributed to direct stimulation of post-synaptic D1 receptors. A cholinomimetic, aniracetam, as well as haloperidol and other neuroleptics, reversed the choice reaction performance deficits, whilst tacrine, a cholinesterase inhibitor, worsened them. The investigators concluded that the cognitive deficits were mediated via a D2 mechanism. Unfortunately, EEGs were not monitored so that it cannot be determined whether this is truly a model for human delirium.

Neurophysiology of ageing and cognitive decline

Many cerebral morphological changes have been described in normal ageing. There is a decrease in total brain volume and weight, reduced number and volume of neurons, and loss of dendrites and synapses (Blennow and Gottfries 1998). However, the human brain has great reserve capacities. Most persons' original numbers of neurons is very large, and function can be maintained even when the number of neurons has greatly been reduced. Also, neurons are capable of increasing their metabolism if necessary, and by producing more neurotransmitters, they may compensate for the loss of other neurons. Furthermore, remaining nerve terminals are able to increase in size, taking over the function of lost neighbouring terminals. And, in spite of a reduction of neurotransmitter release, receptors may continue to respond adequately by increasing their sensitivity (Blennow and Gottfries 1998). When all these compensatory mechanisms are exhausted, symptoms of cerebral insufficiency appear, comprising cognitive dysfunction and psychiatric and behavioural disturbances (Blennow and Gottfries 1998).

Ageing affects the function of neurotransmitter systems. Changes in the cholinergic system include selective cell loss in the basal forebrain, decreased synthetic choline acetyltransferase (CAT) activity, and synthesis of acetylcholine in hippocampal and cortical areas, but unchanged acetylcholinesterase (Gibson et al. 1991; Blennow and Gottfries 1998). This age-related decline in release and synthesis of acetylcholine parallels the decline seen in hypoxia and thiamine deficiency, and can also be related to decreased oxidative metabolism with ageing (Gibson et al. 1991).

Deterioration of the cholinergic system may relate to cognitive decline, especially to memory impairment, both in normal ageing and in Alzheimer's disease (Blennow and Gottfries 1998), and, as described above, imbalance between central cholinergic and noradrenergic activity may play a role in delirium (Eikelenboom and Hoogendijk 1999).

In ageing, loss of dopaminergic and noradrenergic neurons in the substantia nigra and locus ceruleus and reduced concentrations of dopamine, dopamine uptake sites, and noradrenaline have been reported (Blennow and Gottfries 1998; Gibson *et al.* 1991). However, the basal release of dopamine and glutamate, both associated with excitotoxic neuronal damage and cell loss, appears to be increased (Gibson *et al.* 1991; Stahl 1996). These excitotoxic mechanisms may play a role in neurodegenerative disorders like Alzheimer's disease, Parkinson's disease, stroke and Huntington's disease, and possibly in delirium. Increased activity of the surviving locus ceruleus neurons may compensate for the noradrenergic cell loss in Alzheimer's disease (Hoogendijk *et al.* 1999).

Serotonin metabolism is also sensitive to ageing. In certain brain regions, serotonergic neurons and concentrations of serotonin are decreased. Decline of serotonergic metabolism may also be deduced from a reduced activity of the two synthesizing enzymes of serotonin, e.g. tryptophan hydroxylase and carboxylase. Possibly, the turnover of serotonin in the remaining neurons is compensatorily enhanced (Blennow and Gottfries 1998). Thus, deficient serotonergic function may make the elderly more vulnerable for delirium if lowered cerebral serotonin is implicated in its pathophysiology.

Hormonal and neurochemical changes have also been described in normal ageing. The activity of hypothalamic CRH neurons and the HPA axis is increased in elderly people and in Alzheimer's disease (Swaab *et al.* 1994; Blennow and Gottfries 1998), whilst chronic overexposure to elevated levels of cortisol has been associated with cognitive impairment in patients with Cushing's syndrome (Forget *et al.* 2000). It is unknown whether, in the elderly individual, the increased HPA axis activity is due to reduced inhibitory control over the hypothalamus from the neurotransmitter systems or to disturbed feedback from other systems that regulate the hypothalamus, e.g. cortisol (Blennow and Gottfries 1998). Non-suppression of cortisol in response to dexamethasone was related to increased risk for developing delirium during acute illness in the elderly (O'Keeffe and Devlin 1994), suggesting feedback resistance at the various levels of the Limbic HPA axis.

Inflammatory and immune mechanisms may play an important role in the pathophysiology of Alzheimer's disease (Kronfol and Remick 2000). Also, dementia is the most common risk factor for delirium in the elderly. This may be because delirium and Alzheimer's disease are simply different stages of a common pathogenetic process, sharing specific aetiological mechanisms comprising inflammation with a generalized stress response and increased cerebral IL-1 and IL-6; reduced cerebral metabolism; imbalance of noradrenergic and cholinergic neurotransmission; and disturbances in the neuronal systems which regulate stress adaptation and the sleep–wake cycle (Eikelenboom and Hoogendijk 1999).

Thus, age-related changes in cerebral neurotransmission, stress management and hormonal regulation, and immune response are in line with pathophysiological mechanisms supposed to underlie delirium, and may help to explain the vulnerability of the elderly to delirium.

Treatment of delirium and its relationship to neuropathophysiology

Better understanding of the neuropathogenesis of delirium will offer opportunities to improve delirium treatment beyond the current clinical standard of using haloperidol, possibly by targeting multiple receptor subtypes of different neurotransmitters simultaneously. Conventional neuroleptics used to treat delirium are not DA receptor subtype specific. Haloperidol predominantly blocks D2 receptors, although it blocks D1, D3, and D4 receptors to a lesser degree (Piercey et al. 1995). Use of selective dopamine antagonists might help elucidate neural mechanisms underlying delirium. It has been hypothesized that differential effects on D1, D2, and D3 receptors might underlie different psychomotor presentations of delirium (Trzepacz 2000).

Pharmacological treatment with a neuroleptic agent (D2 antagonist) is the clinical standard of delirium treatment, even though there is no FDA-approved drug indicated for treatment of delirium. Such D2 blockade is compatible with the DA excess delirium hypothesis. Alternatively, treatment of delirium with a cholinergic enhancer drug is supported by the cholinergic deficiency hypothesis. Physostigmine and tacrine have reversed cases of anticholinergic delirium (Mendelson 1977; Stern 1983). Donepezil has improved three cases of delirium: postoperative state and co-morbid Lewy body and alcohol dementias (Wengel et al. 1998, 1999; Burke et al. 1999).

Psychostimulants theoretically can worsen delirium related to increased dopaminergic activity, and are not traditionally recommended (Rosenberg et al. 1991; Levenson 1992). However, there is some interest in combining a psychostimulant with a D2 blocker to treat hypoactive delirium in order to simultaneously and differentially affect DA receptors in different brain regions related to psychomotor behaviour, cognition, and thought processes. Recently, methylphenidate 10–20 mg/day was used for hypoactive delirium in a cancer patient whose MDAS and DRS scores went from 21 and 20 points to 4 and 10 points, respectively, after treatment, with improved somnolence noted in one day (Morita et al. 2000).

Mianserin, a serotonergic tetracyclic antidepressant, has been used in Japan in several open label studies (Nakamura et al. 1995, 1997a, 1997b; Uchiyama et al. 1996). Efficacy was considered to be related to effects on the sleep–wake cycle and/or to its weak D2 receptor antagonism in conjunction with blockade of post-synaptic 5-HT$_2$, presynaptic α-adrenergic, and H1 and H2 receptor blockade.

Haloperidol is considered the clinical standard for the treatment of delirium, though no randomized double-blind placebo-controlled studies have been done. Positron emission tomography scans show that haloperidol reduces glucose utilization in thalamus, caudate, and frontal, limbic, and anterior cingulate cortices (Bartlett *et al.* 1994) – areas implicated in delirium neuropathogenesis.

Chlorpromazine reversed behavioural and EEG manifestations of experimental anti-cholinergic drug-induced delirium in one study (Itil and Fink 1966). Haloperidol or chlorpromazine – but not lorazepam – reduced delirium in AIDS patients in a double-blind, randomized controlled design (Breitbart *et al.* 1996). Hypoactive and hyper-active delirium subtypes each improved using haloperidol or chlorpromazine, and improvement was documented within hours of treatment initiation before underlying medical causes were addressed (Platt *et al.* 1994).

Atypical antipsychotic drugs primarily differ from conventionals because they have $5-HT_2$ receptor as well as D2 blocking effects, though each of the atypicals has a unique neuroreceptor profile. Clozapine was reported to cause delirium in 8% of 315 psychi-atric in-patients and in 7/33 of these delirium cases it was the only drug used (Gaertner *et al.* 1989), perhaps related to its anticholinergicity. In fact, clozapine-induced deli-rium was reversed by a cholinergic enhancer drug (Schuster *et al.* 1977). This suggests its anticholinergicity makes it less useful for delirium treatment.

In an open label trial, risperidone (mean dose 1.59 ± 0.8 mg/day) reduced globally measured delirium severity in 8/11 patients, with a maximum response on day 5 Sipahimalani and Masand 1997). However, risperidone was reported to cause delirium in four cases for unclear reasons (Chen and Cardasis 1996; Ravona-Springer *et al.* 1998).

In an open label non-randomized case series (11 cases in each group), olanzapine (mean dose 8.2 ± 3.4 mg qhs) efficacy was comparable to haloperidol (mean dose 5.1 ± 3.5 mg qhs) (Masand and Sipahimalani 1998), as defined by a > 50% reduction on the Delirium Rating Scale. A delirious cancer patient responded to olanzapine 10 mg (Passik and Cooper 1999). Delirious cancer in-patients ($n = 82$; mean age = 60 years), 81% of whom had metastases (20% in the brain), were treated with olanzapine (dose range = 2.5–20 mg) for delirium (Breitbart 2001). Using the Memorial Delirium Assessment Scale serially, they found resolution of delirium with olanzapine treatment in 79% of patients by day 3 with overall good tolerability. Olanzapine significantly increased acetylcholine release measured by *in vivo* microdialysis in both rat prefrontal cortex (Meltzer 1999) and hippocampus (Schirazi *et al.* 2000), consistent with pro-cholinergic activity, exceeding values for haloperidol and the other atypicals tested. Kennedy *et al.* (2001) theorized that presynaptic effects of olanzapine at $5-HT_3$, $5-HT_6$ and m2 receptors may account for this increased acetylcholine release.

A single 8 mg intravenous dose of odansetron, a $5-HT_3$ antagonist, was reported to reduce agitation in delirium patients when a four-point rating scale was applied prospectively in 35 post-cardiotomy patients (mean age = 51 years) (Bayindir *et al.* 2000).

Two delirious patients received 25–50 mg qd of quetiapine and improved on the Delirium Rating Scale-Revised-98 (Torres *et al.* 2001). A retrospective open label case series of 11 delirious patients who either received between 25 and 750 mg qd of queti-apine or 1–10 mg qd of haloperidol found similar response times between drugs, with an average peak response at about 7 days (Schwartz and Masand 2000). Quetiapine 300 mg bid was reported to cause delirium in a 62-year-old man that was associated with EEG slowing compared to a prior normal EEG and that cleared when quetiapine was discontinued (Sim *et al.* 2000). A previous right thalamic lacunar infarct may have increased his risk for delirium.

Though randomized double-blind placebo-controlled trials are needed, reports suggest a role for DA antagonists. Evidence for efficacy of cholinergic enhancers for delirium treatment is even more limited than for DA antagonists.

Conclusions

Certain symptoms of delirium may represent 'core' symptoms, whilst others may be associated symptoms that occur related to particular aetiologies or individual varia-tion. Core symptoms may reflect dysfunction of certain brain regions and neurotrans-mitter systems that comprise a 'final common neural pathway' that represents common symptoms comprising the syndrome of delirium. Regions implicated include prefrontal cortex, thalamus, basal ganglia, temporoparietal cortex, fusiform cortex, and lingual gyri, especially on the right side. A diversity of physiologies related to the wide variety of aetiologies for delirium may funnel into a common neurochemical expres-sion that involves elevated brain DA and reduced Ach activity, or a relative imbalance of these. Serotonin activity may interact to regulate and alter activity of acetylcholine and dopamine, and alterations in serotonin levels or of its precursor have been impli-cated in delirium.

The stress response associated with severe medical illness, surgery, and trauma involves sympathetic and immune system activation, increased activity of the HPA axis, cerebral release of cytokines that can alter neurotransmitter systems, changes in the thryoid axis, and modifications of the blood–brain barrier. These effects may contribute to delirium through several avenues. Age-related changes in central neuro-transmission, stress management, and hormonal regulation, and immune response may underlie the vulnerability of elderly people to delirium.

The clinical standard of treatment involves a dopamine antagonist medication – usually haloperidol – though, theoretically, procholinergic drugs should help. There is a dearth of drug treatment studies for delirium, in particular randomized double-blind trials, and there is none with placebo controls. Open label reports with newer atypical neuroleptics suggest some may have utility in delirium treatment, and deserve more study as well.

References

Accili, D., Fishburn, C. S., Drago, J., Steiner, H., *et al.* (1996). A targeted mutation of the D3 dopamine receptor gene is associated with hyperactivity in mice. *Proceedings of the National Academy of Sciences*, **93**, 1945–1949.

Ames, D., Wirshing, W. C., and Szuba, M. P. (1992). Organic mental disorders associated with bupropion in three patients. *Journal of Clinical Psychiatry*, **53**, 53–55.

Badawy, A. B. (1988). Effects of alcohol on tryptophan metabolism. *Biochemical Society Transactions*, **16**, 254–256.

Baraka, A. and Harik, S. (1977). Reversal of central anticholinergic syndrome by galanthamine. *Journal of the American Medical Association*, **238**, 2293–2294.

Bartlett, E. J., Brodie, J. D., Simkowitz, P., *et al.* (1994). Effects of haloperidol challenge on regional cerebral glucose utilization in normal human subjects. *American Journal of Psychiatry*, **151**, 681–686.

Basile, A. S., Saito, K., Li, Y., *et al.* (1995). The relationship between plasma and brain quinolinic acid levels and the severity of hepatic encephalopathy in animal models of fulminant hepatic failure. *Journal of Neurochemistry*, **64**, 2607–2614.

Bayinder, O., Akpinar, B., Can, E., Guden, M. *et al.* (2000). The use of the 5-HT3 antagonist odansetron for the treatment of post-cardiotomy delirium. *Journal of Cardiothoracic and Vascular Anesthesiology*, **14**, 288–292.

Beasley, B. L., Nutt, J. G., Davenport, R. W., and Chase, T. N. (1980). Treatment with tryptophan of levodopa-associated psychiatric disturbances. *Archives of Neurology*, **37**, 155–156.

Benigmus, V. A. (1984). EEGs as a cross-species indicator of neurotoxicity. *Neurobehavioral Toxicology and Teratology*, **6**, 473–483.

Bertrand, N., Ishii, H., Beley, A., and Spatz, M. (1993). Biphasic striatal acetylcholine release during and after transient cerebral ischemia in gerbils. *Journal of Cerebral Blood Flow and Metabolism*, **13**, 789–795.

Blass, J. P. and Gibson, G. E. (1999). Cerebrometabolic aspects of delirium in relationship to dementia. *Dementia and Geriatric Cognitive Disorders*, **10**, 335–338.

Blennow, K. and Gottfries, C. G. (1998) Neurochemistry of aging. In: *Geriatric psychopharmacology* (ed. J. G. Nelson), pp. 1–27. Marcel Dekker, Inc., New York.

Blumberg, H. P., Stern, E., Ricketts, S., *et al.* (1999). Rostral orbitofrontal prefrontal cortex dysfunction in the manic state of bipolar disorder. *American Journal of Psychiatry*, **156**, 1986–1988.

Bogousslavsky, J., Ferranzzini, M., Regli, F., *et al.* (1988). Manic delirium and frontal-like syndrome with paramedian infarction of the right thalamus. *Journal of Neurology, Neurosurgery and Psychiatry*, **51**, 116–119.

Boiten, J. and Lodder, J. (1989). An unusual sequela of a frequently occurring neurologic disorder: delirium caused by brain infarct (In Dutch). *Nederlands Tijdschrift voor Geneeskunde*, **133**, 617–620.

Breitbart, W. (2001). Consecutive case series of olanzapine treatment of delirium. In: *Symposium presented at Academy of Psychosomatic Medicine Annual Meeting*, Palm Springs, November 2001.

Breitbart, W., Marotta, R., Platt, M. M., *et al.* (1996). A double blind trial of haloperidol, chlorpromazine and lorazepam in the treatment of delirium in hospitalized AIDS patients. *American Journal of Psychiatry*, **153**, 231–237.

Broadhurst, C. (2001). Immunology of delirium: new opportunities for treatment and research. *British Journal of Psychiatry*, **179**, 288–289.

Broderick, P. A. and Gibson, G. E. (1989). Dopamine and serotonin in rat striatum during in vivo hypoxic-hypoxia. *Metabolic Brain Research*, **4**, 143–153.

Burke, W. J., Roccaforte, W. H., and Wengel, S. P. (1999). Treating visual hallucinations with donepezil. *American Journal of Psychiatry*, **156**, 1117–1118.

Burns, M. J., Linden, C. H., Graudins, A., *et al.* (2000). A comparison of physostigmine and benzodiazepines for the treatment of anticholinergic poisoning. *Annals of Emergency Medicine*, **35**, 374–381.

Buydens-Branchey, L., Branchey, M., Worner, T. D., Zucker, D., Aramsombatdee, E., and Lieber, C. S. (1988). Increase in tryptophan oxygenase activity in alcoholic patients. *Alcoholism: Clinical and Experimental Research*, **12**, 163–167.

Camacho, P. M. and Dwarkanathan, A. A. (1999). Sick euthyroid syndrome. What to do when thyroid function tests are abnormal in critically ill patients. *Postgraduate Medicine*, **105**, 215–219.

Cass, W. A. and Gerhardt, G. A. (1995). In vivo assessment of dopamine uptake in rat medial prefrontal cortex: comparison with dorsal striatum and nucleus accumbens. *Journal of Neurochemistry*, **65**, 201–207.

Caston, J. C., Utley, J. R., and Fleming, H. E. (1989). Endocrine marker for l-tryptophan response in cardiopulmonary bypass delirium patients: case reports. *Advances in Therapy*, **6**, 161–179.

Chen, B. and Cardasis, W. (1996). Delirium induced by lithium and risperidone combination. *American Journal of Psychiatry*, **153**, 1233–1234.

Cherem, H. J., Hummel, N. H., Barabejski, G. F., Martinez, C. B. A., and Guizberg, A. L. (1992). Thyroid function and abdominal surgery. A longitudinal study. *Archives of Medical Research*, **23**, 143–147.

Coffman, J. A. and Dilsaver, S. C. (1988). Cholinergic mechanisms in delirium. *American Journal of Psychiatry*, **145**, 382–383.

Cortes, R., Probst, A., Tobler, H. J., *et al.* (1986). Muscarinic cholinergic receptor subtypes in human brain, II: quantitative autoradiographic studies. *Brain Research*, **362**, 239–253.

Cullen, K. M. and Halliday, G. M. (1995). Neurofibrillary tangles in chronic alcoholics. *Neuropathology and Applied Neurobiology*, **21**, 312–318.

Cummings, J. L., Gorman, D. G., and Shapira, J. (1993). Physostigmine ameliorates the delusions of Alzheimer's disease. *Biological Psychiatry*, **33**, 536–541.

Dager, S. R. and Heritch, A. J. (1990). A case of bupropion-associated delirium. *Journal of Clinical Psychiatry*, **51**, 307–308.

Daunderer, M. (1983). Physostigmine as delirium-preventive agent in ambulatory ethanol delirium. *Fortschritte der Medizin*, **101**, 778–780.

De Kloet, E. R., Vreugdenhil, E., Oitzl, M. S., and Joels, M. (1998). Brain corticosteroid receptor balance in health and disease. *Endocrine Reviews*, **19**, 269–301.

Denicoff, K. D., Rubinow, D. R., and Papa, M. Z. (1987). The neuropsychiatric effects of treatment with interleukin-2 and lymphokine-activated killer cells. *Annals of Internal Medicine*, **107**, 293–300.

Dixon, C. E., Hamm, R. J., Taft, W. C., *et al.* (1994). Increased anticholinergic sensitivity following closed skull impact and controlled cortical impact traumatic brain injury in the rat. *Journal of Neurotrauma*, **11**, 275–287.

D'Orlando, K. J. and Sandage, B. W., Jr. (1995). Citicoline (CDP-choline): mechanisms of action and effects in ischemic brain injury. *Neurological Research*, **17**, 281–284.

Dringenberg, H. C. and Vanderwolf, C. H. (1995). Some general anesthetics reduce serotonergic neocortical activation and enhance the action of serotonergic antagonists. *Brain Research Bulletin*, **36**, 285–292.

Dunne, J. W., Leedman, P. J., and Edis, R. H. (1986). Inobvious stroke: a cause of delirium and dementia. *Australian and New Zealand Journal of Medicine*, **16**, 771–778.

Ehlert, F. J., Roeske, W. R., and Yamamura, H. I. (1995). Molecular biology, pharmacology, and brain distribution of subtypes of the muscarinic receptor. In: *Psychopharmacology: the fourth generation of progress* (eds F. E. Bloom and D. J. Kupfer), pp. 111–124. Raven Press, New York.

Eikelenboom, P. and Hoogendijk, W. J. (1999). Do delirium and Alzheimer's dementia share specific pathogenetic mechanisms? *Dementia and Geriatric Cognitive Disorders*, **10**, 319–324.

Factor, S. A., Molho, E. S., and Brown, D. L. (1998). Acute delirium after withdrawal of amantadine in Parkinson's disease. *Neurology*, **50**, 1456–1458.

Felicetta, J. V. (1989). Effects of illness on thyroid function tests. *Postgraduate Medicine*, **85**, 213–220.

Fernström, J. D. and Wurtman, R. J. (1972). Brain serotonin content: physiological regulation by plasma neutral amino acids. *Science*, **178**, 414–416.

Figiel, G. S., Hassen, M. A., Zorumski, C., *et al.* (1991). ECT-induced delirium in depressed patients with Parkinson's disease. *Journal of Neuropsychiatry and Clinical Neuroscience*, **3**, 405–411.

Figiel, G. S., Krishman, K. R., Breitner, J. C., *et al.* (1989). Radiologic correlates of antidepressant-induced delirium: the possible significance of basal ganglia lesions. *Journal of Neuropsychiatry and Clinical Neuroscience*, **1**, 188–190.

Fischer, P. (2001). Successful treatment of nonanticholinergic delirium with a cholinesterase inhibitor. *Journal of Clinical Psychopharmacology*, **21**, 118.

Flacker, J. M. and Lipsitz, L. A. (1999). Neural mechanisms of delirium: current hypotheses and evolving concepts. *Journal of Gerontology Biological Sciences*, **54A**, B239–B246.

Flacker, J. M. and Lipsitz, L. A. (2000). Large neutral amino acid changes and delirium in febrile elderly medical patients. *Journal of Gerontology Biological Sciences*, **55A**, B249–B252.

Flacker, J. M., Cummings, V., Mach, J. R. Jr, Bettin, K., Kiely, D. K., and Wei, J. (1998). The association of serum anticholinergic activity with delirium in elderly medical patients. *American Journal of Geriatric Psychiatry*, **6**, 31–41.

Fogel, B. S., Schiffer, R. B., and Rao, S. M. R. (1996). *Neuropsychiatry*. Williams & Wilkins, Baltimore.

Forget, H., Lacroix, A., Somma, M. and Cohen, H. (2000). Cognitive decline in patients with Cushing's syndrome. *Journal of the International Neuropsychologic Society*, **6**, 20–29.

Friedman, J. H. (1985). Syndrome of diffuse encephalopathy due to nondominant thalamic infarction. *Neurology*, **35**, 1524–1526.

Gaertner, H. J., Fischer, E., and Hoss, J. (1989). Side effects of clozapine. *Psychopharmacology*, **99**, S97–S100.

Ghajar, J. B., Gibson, G. E., and Duffy, T. E. (1985). Regional acetylcholine metabolism in brain during acute hypoglycemia. *Journal of Neurochemistry*, **44**, 94–98.

Gibson, G. E., Jope, R., and Blass, J. P. (1975). Decreased synthesis of acetylcholine accompanying impaired oxidation of pyruvate in rat brain slices. *Biochemical Journal*, **26**, 17–23.

Gibson, G. E., Barclay, L. L., and Blass, J. P. (1982). The role of the cholinergic system in thiamine deficiency, thiamine: 20 years of progress. *Annals of the New York Academy of Sciences*, **378**, 382–403.

Gibson, G. E., Blass, J. P., Huang, H. M. and Freeman, G. B. (1991) The cellular basis of delirium and its relevance to age-related disorders including Alzheimer's Disease. In: *Delirium. Advances in research and clinical practice* (eds N. E. Miller, Z. J. Lipowski, and B. D. Lebowitz). *International Psychogeriatrics*, **3**, 135–149.

Gillman, P. K. (1998). Serotonin syndrome: history and risk. *Fundamental Clinical Pharmacology*, **12**, 482–491.

Gillman, P. K. (1999). The serotonin syndrome and its treatment. *Journal of Psychopharmacology*, **13**, 100–109.

Glick, S. D., Ross, D. A., and Hough, L. B. (1982). Lateral asymmetry of neurotransmitters in human brain. *Brain Research*, **234**, 53–63.

Goldberg, E. L. (1998). Lateralization of frontal lobe functions and cognitive novelty. *Journal of Neuropsychiatry and Clinical Neuroscience*, **6**, 371–378.

Goldberg, R. J. and Huk, M. (1992). Serotonergic syndrome from trazodone and buspirone (letter). *Psychosomatics*, **33**, 235–236.

Goldman-Rakic, P. S. (1998). The cortical dopamine system: role in memory and cognition. *Advances in Pharmacology*, **42**, 707–711.

Goldman-Rakic, P. S., Lidow, M. S., Smiley, J. F., and Williams, M. S. (1992). The anatomy of dopamine in monkey and human prefrontal cortex. *Journal of Neural Transmission*, **36**, 163–177.

Goldsmith, S. K., Shapiro, R. M., and Joyce, J. N. (1997). Disrupted pattern of D2 dopamine receptors in the temporal lobe in schizophrenia. A postmortem study. *Archives of General Psychiatry*, **54**, 649–658.

Golinger, R. C., Peet, T., and Tune, L. E. (1987). Association of elevated plasma anticholinergic activity with delirium in surgical patients. *American Journal of Psychiatry*, **144**, 1218–1220.

Gustafson, Y., Berggren, D., Brannstrom, B., *et al.* (1988). Acute confusional states in elderly patients treated for femoral neck fracture. *Journal of the American Geriatrics Society*, **36**, 525–530.

Gustafson, Y., Olsson, T., Eriksson, S., *et al.* (1991). Acute confusional state (delirium) in stroke patients. *Cerebrovascular Disease*, **1**, 257–264.

Han, L., McCusher, J., Cole, M., *et al.* (2001). Use of medications with anticholinergic effect predicts clinical severity of delirium symptoms in older medical inpatients. *Archives of Internal Medicine*, **161**, 1099–1105.

Hart, R. P., Best, A. M., Sessler, C. N., and Levenson, J. L. (1997). Abbreviated Cognitive Test for Delirium. *Journal of Psychosomatic Research*, **43**, 417–423.

Henon, H., Lebert, F., Durieu, I., *et al.* (1999). Confusional state in stroke. Relation to preexisting dementia, patient characteristics and outcome. *Stroke*, **30**, 773–779.

Hirano, H., Day, J., and Fibiger, H. C. (1995). Serotonergic regulation of acetylcholine release in rat frontal cortex. *Journal of Neurochemistry*, **65**, 1139–1145.

Hoogendijk, W. J., Feenstra, M. G., Botterblom, M. H., *et al.* (1999). Increased activity of surviving locus ceruleus neurons in Alzheimer's disease. *Annals of Neurology*, **45**, 82–91.

Hopkins, S. J. and Rothwell, N. J. (1995). Cytokines and the nervous system: I. Expression and recognition. *Trends in Neurosciences*, **18**, 83–88.

Horenstein, S., Chamberlin, W., and Conomy, J. (1967). Infarction of the fusiform and calcarine regions: agitated delirium and hemianopia. In: *Transactions of the American Neurological Association* (ed. M. D. Yahr), **92**, 85–89. Springer, New York.

Ikarashi, Y., Takahashi, A., Ishimaru, H., *et al.* (1997). Regulation of dopamine D1 and D2 receptors on striatal acetylcholine release in rats. *Brain Research Bulletin*, **43**, 107–115.

Irwin, M., Fuentenebro, F., Marder, S. R., *et al.* (1986). L-5-Hydroxytryptophan-induced delirium. *Biological Psychiatry*, **21**, 673–676.

Ishikara, K. and Sasa, M. (1999). Mechanism underlying the therapeutic effects of electroconvulsive therapy (ECT) on depression. *Japanese Journal of Pharmacology*, **80**, 185–189.

Ishimaru, H., Takahashi, A., Ikarashi, Y., and Maruyama, Y. (1995). Pentobarbital protects against CA1 pyramidal cell death but not dysfunction of hippocampal cholinergic neurons following transient ischemia. *Brain Research*, **673**, 112–118.

Ismail, K. and Wessely, S. (1995). Psychiatric complications of corticosteroid therapy. *British Journal of Hospital Medicine*, **53**, 495–499.

Itil, T. and Fink, M. (1966). Anticholinergic drug-induced delirium: experimental modification, quantitative EEG and behavioral correlations. *Journal of Nervous and Mental Disorders*, **143**, 492–507.

Itil, T. M. (1966). Quantitative EEG changes induced by anticholinergic drugs and their behavioral correlates in man. *Recent Advances in Biological Psychiatry*, **8**, 151–173.

Jaber, M., Robinson, S. W., Missale, C., and Caron, M. G. (1996). Dopamine receptors and brain function. *Neuropharmacology*, **35**, 1503–1509.

James, J. H., Ziparo, V., Jeppsson, B., and Fischer, J. E. (1979). Hyperammonaemia, plasma aminoacid imbalance, and blood–brain aminoacid transport: a unified theory of portal-systemic encephalopathy. *Lancet*, **ii**, 772–775.

Joyce, J. N. J., Janowsky, A., and Neve, K. A. (1991). Characterization and distribution of [^{125} I] epidepride binding to dopamine D2 receptors in basal ganglia and cortex of human brain. *Journal of Pharmacological Experiment and Therapeutics*, **257**, 1253.

Kalmijn, S., Launer, L. J., Stolk, R. P., *et al.* (1998). A prospective study on cortisol, dehydroepian-rosterone sulfate, and cognitive function in the elderly. *Journal of Clinical Endocrinologic Metabolism*, **83**, 3487–3492.

Kandel, E. R. (2000). *The brain and behavior*. McGraw-Hill, New York.

Kaufer, D. I., Catt, K. E., Lopez, O. L., *et al.* (1998). Dementia with Lewy bodies: response of delirium-like features to donepezil. *Neurology*, **51**, 1512–1513.

Keane, P. E. and Neal,H. (1981). The effect of injections of dopaminergic agonists into the caudate nucleus on the electrocortigram of the rat. *Journal of Neuroscience Research*, **6**, 237–241.

Kennedy, J. S., Zagar, A., Bymaster, F., *et al.* (2001). The central cholinergic system profile of olanzapine compared with placebo in Alzheimer's disease. *International Journal of Geriatric Psychiatry*, **16**, S24–S32.

Knell, A. J., Davidson, A. R., Williams, R., *et al.* (1974). Dopamine and serotonin metabolism in hepatic encephalopathy. *British Medical Journal*, **i**, 549–551.

Kondo, Y., Ogawa, N., Asanuma, M., *et al.* (1995). Cyclosporin A prevents ischemia-induced reduction of muscarinic acetylcholine receptors with suppression of microglial activation in gerbil hippocampus. *Neuroscience Research*, **22**,123–127.

Kopf, S. R. and Baratti, C. M. (1994). Memory-improving actions of glucose: involvement of a central cholinergic muscarinic mechanism. *Behavioral and Neural Biology*, **62**, 237–243.

Koponen, H., Hurri, L., Stenback, U., *et al.* (1989). Computed tomography findings in delirium. *Journal of Nervous and Mental Disorders*, **177**, 226–231.

Koponen, H. J., Sirvio, J., Reinkainen, K. J. and Riekkinen, P. J. (1991). A longitudinal study of CSF acetylcholinesterase in delirium: changes at the acute stage and at one year follow up. *Psychiatry Research*, **38**, 135–142.

Koponen, H., Sirvio, J., Lepola, U., *et al.* (1994). A long-term follow-up study of cerebrospinal fluid acetylcholinesterase in delirium. *European Archives of Psychiatry and Clinical Neuroscience*, **243**, 347–351.

Kreis, R., Farrow, N., and Ross, B. N. (1991). Localized NMR spectroscopy in patients with chronic hepatic encephalopathy: analysis of changes in cerebral glutamine, choline, and inositols. *NMR Biomedicine*, **4**, 109–116.

Kronfol, Z. and Remick, D. G. (2000). Cytokines and the brain: implications for clinical psychiatry. *American Journal of Psychiatry*, **157**, 683–694.

Leavitt, M., Trzepacz, P. T., and Ciongoli, K. (1994). Rat model of delirium: atropine dose-response relationships. *Journal of Neuropsychiatry and Clinical Neuroscience*, **6**, 279–284.

Lehman, J. (1982). Tryptophan deficiency stupor: a new psychiatric syndrome. *Acta Psychiatrica Scandinavica*, **300** (supplement), 1–46.

Leonard, B. E. (1992). *Fundamentals of psychopharmacology*. John Wiley & Sons Ltd., Chichester.

Lesch, K. P., Wolozin, B. L., Murphy, D. L., and Reiderer, P. (1993). Primary structure of the human platelet serotonin uptake site: identity with the brain serotonin transporter. *Journal of Neurochemistry*, **60**, 2319–2322.

Levenson, J. A. (1992). Should psychostimulants be used to treat delirious patients with depressed mood? (Letter) *Journal of Clinical Psychiatry*, **53**, 69.

Lin, S. C., Olson, K., Okazaki, H., *et al.* (1986). Studies on muscarinic binding sites in human brain identified with [³H] pirenzepine. *Journal of Neurochemistry*, **46**, 274–290.

Lyeth, B. G., Dixon, C. E., Jenkins, L. W., *et al.* (1988). Effects of scopolamine treatment on long-term behavioral deficits following concussive brain injury to the rat. *Brain Research*, **452**, 39–48.

Mach, J. R., Dysken, M. W., Kuskowski, M., *et al.* (1995). Serum anticholinergic activity in hospitalized older persons with delirium: a preliminary study. *Journal of the American Geriatrics Society*, **43**, 491–495.

Maes, M., Scharpe, S., Meltzer, H. Y., *et al..* (1994). Increased neopterin and interferon-gamma secretion and lower availability of L-tryptophan in major depression: further evidence for an immune response. *Psychiatry Research*, **54**, 143–160.

Maes, M., Verkerk, R., Vandoolaeghe, E., *et al.* (1997). Serotonin-immune interactions in major depression: lower serum tryptophan as a marker of an immune-inflammatory response. *European Archives of Psychiatry and Clinical Neurosciences*, **247**, 154–161.

Martin, M., Figiel, G., Mattingly, G., *et al.* (1992). ECT-induced interictal delirium in patients with a history of a CVA. *Journal of Geriatric Psychiatry and Neurology*, **5**, 149–155.

Masand, P. S. and Sipahimalani, A. (1998). Olanzapine in the treatment of delirium. *Psychosomatics*, **39**, 422–430.

McEntee, W. J., Mair, R. G., and Langlais, P. J. (1987). Neurochemical specificity of learning: dopamine and motor learning. *The Yale Journal of Biology and Medicine*, **60**, 187–193.

McIver, B. and Gorman, C. (1997). Euthyroid sick syndrome: an overview. *Thyroid*, **7**, 125–132.

Medina, J. L., Rubino, F. A., and Ross, E. (1974). Agitated delirium caused by infarctions of the hippocampal formation and fusiform and lingual gyri. *Neurology*, **24**, 1181–1183.

Medina, J. L., Sudhansu, C., and Rubino, F. A. (1977). Syndrome of agitated delirium and visual impairment: a manifestation of medial temporo-occipital infarction. *Journal of Neurology, Neurosurgery and Psychiatry*, **40**, 861–864.

Meijer, O. C. and de Kloet, E. R. (1998). Corticosterone and serotonergic neurotransmission in the hippocampus: functional implications of central corticosteroid receptor diversity. *Critical Reviews in Neurobiology*, **12**, 1–20.

Meltzer, H. Y. (1993). Serotonin and dopamine interactions and atypical antipsychotic drugs. *Psychiatric Annals*, **23**, 193–200.

Meltzer, H. Y., O'Laughlin, I. A., Dai, J., *et al.* (1999). Atypical antipsychotic drugs but not typical increased extracellular acetylcholine levels in rat medial prefrontal cortex in the absence of acetylcholinesterase inhibition. *Society of Neuroscience Abstracts*, **25**, 452.

Mendelson, G. (1977). Pheniramine aminosalicylate overdosage – reversal of delirium and choreiform movements with tacrine treatment. *Archives of Neurology*, **34**, 313.

Mesulam, M.-M., Waxman, S. G., Geschwind, N., *et al.* (1979). Acute confusional states with right middle cerebral artery infarction. *Journal of Neurology, Neurosurgery and Psychiatry*, **39**, 84–89.

Miller, P. S., Richardson, J. S., Jyu, C. A., *et al.* (1988). Association of low serum anticholinergic levels and cognitive impairment in elderly presurgical patients. *American Journal of Psychiatry*, **145**, 342–345.

Miyasaki, J. M., Grimes, D., and Lang, A. E. (1999). Acute delirium after withdrawal of amantadine in Parkinson's disease. *Neurology*, **52**, 1717–1720.

Mizock, B. A., Sabelli, H. C., Dubin, A., *et al.* (1990). Septic encephalopathy: evidence for altered phenylalanine metabolism and comparison with hepatic encephalopathy. *Archives of Internal Medicine*, **150**, 443–449.

Molchan, S. E., Martinez, R. A., Hill, J. L., *et al.* (1992). Increased cognitive sensitivity to scopolamine with age and perspective on the scopolamine model. *Brain Research Reviews*, **17**, 215–226.

Mondimore, F. M., Damlouji, N., Folstein, M. F., and Tune, L. (1983). Post-ECT confusional states associated with elevated serum anticholinergic levels. *American Journal of Psychiatry*, **140**, 930–931.

Monsoma, F. J. Jr, Shen, Y., Ward, R. P., Hamblin, M. W., and Sibley, D. R. (1993). Cloning and expression of a novel serotonin receptor with high affinity for tricyclic psychotropic drugs. *Molecular Pharmacology*, **43**, 320–327.

Montague, D. M., Lawler, C. P., Mailman, R. B., and Gilmore, J,H. (1999). Developmental regulation of the dopamine D1 receptor in human caudate and putamen. *Neuropsychopharmacology*, **21**, 641–649.

Morita, T., Otani, H., Tsunoda, J., *et al.* (2000). Successful palliation of hypoactive delirium due to multi-organ failure by oral methylphenidate. *Support Care Cancer*, **8**, 134–137.

Mousseau, D. D. and Butterworth, R. F. (1994). Current theories on the pathogenesis of hepatic encephalopathy. *Proceedings of the Society of Experimental Biology and Medicine*, **206**, 329–344.

Mrzljak, L. and Goldman-Rakic, P. (1992). Acetylcholinesterase reactivity in the frontal cortex of human and monkey: contribution of AChE-rich pyramidal neurons. *Journal of Comparative Neurology*, **324**, 261–281.

Mullaly, W., Huff, K., Ronthal, M., *et al.* (1982). Frequency of acute confusional states with lesions of the right hemisphere. *Annals of Neurology*, **12**, 113.

Müller, N. (1997). Role of the cytokine network in the CNS and psychiatric disorders [in German]. *Nervenarzt*, **68**, 11–20.

Müller, U., von Cramon, D. Y., and Pollmann, S. (1998). D1- versus D2-receptor modulation of visuospatial working memory in humans. *Journal of Neuroscience*, **18**, 2720–2728.

Müller, W. E., Stoll, L., Schubert, T., and Gelbmann, C. M. (1991). Central cholinergic functioning and aging. *Acta Psychiatrica Scandinavica*, **366** (supplement), 34–39.

Mussi, C., Ferrari, R, Ascari, S., and Salvioli, G. (1999). Importance of serum anticholinergic activity in the assessment of elderly patients with delirium. *Journal of Geriatric Psychiatry and Neurology*, **12**, 82–86.

Nagasawa, H., Araki, T., and Kogure, K. (1994). Alteration of muscarinic acetylcholine binding sites in the postischemic brain areas of the rat using in vitro autoradiography. *Journal of Neurological Sciences*, **121**, 27–31.

Nakamura. J., Uchimura, N., Yamada, S., *et al.* (1995). The effect of mianserin hydrochloride on delirium. *Human Psychopharmacology*, **10**, 289–297.

Nakamura, J., Uchimura, N., Yamada, S., *et al.* (1997a). Mianersin suppositories in the treatment of post-operative delirium. *Human Psychopharmacology*, **12**, 595–599.

Nakamura, J., Uchimura, N., Yamada, S., and Nakazawa, Y. (1997b). Does plasma free-3-methoxy-4-hydroxyphenyl(ethylene)glycol increase the delirious state? A comparison of the effects of mianserin and haloperidol on delirium. *International Clinical Psychopharmacology*, **12**, 147–152.

Nakamura. K., Kurasawa, M., and Tanaka, Y. (1998). Apomorphine-induced hypoattention in rats and reversal of the choice performance impairment by aniracetam. *European Journal of Pharmacology*, **342**, 127–138.

Nausieda, P. A., Weiner, W. J., Kaplan, L. R., Weber, S., and Klawans, H. L. (1982). Sleep disruption in the course of chronic levodopa therapy: an early feature of the levodopa psychosis. *Clinical Neuropharmacology*, **5**, 183–194.

Nighoghossian, N., Trouillas, P., Vighetto, A., *et al.* (1992). Spatial delirium following a right subcortical infarct with frontal deactivation. *Journal of Neurology, Neurosurgery and Psychiatry*, **55**, 334–335.

Nymeyer, L. and Grossberg, G. T. (1997). Delirium in a 75 year old woman receiving ECT and levodopa. *Convulsive Therapy*, **13**, 114–116.

O'Hare, E., Weldon, D. T., Bettin, K., Cleary, J., and Mach, J. R. Jr. (1997). Serum anticholinergic activity and behavior following atropine sulfate administration in the rat. *Pharmacology, Biochemistry and Behavior*, **56**, 151–154.

O'Keeffe, S. T. and Devlin, J. G. (1994). Delirium and the dexamethasone suppression test in the elderly. *Neuropsychobiology*, **30**, 153–156.

Ongini, E., Caporali, M. G., and Massotti, M. (1985). Stimulation of dopamine D-1 receptors by SKF 38393 induces EEG desynchronization and behavioral arousal. *Life Sciences*, **37**, 2327–2333.

Passik, S. D. and Cooper, M. (1999). Complicated delirium in a cancer patient successfully treated with olanzapine. *Journal of Pain Symptom Management*, **17**, 219–223.

Perry, E. K. and Perry, R. H. (1995). Acetylcholine and hallucinations: disease-related compared to drug-induced alterations in human consciousness. *Brain and Cognition*, **28**, 240–258.

Piercey, M. F., Camacho-Ochoa, M., and Smith, M. W. (1995). Functional roles for dopamine-receptor subtypes. *Clinical Neuropharmacology*, **18**, S34–S42.

Platt, M. M., Breitbart, W., Smith, M., *et al.* (1994). Efficacy of neuroleptics for hypoactive delirium. *Journal of Neuropsychiatry and Clinical Neurosciences*, **6**, 66.

Posner, M. L. and Bois, S. J. (1971). Components of attention. *Psychology Review*, **78**, 391–408.

Powers, J. S., Decoskey, D., and Kahrilas, P. J. (1981). Physostigmine for treatment of delirium tremens. *Journal of Clinical Pharmacology*, **21**, 57–60.

Price, B. H. and Mesulam, M. (1985). Psychiatric manifestations of right hemisphere infarctions. *Journal of Nervous and Mental Disorders*, **173**, 610–614.

Quirion, R., Richard, J., and Dam, T. V. (1985). Evidence for the existence of serotonin type-2 receptors on cholinergic terminals in rat cortex. *Brain Research*, **333**, 345–349.

Ramirez, M. J., Cenarruzabeitia, E., Lasheras, B., and Del Rio, J. (1996). Involvement of GABA systems in acetylcholine release induced by 5-HT3 receptor blockade in slices from rat entorhinal cortex. *Brain Research*, **712**, 274–280.

Ravona-Springer, R., Dohlberg, O. T., Hirschman, S., *et al.* (1998). Delirium in elderly patients treated with risperidone: a report of three cases. *Journal of Clinical Psychopharmacology*, **18**, 171–172.

Ray, P. G., Meador, K. J., Loring, D. W., *et al.* (1992). Central anticholinergic hypersensitivity in aging. *Journal of Geriatric Psychiatry and Neurology*, **5**, 72–77.

Reiner, P. B. and Fibiger, H. C. (1995). Functional heterogeneity of central cholinergic systems. In: *Psychopharmacology: the fourth generation of progress* (eds F. E. Bloom and D. J. Kupfer), pp 147–153. Raven Press, New York.

Reinhardt, W., Mocker, V., Jockenhovel, F., *et al.* (1997). Influence of coronary artery bypass surgery on thyroid hormone parameters. *Hormone Research*, **47**, 1–8.

Renault, P. F. and Hoofnagle, J. H. (1989). Side effects of alpha interferon. *Seminars in Liver Disease*, **9**, 273–277.

Richardson, M. A. (Ed.). (1990). *Amino acids in psychiatric disease*, Vol. 22. American Psychiatric Press, Washington, DC.

Ritchie, J., Steiner, W., and Abrahamowicz, M. (1996). Incidence of and risk factors for delirium among psychiatric patients. *Psychiatric Services*, **47**, 727–730.

Robertsson, B., Blennow, K., Gottfries, C. G., *et al.* (1998). Delirium in dementia. *International Journal of Geriatric Psychiatry*, **13**, 49–56.

Rodriguez, G., Testa, R., Celle, G., *et al.* (1987). Reduction of cerebral blood flow in subclinical hepatic encephalopathy and its correlation with plasma free tryptophan. *Journal of Cerebral Blood Flow and Metabolism*, **7**, 768–772.

Rosenberg, P. B., Ahmed, I., and Hurwitz, S. (1991). Methylphenidate in depressed medically ill patients. *Journal of Clinical Psychiatry*, **52**, 263–267.

Ross, C. A. (1991). CNS arousal systems: possible role in delirium. In: *Delirium. Advances in research and clinical practice* (eds N. E. Miller, Z. Lipowski, and B. Lebowitz). *International Psychogeriatrics*, **3**, 353–371.

Rovner, B. W., David, A., Lucas-Blaustein, M. J., et al. (1988). Self care capacity and anticholinergic drug levels in nursing home patients. *American Journal of Psychiatry*, **145**, 107–109.

Rudrofer, M. V., Manji, H. K., and Potter, W. J. (1991). Bupropion, ECT, and dopapminergic overdrive (letter). *American Journal of Psychiatry*, **148**, 1101–1102.

Saija, A., Hayes, R. L., Lyeth, B. G., et al. (1988). The effect of concussive head injury on central cholinergic neurons. *Brain Research*, **452**, 303–311.

Sander, T., Harms, H., Podschus, J., et al. (1997). Allelic association of a dopamine transporter gene polymorphism in alcohol dependence with withdrawal seizures or delirium. *Biological Psychiatry*, **41**, 299–304.

Santamaria, J., Blesa, R., and Tolosa, E. S. (1984). Confusional syndrome in thalamic stroke. *Neurology*, **34**, 1618.

Sawaguchi, T. and Goldman-Rakic, P. S. (1991). D1 receptors in prefrontal cortex: involvement in working memory. *Science*, **251**, 947–950.

Schirazi, S., Rodrigue, D., and Nomikos, G. G. (2000). Effects of typical and atypical antipsychotic drugs on acetylcholine release in the hippocampus. *Society for Neuroscience Abstracts*, **26**, 2144.

Schmidley, J. W. and Messing, R. O. (1984). Agitated confusional states with right hemisphere infarctions. *Stroke*, **5**, 883–885.

Schuster, P., Gabriel, E., Kufferle, B., et al. (1977). Reversal by physostigmine of clozapine-induced delirium. *Clinical Toxicology*, **10**, 437–441.

Schwartz, J. C., Diaz, J., Bordet, R., et al. (1998). Functional implications of multiple dopamine receptor subtypes: the D1/D3 receptor coexistence. *Brain Research*, **26**, 235–242.

Schwartz, T. L. and Masand, P. S. (2000). Treatment of delirium with quetiapine. *Primary Care Companion. Journal of Clinical Psychiatry*, **2**,10–12.

Scremin, O. U. and Jenden, D. J. (1989). Effects of middle cerebral artery occlusion on cerebral cortex choline and acetylcholine in rats. *Stroke*, **20**, 1524–1530.

Seamens, J. K., Floresco, S. B., and Phillips, A. G. (1998). D1 receptor modulation of hippocampal-prefrontal cortical circuits integrating spatial memory with executive functions in rat. *Journal of Neuroscience*, **18**, 1613–1621.

Selden, N. R., Gitelman, D. R., Salamon-Murayama, N., Parrish, T. B., and Mesulam, M.-M. (1998). Trajectories of cholinergic pathways within the cerebral hemispheres of the human brain. *Brain*, **121**, 2249–2257.

Sherman, S. M. and Kock, C. (1990). Thalamus. In: *The synaptic organization of the brain* (ed. G. M. Shepherd), 3rd edn, pp. 246–278. Oxford University Press, New York.

Sim, F. H., Brunet, D. G., and Conacher, G. N. (2000). Quetiapine associated with acute mental status changes. *Canadian Journal of Psychiatry*, **3**, 299.

Sipahimalani, A. and Masand, P. S. (1997). Use of risperidone in delirium: case reports. *Annals of Clinical Psychiatry*, **9**, 105–107.

Skaug, O. E. (1984) Postoperative delirium. A stress reaction due to cerebral tryptophan deficiency? Report of a case successfully treated with tryptophan [in Norwegian]. *Tidsskrift for den Norske Laegeforening*, **104**, 97–98.

Sleight, A. J., Boess, F. G., Bos, M., and Bourson, A. (1998). The putative 5-HT6 receptor: localization and function. *Annals of the New York Acadamy of Sciences*, **861**, 91–96.

Sloan, E. P., Fenton, G. W., and Standage, K. P. (1992). Anticholinergic drug effects on quantitative EEG, visual evoked potentials, and verbal memory. *Biological Psychiatry*, **31**, 600–606.

Smith, S., Lindefors, N., Hurd, Y., and Sharp, T. (1995). Electroconvulsive shock increases dopamine D1 and D2 receptor mRNA in the nucleus accumbens of the rat. *Psychopharmacology*, **120**, 333–340.

Stahl, S. M. (1996). *Essential psychopharmacology. Neuroscientific basis and practical applications.* Cambridge University Press, Cambridge.

Stefano, G. B., Bilfinger, T. V., and Fricchione, G. L. (1994). The immune-neuro-link and the macrophage: post-cardiotomy delirium, HIV-associated dementia and psychiatry. *Progress in Neurobiology*, **42**, 475–488.

Stern, T. A. (1983). Continuous infusion of physostigmine in anticholinergic delirium: a case report. *Journal of Clinical Psychiatry*, **44**, 463–464.

Sternbach, H. (1991). The serotonin syndrome. *American Journal of Psychiatry*, **148**, 705–713.

Summers, W. K. (1978). A clinical method of estimating risk of drug induced delirium. *Life Sciences*, **22**, 1511–1516.

Swaab, D. F., Raadsheer, F. C., Endert, E., Hofman, M. A., Kamphorst, W., and Ravid, R. (1994). Increased cortisol levels in aging and Alzheimer's disease in postmortem cerebrospinal fluid. *Journal of Neuroendocrinology*, **6**, 681–687.

Tam, S. Y. and Roth, R. H. (1997). Mesoprefrontal dopaminergic neurons: can tyrosine availability influence their function? *Biochemical Pharmacology* , **53**, 441–453.

Tanda. G., Carboni, E., Frau, R., and DiChiara, G. (1994). Increase of extracellular dopamine in the PFC: a trait of drugs with antidepressant potential? *Psychopharmacology*, **115**, 285–288.

Tassin, J-P. (1998). Norepinephrine-dopamine interactions in the prefrontal cortex and the ventral tegmental area: relevance to mental diseases. *Advances in Pharmacology*, **42**, 712–716.

Tollefson, G. D., Montague-Clouse, J., and Lancaster, S. P. (1991). The relationship of serum anticholinergic activity to mental status performance in an elderly nursing home population. *Journal of Neuropsychiatry and Clinical Neuroscience*, **3**, 314–319.

Torres, R., Mittal, D., and Kennedy, R. (2001). Use of quetiapine in delirium: case reports. *Psychosomatics*, **42**, 347–349.

Trzepacz, P. T. (1994). Neuropathogenesis of delirium: a need to focus our research. *Psychosomatics*, **35**, 374–391.

Trzepacz, P. T. (1996). Anticholinergic model for delirium. *Seminars in Clinical Neuropsychiatry*, **1**, 294–303.

Trzepacz, P. T. (1999). Update on the neuropathogenesis of delirium. *Dementia and Geriatric Cognitive Disorders*, **10**, 330–334.

Trzepacz, P. T. (2000). Is there a final common neural pathway in delirium? Focus on acetylcholine and dopamine. *Seminars in Clinical Neuropsychiatry*, **5**, 132–148.

Trzepacz, P. T., Leavitt, M., and Ciongoli, K. (1992). An animal model for delirium. *Psychosomatics*, **33**, 404–415.

Trzepacz, P. T., Meager, D. J., and Wise, M. G. (2002). Neuropsychiatry of delirium. In: *American Psychiatric Textbook of Neuropsychiatry* (eds S. Yudfosky and R. M. Hales), 4th edition. American Psychiatric Press Inc, Washington, DC, pp. 525–564.

Tune, L. E. (2000). Serum anticholinergic activity levels and delirium in the elderly. *Seminars in Clinical Neuropsychiatry*, **5**, 149–153.

Tune, L. E., Holland, A., Folstein, M. F., *et al.* (1981). Association of postoperative delirium with raised serum levels of anticholinergic drugs. *Lancet*, **ii**, 651–652.

Tune, L. E., Carr, S., Hoag, E., *et al.* (1992). Anticholinergic effects of drugs commonly prescribed for the elderly: potential means for assessing risk of delirium. *American Journal of Psychiatry*, **149**, 1393–1394.

Tune, L. E., Carr, S., Cooper, T., *et al.* (1993). Association of anticholinergic activity of prescribed medications with postoperative delirium. *Journal of Neuropsychiatry and Clinical Neuroscience*, **5**, 208–210.

Uchiyama, M., Tanaka, K., Isse, K., *et al.* (1996). Efficacy of mianserin on symptoms of delirium in the aged: an open trial study. *Progress in Neuro-Psychopharmacology and Biological Psychiatry* **20**, 651–656.

Valphiades, M. S., Celesia, G. G., and Brigell, M. G. (1996). Positive spontaneous visual phenomena limited to the hemianopic field in lesions of central visual pathways. *Neurology*, **47**, 408–417.

Van den Berghe, G. (2000). Novel insights into the neuroendocrinology of critical illness. *European Journal of Endocrinology*, **143**, 1–13.

Van den Berghe, G., de Zegher, F., and Bouillon, R. (1998). Clinical review 95: acute and prolonged critical illness as different neuroendocrine paradigms. *Journal of Clinical Endocrinology and Metabolism*, **83**, 1827–1834.

Van der Mast, R. C. (1998). Pathophysiology of delirium. *Journal of Geriatric Psychiatry and Neurology*, **11**, 138–146.

Van der Mast, R. C. (2000). Do aminoacids play a role in the pathophysiology of delirium? *Journal of Gerontology: Biological Sciences*, **55A**, B253–B254.

Van der Mast, R. C. and Fekkes, D. (2000). Serotonin and amino acids: partners in delirium pathophysiology? *Seminars in Clinical Neuropsychiatry*, **5**, 125–131.

Van der Mast, R. C., Fekkes, D., Moleman, P., and Pepplinkhuizen, L. (1991). Is postoperative delirium related to reduced plasma tryptophan? *Lancet*, **338**, 851–852.

Van der Mast, R. C., Fekkes, D., van den Broek, W. W., *et al.* (1994). Reduced cerebral tryptophan availability as a possible cause for post-cardiotomy delirium. *Psychosomatics*, **35**, 195.

Van der Mast, R. C., van den Broek, W. W., Fekkes, D., Pepplinkhuizen, L., and Habbema, J. D. F. (1999). Incidence of and preoperative predictors for delirium after cardiac surgery. *Journal of Psychosomatic Research*, **46**, 479–483.

Van der Mast, R. C., van den Broek, W. W., Fekkes, D., Pepplinkhuizen, L., and Habbema, J. D. (2000). Is delirium after cardiac surgery related to plasma amino acids and physical condition? *Journal of Neuropsychiatry and Clinical Neurosciences*, **12**, 57–63.

Vincent, F. M. (1995). The neuropsychiatric complications of corticosteroid therapy. *Comprehensive Therapy*, **21**, 524–528.

Vitiello, B., Martin, A., Hill., J., *et al.* (1997). Cognitive and behavioral effects of cholinergic, dopaminergic, and serotonergic blockade in humans. *Neuropsychopharmacology*, **16**, 15–24.

Volkow, N. D., Gu, R. C., Wang, G-J., *et al.* (1998). Association between decline in brain dopamine activity with age and cognitive and motor impairment in healthy individuals. *American Journal of Psychiatry*, **155**, 344–349.

Wengel, S. P., Roccaforte, W. H., and Burke, W. J. (1998). Donepezil improves symptoms of delirium in dementia: *Journal of Geriatric Psychiatry and Neurology*, **11**, 159–161.

Wengel, S. P., Burke, W. J., and Roccaforte, W. H. (1999). Donepezil for postoperative delirium associated with Alzheimer's disease. *Journal of the American Geriatrics Society*, **47**, 379–380.

Wetli, C. V., Mash, D., and Karch, S. B. (1996). Cocaine-associated agitated delirium and the neuroleptic malignant syndrome. *American Journal of Emergency Medicine*, **14**, 425–428.

Wilkinson, L. S. (1997). The nature of interactions involving prefrontal and striatal dopamine systems. *Journal of Psychopharmacology*, **11**, 143–150.

Wilson, J. M., Sanyal, S., and Van Tol, H. H. M. (1998). Dopamine D2 and D4 receptor ligands: relation to antipsychotic action. *European Journal of Pharmacology*, **351**, 273–286.

Wurtman, R. J., Hefti, F., and Melamed, E. (1980). Precursor control of neurotransmitter synthesis. *Pharmacological Reviews*, **32**, 315–335.

Yamaguchi, T., Suzuki, M., and Yamamoto, M. (1997). Evidence for 5-HT4 receptor involvement in the enhancement of acetylcholine release by *p*-chloroamphetamine in rat frontal cortex. *Brain Research*, **772**, 95–101.

Yamamoto, T., Lyeth, B. G., Dixon, C. E., *et al.* (1988). Changes in regional brain acetylcholine content in rats following unilateral and bilateral brainstem lesions. *Journal of Neurotrauma*, **5**, 69–79.

Yoshida, K., Higuchi, H., Kamata, M., Yoshimoto, M., Shimizu, T., and Hishikawa, Y. (1998). Single and repeated electroconvulsive shocks activate dopaminergic and 5-hydroxytryptaminergic neurotransmission in the frontal cortex of rats. *Progress in Neuro-Psychopharmacology and Biological Psychiatry*, **22**, 435–444.

Chapter 5

Clinical assessment and diagnosis

Hannu Koponen, Kenneth Rockwood, and
Colin Powell

Delirium is a common, costly, and potentially devastating condition for hospitalized older patients. Delirium is a multifactorial syndrome, involving the interrelationship between patient vulnerability, predisposing factors at admission, and the noxious insults and aggravating factors during hospitalization. Despite the prevalence of delirium in hospitals, modern hospital staff tend to be preoccupied with the technological aspects of their practice, and commonly overlook the cognitive and emotional problems of their patients and their carers. No specific diagnostic test for delirium exists, and the diagnosis is made on the basis of its key features. The main challenge in diagnosing delirium is to detect the great variety of fluctuating signs and symptoms of the disorder and to organize them into a definable set of symptoms and signs that span a spectrum of manifestations. The challenge of recognizing delirium is an important one, not just because there are many phenotypes of delirium across this spectrum, from lethargy bordering on coma to agitation bordering on mania, but because the individual features fluctuate. The differential diagnosis of delirium begins with its syndromic distinction and then seeks an aetiological cause. In most cases, the delirium can be distinguished clinically by its unique set of symptoms, its acute onset, and its fluctuating and transient course (Inouye 1994; Meagher 2001).

This chapter seeks to bridge information on instrumentation and on management by proposing one means of thinking about delirium that does not do violence to its essentially complex and protean nature. Experienced physicians will, of course, usually detect delirium very quickly, typically within a few seconds, and modify their approach accordingly. This is not unique to delirium but, rather, is the case for most diagnoses, especially syndromic diagnoses, made by experts (Sackett *et al.* 1991).

Commonly, physicians less experienced in the diagnosis of delirium encounter the gestalt in an altogether different guise: that of the 'confused' patient or of the 'poor historian'. Confusion is a most unhelpful term. Simpson (1984) showed complete lack of correlation between the standard definitions of 'confusion' (e.g. both including and not including disorientation as part of the definition) by the various professionals (internists, psychiatrists, registered nurses, mental health nurses) who use these terms. Moreover, given that a historian collects data from primary sources, and then analyses and presents these to others, makes one wonder who is the poor historian in this particular patient–doctor encounter. At the heart of this label is the recognition that the patient is cognitively impaired, but unfortunately this impairment is seen as the patient's problem rather than the physician's opportunity for diagnosis and management. From this it should be only a short step first to consider the syndromic diagnosis (delirium, dementia, depression, a delusional disorder, dysphasia) and then to determine the cause, but in many settings this convention is honoured more in the breach than in the observance.

It is not clear why physicians should react to the delirious patient as though the encounter were a social and not a professional one. Again, this is not unique to delirium. For example, Goodwin *et al.* (1979) reported that when four rheumatologists were asked to quantify their emotional response to 22 patients with SLE in terms of the patients' 'likeability', the 10 patients 'most disliked' included all those with cognitive impairment. The editorialist commented: 'the intensity of the physician's dislike thus provided a clue to diagnosing serious organic brain disease' (Vaisrub 1979). Another editorial commented that: 'irritability in the physician may be a useful sign of brain damage in the patient', although a correspondent pondered the converse (Powell 1979). In other settings we recognize that transference can sometimes be diagnostic; if a non-depressed doctor interviews a depressed patient and concludes the examination feeling sad, then the patient may well be depressed (Powell 1979).

Psychopathological manifestations of cerebral dysfunction in delirium include:

- impairment of cognitive functions, e.g. thinking, memory and perception;
- disorders of consciousness, wakefulness and attention;
- personality change; and
- compensatory and protective strategies.

Elderly people with delirium usually show some of the central features of the syndrome (see also Table 5.1), but it is important to bear in mind that the clinical picture may be less complete and characteristic than it is in younger people. For example, unlike the florid disturbances that often accompany delirium in younger adults, delirium in older adults may be quiet and easily overlooked by those who do not know the person well. For this reason, the clinical assessment of delirium requires a precise approach. It is wrong, however, to presume that one arrives at a diagnosis of delirium after the mythical 'complete history and physical examination'. This is an unsatisfactory creed on many grounds: it is not the case; it misleads trainees; it promotes inappropriate investigations; it impedes research; and, even if it were true, the traditional medical encounter ignores many important aspects of a patient's presentation (e.g. the evaluation of physical function), which will be essential to management. But how is delirium assessed?

History

The patient's own account of events will nearly always be unreliable or incomplete, and a collateral history from other sources is mandatory. Family members and informal

Table 5.1 Essential features of delirium (Lipowski 1990)

- Impaired awareness of self and surroundings
- Impairment of directed thinking
- Disorders of attention, with hypo- or hyperalertness
- Impairment of memory
- Diminished perceptual discrimination, with a tendency toward misperceptions, i.e. illusions and hallucinations
- Impairment of spatio-temporal orientation
- Disturbance of psychomotor behaviour, with hypo- or hyperactivity, both verbal and nonverbal
- Disordered sleep–wake cycle, usually marked drowsiness and naps during the day, insomnia at night, or both
- Unpredictable fluctuations in alertness and in severity of cognitive impairment during the day and overall exacerbation of symptoms at night and upon waking
- Acute onset and relatively brief duration
- Laboratory evidence of widespread cerebral dysfunction, especially diffuse changes (slowing or fast activity) of background activity on the EEG

and formal carers should be interviewed, and nursing notes should be reviewed for evidence of disorientation or inappropriate communication, unusual behaviours and illusions or hallucinations. The onset of delirium is typically rapid, and one should examine any recent change in the patient's observable behaviour and cognitive functioning (see also Table 5.2).

Delirium can develop more insidiously in some cases, such as slowly developing drug toxicity, but the history of problems will rarely be more than a few weeks. One can often distinguish a prodromal stage, during which the patient tends to have some difficulty in concentrating and thinking clearly; they may feel restless and anxious, and may complain of irritability, fatigue, malaise, hypersensitivity to lights and sounds, drowsiness, insomnia, vivid dreams or nightmares, and even transient illusions and hallucinations. Informants should always be asked about similar episodes in the past, their cause, treatment, and outcome. In elderly delirious patients, it is important to determine the extent of any pre-existing cognitive deficit, since it is from this prior level of cognitive function that the recent decrement must be assessed. Similarly, the development of delirium in an otherwise apparently well elderly person should alert health-care professionals of an increased risk of dementia, even when recovery appears complete.

Examination of the mental state

In the prodromal phase of delirium, the patient may complain of muddled thinking, and there is increasing difficulty with concentrating and judging the passage of time. The patient becomes irritable and restless, or lethargic and withdrawn.

Table 5.2 Features indicating delirium (Lipowski 1990)

- A relatively acute change in the patient's behaviour and mental functioning
- Appearance of symptoms suggestive of impaired thinking, recent memory, perceptual clarity, and orientation for time and place
- Observable evidence of distractibility, i.e. difficulty in mobilizing, shifting, maintaining, and focusing attention in response to questions
- Irregular and unpredictable fluctuation in previously mentioned cognitive and attentional deficits during daytime and their worsening during a sleepless night
- Reduced accessibility of the patient to verbal communication as a result of a reduced or abnormally heightened alertness, i.e. impaired readiness to respond
- Appearance of visual illusions and hallucinations to which the patient tends to respond with fear or anger and agitation
- Markedly increased or reduced psychomotor, i.e. both verbal and non-verbal behaviour, with a tendency to display incoherent speech
- Appearance of fleeting, mostly persecutory, delusions that tend to accompany hallucinations and shift in content in response to environmental stimuli
- Disrupted sleep–wake cycle, with insomnia at night and excessive drowsiness during the day, or complete sleep loss, or reversal of the circadian sleep–wake cycle
- A tendency to exhibit at any time so-called lucid intervals, marked by improved accessibility, attention, and grasp of the situation

Mood disturbance is common, particularly if the patient is aware that something is the matter. Hypersensitivity to stimuli may be reported, and the same is true for perceptual distortions, or the evident effort needed to maintain normal perceptions. The sleep–wake cycle often shows early signs of disturbance, with insomnia by night and drowsiness by day. Sleep can be accompanied by vivid dreams or hallucinations, especially on falling asleep or on waking up. In an attempt to maintain a façade of normality in the face of cognitive testing, the subject may be evasive, refuse to cooperate, or respond with a catastrophic reaction when pressed. In demented elderly people, the onset of a delirium may be heralded by sudden changes in behaviour, or sudden deterioration of self-care capacity, mobility, or urinary continence.

When taking history from the patients themselves, attention should be paid to how recent events are recalled, sequenced, and made sense of, since this provides a good opportunity to make an unobtrusive assessment of alertness, memory, and thinking. Where the delirium is severe, formal assessment of the mental state may be impossible, but in moderate and doubtful cases brief cognitive function tests are helpful, particularly those that are sensitive to attentional deficits, such as tests of attention and concentration, temporo-spatial orientation and arithmetical function. When testing memory function in delirium, it is new learning ability that is most important. Asking the subject to name objects and obey commands may briefly test language function. Visuo-spatial function is commonly disturbed in delirium, and may be tested by asking the subject to draw a clock and copy a diagram. Sometimes delirium only becomes apparent if the doctor–patient conversation is sufficiently long to detect inconsistencies in temporal recall, subtle changes of attention, and eventual inability of the patient to sustain a wholly coherent conversation.

Central features of delirium are a reduced ability to focus, sustain, and shift attention to external stimuli, and disorganized thinking, manifested as global cognitive impairment. There is a rapidly developing disorientation in time and place, together with disorientation in person if the delirium is severe. The attentional deficit results in impaired concentration and ready distractibility. Typically, the cognitive impairment fluctuates over time, with lucid intervals in the morning and maximum disturbance at night when the patient is fatigued and sensory input is reduced. However, 'morning delirium' has been described in some patients (Edlund *et al.* 1999). Delirium often makes its first appearance as an episode of nocturnal disturbance.

In delirium, thinking is progressively disturbed. If the delirium is mild, the only abnormality may be slowing down or speeding up of the stream of thought. As the delirium becomes more severe, the capacity to make judgements, to grasp abstract concepts, and to reason logically are all impaired. The thinking eventually becomes undirected, disorganized, and incoherent. As the patient's awareness of the external environment diminishes, so the significance of the internal world increases, and the patient loses the ability to distinguish between them. False perceptions and misinterpretations of the outside world combine with intrusive private fantasies and dreams, and this can result in the sudden and powerful formation of delusions. These delusions are usually described as persecutory, but compared with schizophrenic delusions, organic delusions may be more likely to involve others as victims of the imagined drama. However, delirious delusions are for the most part transient, poorly systematized, inconsistent, and stimulus-bound, and only very seldom do they persist and become more systematized following recovery from the delirium. Nevertheless, patients usually perceive (and may remember) hallucinations as frightening, threatening, and unpleasant. This adds to their psychic distress and consequent agitation, and fuels reactive aggression.

In delirium, the registration, retention, and recall of experience is disturbed. In particular, the impaired registration results in new learning deficits and anterograde amnestic gaps, and these provide sensitive clinical indicators of mild and early delirium. There is usually a partial or complete amnesia for the period of the delirium once it has remitted, but certain psychotic experiences may be recalled (see Chapter 9). Impairment of remote memory is less common, but recall is inevitably disturbed in more severe cases.

A wide range of perceptual distortions, illusions, and hallucinations have been described in association with delirium. They occur in all sensory modalities, but visual, auditory, and visual-plus-auditory disturbances are most common. Although hallucinations are common in delirium, they are not a core feature of the syndrome.

Delirious patients may be hyperactive, hypoactive, or both, with behaviour oscillating rapidly and unpredictably between the two conditions (O'Keeffe 1999). Hypoactivity with reduced spontaneous and purposeful motor activity, and slowing, hesitation, and perseveration of movements and speech, is the form more commonly encountered in the elderly. It is not dramatic and can easily be missed, particularly if the patient already has a degree of cognitive impairment due to dementia. Much more dramatic, albeit less common, is the hyperactive delirium associated with drug withdrawal states and certain systemic infections. Semi-purposeful overactivity in delirium is less common and is usually inappropriate and clumsy. However, it results in wandering and searching, and ultimately the verbal and physical aggressive outbursts that cause the greatest management problems, particularly in hospital and residential environments. Violent behaviour is not common in elderly delirious patients. The greatest risk to elderly delirious patients are themselves, who may become exhausted, or fall, risking hip fractures and head injury.

Delirium is usually accompanied by profound affective changes. When hypoactive, patients appear apathetic and show little affective responsiveness, but assessment of their state is rarely possible and it may be that they are in fact significantly distressed. The distress associated with delirium is more apparent in hyperactive patients, who typically display fear, depression, and rage in response to their hallucinations and imagined persecutions. Vocalizations may indicate the emotional state and prominent crying may be a sign of delirium. Profoundly distressed patients may attempt to kill themselves, but fortunately delirium seems to interfere with the successful completion of suicide. The patient's pre-morbid personality, mood state, life events, and relationships all have an impact on the nature and extent of affective responses in delirium (see Chapter 9).

Hyperactive and fearful patients are often autonomically aroused. Neurological symptoms occurring in delirium include motor abnormalities such as tremor, myoclonus, ataxia, choreiform movements, asterixis, and dysarthria, and cortical signs such as dysphasia and dyspraxia. Elderly patients may become incontinent of both urine and faeces when delirious. In all cases, physical symptoms due to delirium must be distinguished from those caused by any underlying physical illness or intoxication.

Rating scales and assessment tools in the diagnosis of delirium

As reviewed in detail in Chapter 2, brief cognitive tests, for example, Mini-Mental State Examination (MMSE, Folstein *et al.* 1975), Short Portable Mental Status Questionnaire (Pfeiffer 1975), Mental Status Questionnaire (Kahn *et al.* 1960), Trail Making Test (Lezak 1983), and Clock Drawing Test (Sunderland *et al.* 1989), have been used as instruments for delirium evaluation. They are quite easy to administer, and include precise instructions how to score the patient's answers to the individual specific test questions or his/her performance of a special task. In delirium research, such brief cognitive tests have been, and still are, used for screening, i.e. for identifying subjects with cognitive impairment; Before delirium-specific instruments were developed, these cognitive tests were also used in follow-up studies.

In research and in clinical practice, instruments assessing symptoms of delirium are of value in the diagnostic process, in the evaluation of interventions, and in the care of patients. Most of the instruments developed are screening instruments or diagnostic tools. The use of scores of diagnostic rating scales remains unsatisfactory as a measure of the severity of the disorder. For example, many diagnostic scales contain items not only of symptoms but also of onset of symptoms, fluctuations of symptoms, and 'organic' aetiology that do not contribute to the severity of the disorder. The total score may thus not be a measure of severity of the disorder but may rather reflect the degree of confidence in the diagnosis (Robertsson 2000).

An important clinical and research issue in this regard, which has received little attention, is how best to track the course of delirium. Given that individual symptoms fluctuate and that many persist even in patients who no longer meet delirium diagnostic criteria (Levkoff et al. 1992; Rockwood 1993), many current measures are inadequate for tracking recovery of cognitive function. Two approaches that are useful and can be complementary are to track attention and concentration alone, and also to track mobility and balance in patients in whom it was impaired. With regard to the former, there is anecdotal experience to support the use of Axis I of the Brief Cognitive Rating Scale (Reisberg et al. 1988). Axis I ranks tests in decreasing difficulty as serial 7s from 100, serial 4s from 40, serial 2s from 20, counting 10 to 1, and finally 1 to 10. While also prone to fluctuation, this shows a trend that appears to correlate well with other clinical markers of recovery or worsening.

Many older adults who develop delirium are frail, and in many such patients, delirium coexists with impaired mobility (Jarrett et al. 1995). In such patients, tracking of mobility and balance has shown promise as a means of understanding the patient's overall clinical state (MacKnight and Rockwood 1995, 2000). That this should be so is perhaps best understood by thinking about delirium less as a specific brain disease and more as a manifestation of the failure of a highest order variable (cognition) in a complex system at the edge of failure. From this standpoint, that it should track with another high order variable (mobility and balance) makes a certain sense.

Differential diagnosis

The differential diagnosis of delirium in the elderly patient includes most other organic and functional psychiatric disorders in this age group (Lindesay 1997). Many of these conditions are direct or indirect predisposing factors for delirium in the elderly, so it is important to bear in mind that their presence does not exclude the possibility that the subject is delirious as well. A few points of emphasis in assessment are reviewed here.

Distinguishing between delirium and dementia in an elderly patient is important because of grave consequences of misdiagnosis if the subject is only suffering from a potentially reversible delirium without an underlying dementia. Dysphasia due to a cerebrovascular accident is a disorder of language that can be mistaken for delirium. The mental state in severe late life depression may at times resemble that of delirium, with agitation, retardation, persecutory auditory hallucinations and delusions, slowed thinking, impaired concentration, disturbed sleep, and disorders of behaviour, such as incontinence and screaming. Furthermore, any diurnal variation in the severity of depressive symptoms may be mistaken for delirious fluctuation of cognitive impairment. It is sometimes difficult to distinguish clinically between severe depression and delirium, but as a rule, if clinical and psychological testing show that the cognitive impairment is mild compared with disturbances of mood, psychotic symptoms, and psychomotor behaviour, it is likely that the patient is depressed rather than delirious. Collateral history may also be helpful as the onset of depression is typically more insidious and there may be a history of previous depression, often presenting in this fashion (Lindesay *et al.* 1990).

In old age, it is not uncommon for delirium and depression to occur together in the same patient. Late life depression is associated with physical illness and self-neglect, so depressed elderly people are at increased risk for delirium. Antidepressants may also induce delirium.

Episodes of mania are less common than depression in old age, but when they occur they can closely resemble hyperactive delirium. Subjects are distractible, irritable, agitated, overactive, and they may have hallucinations and be deluded. The mood is usually labile and mixed rather than euphoric. In most cases there is a personal or family history of affective disorder, but in others the mania is of late onset, possibly secondary to some cerebral insult or overtreatment with antidepressant drugs or ECT.

Summary

In general, acute onset of cognitive and attentional deficits and abnormalities, whose severity fluctuates during the day and tends to increase at night, is practically diagnostic for delirium. However, several factors appear to be responsible for the reportedly frequent non-recognition of delirium by physicians. Its clinical manifestations are protean, and it may at times mimic other mental disorders such as mania, depression, or schizophrenia. A patient experiencing prodromal or early signs of delirium is likely to look normal and behave appropriately and might thus be overlooked or ignored by the medical staff. On the other hand, many of even severely cognitively impaired patients are quiet, listless, or just drowsy, and a skewed conception of delirium is liable to result in missing the diagnosis in a quiet, undisturbing, and inconspicuous patient. The severity of the psychopathological disturbance may not correlate positively with the severity of the cognitive-attentional deficits and with objective indices of cerebral dysfunction, such as EEG abnormality. The presence of psychotic features or abnormal emotions neither increases nor decreases the probability that the patient is suffering from delirium.

There has been a prolonged disagreement and confusion in the medical literature with regard to the proper identification and diagnostic criteria for this syndrome. The existence, the clinical criteria, and the clinical importance of delirium have not been successfully emphasized in the teaching of medical students and residents. All these factors contribute to the common failure to diagnose the syndrome. Yet to diagnose it is relatively easy, especially once its symptoms have reached a certain degree of severity, and provided that the clinical team is familiar with them. Moreover, it is important to make the diagnosis early in order to initiate a search for the underlying aetiological factor (or factors), and to start appropriate, cause-related treatment. Early recognition, appropriate investigation, and treatment will help patients to emerge as quickly as possible from the hell of delirium.

References

Edlund, A., Lundström, M., Lundström, G., Hedqvist, B., And Gustafson, Y. (1999) Clinical profile of delirium in patients treated for femoral neck fracture. *Dementia and Geriatric Cognitive Disorders,* **10**, 325–329.

Folstein, M. F., Folstein, S. E., and McHugh, P. R. (1975) 'Mini-Mental State'. A practical method for grading the cognitive state of patients for the clinician. *Journal of Psychiatric Research,* **12**, 189–198.

Goodwin, J. M., Goodwin, J. S., and Kellner, R. (1979) Psychiatric symptoms in disliked medical patients. *Journal of the American Medical Association,* **241**, 1117–1118 .

Inouye, S. K. (1994) The dilemma of delirium: clinical and research controversies regarding diagnosis and evaluation of delirium in hospitalized elderly medical patients. *American Journal of Medicine,* **97**, 278–288.

Jarrett, P., Rockwood, K., Stolee, P., Carver, D., and Cosway, S. (1995) Illness presentation in elderly patients. *Archives of Internal Medicine,* **155**, 1000–1004.

Kahn, R. L., Goldfarb, A. I., Polack, M., and Peck, A. (1960) Brief objective measures for the determination of mental status in the aged. *American Journal of Psychiatry,* **117**, 326–328.

Levkoff, S. E., Evans, D. A., Liptzin, B., *et al.* (1992). Delirium. The occurrence and persistence of symptoms among elderly hospitalized patients. *Archives of Internal Medicine,* **152**, 334–340.

Lezak, M. D. (1983) *Neuropsychological assessment.* Oxford University Press, Oxford.

Lindesay, J. (1997) Delirium – the psychiatrist's perspective. In: *Psychiatry in old age* (eds R. Jacoby and C. Oppenheimer), pp 527–535. Oxford University Press, Oxford.

Lindesay, J., Macdonald, A., and Starke, I. (1990) *Delirium in the elderly.* Oxford University Press, Oxford.

Lipowski, Z. J. (1990) *Delirium: acute confusional states.* Oxford University Press, Oxford.

MacKnight, C. and Rockwood, K. (1995) A hierarchic assessment of balance and mobility. *Age and Ageing,* **24**, 126–130.

MacKnight, C. and Rockwood, K. (2000) Rasch analysis of the hierarchical assessment of balance and mobility (HABAM). *Journal of Clinical Epidemiology,* **53**, 1242–1247.

Meagher, D. J. (2001) Delirium: optimising treatment. *British Medical Journal,* **322**, 144–149.

O'Keeffe, S. T. (1999) Clinical subtypes of delirium in the elderly. *Dementia and Geriatric Cognitive Disorders,* **10**, 380–385.

Pfeiffer, E. (1975) A short portable mental status questionnaire for the assessment of organic brain deficit in elderly patients. *Journal of the American Geriatrics Society,* **23**, 433–441.

Powell, C. (1979) Irritability in patient and physician. *Lancet*, **ii**, 159.

Reisberg, B., Ferris, S. H., deLeon, M. J., and Crook, T. (1988) Global Deterioration Scale (GDS). *Psychopharmacology Bulletin*, **24**, 661–663.

Robertsson, B. Delirium in the elderly. The construction of a rating scale and aspects on risk factors and treatment. Thesis, University of Gothenburg.

Rockwood, K. (1993) The occurrence and duration of symptoms in elderly patients with delirium. *Journal of Gerontology*, **48**, M162–M166.

Sackett, D. L., Hayes, R. B., Guyatt, G. H., *et al.* (1991) *Clinical epidemiology: a basic science for clinical medicine*, 2nd edn. Little, Brown, Boston.

Simpson, C. J. (1984) Doctors' and nurses' use of the word confusion. *British Journal of Psychiatry*, **145**, 441–443.

Sunderland, T., Hill, J. L., Mellow, *et al.* (1994) Clock drawing in Alzheimer's disease. A novel measurement of dementia severity. *Cleveland Clinical Journal of Medicine*, **61**, 258–262.

Vaisrub, S. (1979) Helpful hate. *Journal of the American Medical Association*, **241**, 1157.

Chapter 6

The causes of delirium

Darryl Rolfson

Even for the experienced clinician, delirium in an older person can be a perplexing clinical challenge. The syndrome may develop insidiously, progress with periods of lucidity, and masquerade as a less acute cognitive syndrome. When recognized, the job has only just begun. Considering that the management of delirium is first and foremost to 'treat the underlying cause'; a sometimes exhaustive search then ensues to identify this. In fact, finding the causes of a delirious state becomes the central activity of a health-care provider who is interested in its resolution. Failure to address causation may reflect a serious uncertainty about the diagnosis, and will result in prolongation of the delirium and its consequences.

Inadequate recognition and treatment of delirium may be due to:

- problems with distinguishing it from other causes of confusion;
- difficulties in characterizing atypical manifestations such as hypoactive delirium;
- inadequate documentation of the fluctuating course; and
- inability to appreciate that the syndrome is a potential medical emergency.

However, the under-recognition of delirium may also reflect a more basic discomfort with how to proceed with its investigation. Even worse, when delirium is viewed only as a 'behavioural problem', the diagnosis and necessary exploration for the underlying cause may be replaced with quick fix solutions such as the prescription of a sedative without identification of the cause.

Is it possible that barriers to the investigation of delirium exist at a more basic level? Perhaps the very model of causation used by clinicians to assign aetiology to other diagnoses is inadequate when applied to 'geriatric syndromes' such as delirium, falls, immobility, functional breakdown, acute urinary incontinence, and dehydration. Traditional medical dogma rests on such concepts as 'Occam's razor', wherein there is parsimony in diagnosis. As stated in the fourteenth century by William of Occam himself: 'plurality must not be posited without necessity'. Since then, this concept has become well engrained in the practice patterns of clinician-scientists (Drachman 2000). Cartesian philosophy encourages scientists to explain complex phenomenon in the simplest way possible (i.e. the whole is equal to sum of the parts). Ideally, disease manifestations would then be explained by a single aetiology.

By contrast, research into the causation of delirium in the elderly over the past decade has illuminated an extremely powerful model with different philosophical under-pinnings. In this model, clinicians are encouraged to delineate multiple predisposing factors or aspects of vulnerability, and also to clearly enumerate acute precipitating factors, 'stressors', or insults. This model welcomes the possibility of multifactorial processes. It also naturally leads to the opportunity for prevention. Tragically, clinicians who jealously hold to the 'single disease entity' model when attempting to prevent or explain delirium in the frail elderly will, like Don Quixote, frequently return frustrated despite their best efforts.

Diversity in the literature in terms of the populations and aetiologies examined, the delirium subtypes considered, and the quality of the evidence, makes a review of causation challenging. Delirium has been described in various medical, surgical, and psychiatric populations. Some authors have contended that unique delirium subtypes reflect specific aetiologies. In 1998, the quality of the existing evidence for delirium risk factors was systematically examined by Elie *et al.* (1998) and, as in other systematic reviews of the delirium literature, few articles met all the quality criteria selected.

Our first task, then, is to anticipate these diversities. Next, a multifactorial model of causation is outlined. Finally, the potential causes of delirium are reviewed based on an evidence-based review of the literature.

Diversity in the delirium literature

Populations

A cluster of signs and symptoms consistent with the Diagnostic and Statistical Manual of Mental Disorders, 4th edition (DSM-IV) definition of delirium (American Psychiatric Association 1994) have been described in numerous diverse populations. Frequently, the clinical cluster is portrayed as being peculiar to the setting, the underlying disease entity, or the type of medication used. However, as McGuire argues, such a practice may be misleading if not dangerous (McGuire *et al.* 2000). For example, delirium in the intensive care setting is often labelled 'ICU psychosis' or the 'ICU syndrome'. An anaesthesiologist may distinguish 'emergent delirium' from 'interval delirium'. Delirium after surgery is 'postoperative delirium'. Delirium after cardiac surgery may be named 'cardiac psychosis' or the 'post-pump syndrome'. The syndrome of delirium in one large cohort of patients presenting with hip fracture was described as being unique in its phenomenology and course (Brauer *et al.* 2000). Delirium in the context of terminal illness may be labelled 'terminal delirium' (Breitbart and Strout 2000). Delirium attributable to suspect medications is 'drug-induced delirium' (Gray *et al.* 1999; Karlsson 1999) and 'substance intoxication delirium' (American Psychiatric Association 1994). In the case of benzodiazepine or alcohol withdrawal, it is 'substance withdrawal delirium' (American Psychiatric Association 1994). In the context of hepatic failure, delirium is 'hepatic encephalopathy'. More broadly, 'metabolic encephalopathy' is distinguished from 'hypoxic encephalopathy'.

It may be argued that such nosological distinctions allow for focused identification and treatment. However, delirium, when cloaked by any other name, may not be recognized as such nor its potential impact appreciated. Similarly, when delirium is viewed as being specific to a particular aetiology or setting, concurrent aetiological factors thought to be atypical to the setting may not be considered. Furthermore, future gains in educating clinicians to recognize delirium, appreciate its impact, and identify the most likely predisposing and precipitating factors may be lost when the full impact of the syndrome is softened with claims that delirium in a specific clinical setting is substantially different.

Epidemiologically, it cannot be denied that the suspected aetiologies of delirium become a fingerprint for the clinical setting in which it occurs. For example, this will affect how broadly prediction rules, which have been validated in specific settings, can be generalized. For the purpose of this chapter, however, delirium will be considered to be one phenomenological entity.

Delirium subtypes

The prevalence of delirium and its symptoms were recorded by Sandberg *et al.* (1999) in 717 seniors representing the hospital, nursing home, and supportive housing and home environments. In the 315 delirious subjects, diversity of symptoms was evident, with hypoactive, hyperactive, and mixed symptoms found in 26%, 22%, and 42% respectively. The remaining 11% had none of these features. Pronounced emotional symptoms were seen in 77% and pronounced psychotic symptoms were seen in 43%. The group concluded that such disparity in clinical profiles may warrant 'different treatment strategies for patients with different types of delirium'. In this cohort, there was no attempt to link these subtypes with suspected aetiologies.

Aetiological subgroups may differ in the duration of the delirium. Brauer *et al.* (2000) have contended that, unlike delirium in medical populations, delirium in their hip fracture population had resolved without a focused intervention in the majority of cases before discharge. In contrast, Trzepacz (1999) has noted that resolution of delirium in the non-dominant middle cerebral artery stroke syndrome is prolonged. It can be stated that the prolonged delirium in the setting of non-dominant stroke may be also explained by the added effect of perceptual disturbances that hinder a return to normal function. Still, between aetiological subgroups, the timing and severity of delirious episodes clearly will differ. Whether it necessarily follows that the core clinical features reflect different aetiologies is still a matter of some interest.

More compelling evidence for the existence of true delirium subtypes arises from the work of Meagher and colleagues who have made use of the Delirium Rating Scale developed by Trzepacz (Trzepacz *et al.* 1988) to examine symptom-based subscores in comparison to the suspected aetiologies in delirious patients. Delirium in closed head injuries and anticholinergic drug exposure was more likely to be hyperactive, whilst delirium due to metabolic causes and alcohol withdrawal were more likely to be hypoactive (Meagher and Trzepacz 1998). It is also appears that the severity of delirium declines with advancing age (Meagher *et al.* 1998) and is increased when medications are the suspected aetiology.

Ross *et al.* (1991) also found that delirium was more likely to be hyperactive when medication-related, and more commonly hypoactive with infectious and metabolic causes. However, O'Keefe showed that while patients with hypoactive delirium were more severely ill on admission, there were no differences in aetiological factors (medications, infections, metabolic disturbances, and cardiorespiratory factors) between subgroups (O'Keefe and Lavan 1999).

The DSM-IV classification of delirium subdivides delirium based on aetiology (general medical condition, substance induced, multiple aetiologies), while acknowledging that there is a 'common symptom presentation' in all subtypes.

In the minds of some, the examination of delirium subtypes to aid in the recognition of possible causes seems to be a promising future research endeavour. However, so far, the existing medical literature cannot yet help a clinician separate any clear aetiological signal from the noise of delirium subtypes and severities.

Quality of the literature

The most recent systematic review of the risk factors associated with delirium has been conducted by Elie *et al.* (1998), based on the literature from 1966 to 1995. At least 20 well-designed prospective cohort trials have appeared since then. This review includes but does not limit itself to the significant conclusions suggested by Elie *et al.*

The following features of primary articles will be considered as necessary for them to be included as evidence. First, valid criteria for the screening or diagnosis of delirium must have been used. Second, only properly designed prospective cohort trials will be included. If there is a retrospective design, the study populations and selection process (case or control) must have been well described. Third, for the populations studied, a generous minimum age 50 will have been used. Ideally, in risk factor analysis, associations based on multivariate analysis will have been highlighted. Of course, the associations which arise from such analysis are truly independent only to the degree to which all other relevant variables are also considered in the analysis.

A conceptual model for delirium causation

The idea that delirium is in fact an atypical manifestation of physical illness is not new. However, what has become increasingly obvious is that delirium in old age may have more in common with such entities as falls, immobility, acute urinary incontinence, dehydration, and functional decline than with other primary diseases of the central nervous system.

Jarrett *et al.* (1995) demonstrated that in frail elderly people who develop acute illness, these manifestations (delirium, falls, immobility, functional decline, etc.) are actually typical. Furthermore, there are remarkable similarities between delirium and the other 'atypical disease manifestations'. All of these acute geriatric syndromes represent a failure of those complex human behaviours, which require higher order integration of multiple body systems and external factors. For this reason, the causes are likely to be multifactorial. In fact, there is remarkable homology between these 'atypical disease manifestations' in terms of the actual lists of predisposing and precipitating factors. For example, Tinetti *et al.* (1995) argue for a shared list of risk factors for falls, incontinence, and functional dependence. In a systematic review of the risk factors associated with functional status decline in community-dwelling elderly people (Stuck *et al.* 1999), the profile of primary contributors remarkably resembles that of delirium.

In the context of the acute development of delirium, falls, immobility, urinary incontinence, functional dependence, and dehydration, the clinician who would find an acute aetiology seems to be led down different paths depending on the relative burden of predisposing problems. For example, these syndromes in an otherwise vigorous individual with few if any co-morbidities likely represent a severe single insult involving the obvious body system. Thus in this setting, delirium may reflect CNS pathology, dehydration may suggest circulatory or nutritional pathology, and urinary incontinence undoubtedly reflects urinary tract pathology.

However, in the frail elderly patient where there is a complex mixture of co-morbidities and vulnerabilities, the same manifestations of illness have an entirely different aetiological meaning. These manifestations at once reflect multiple acute insults, which can be located outside the obvious body system yet, at the same time, reflecting the 'weakest links' or predisposing variables within the obvious body system. An example is that while delirium in the frail elderly patient can only uncommonly be attributed to an acute central nervous system event, a previously unrecognized dementia often is uncovered as the more common acute causes of the delirium are recognized and successfully treated.

A dynamic model of frailty has been proposed to better understand acute functional breakdown in the elderly (Brocklehurst 1985; Rockwood *et al.* 1994). Frailty has also been conceptualized as being distinct from traditional models of ageing and disability (Rockwood *et al.* 2000). By way of analogy, such a model of causation would envisage the predisposition to delirium and other geriatric syndromes as a balance scale in which pre-existing factors which strengthen the possibility of independent community living are found on one side and factors which threaten such independence are on the other. In this model, the extent to which independence 'hangs in the balance' represents frailty (Figure 6.1). In such a precarious state of frailty, it not surprising to see that less severe insults (stressors) are sufficient to tip the scale toward functional breakdown and acute geriatric syndromes. In another model of frailty, Carlson *et al.* (1998) have described 'functional homeostasis' as 'the ability of an individual to withstand illness without loss of function'. A closely related concept familiar to many physicians is 'failure to thrive'. Like frailty, 'failure to thrive' does not conform to any disease construct, and suggests multifactorial syndromes such as impaired physical functioning, malnutrition, depression, and cognitive impairment (Sarkisian and Lachs 1996).

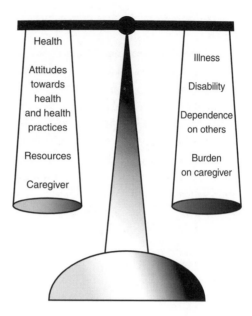

Fig. 6.1 Dynamic model of frailty.

A multifactorial model of delirium

Over the past decade, powerful concepts such as frailty and atypical disease manifestations (acute geriatric syndromes) have been brought to focus in the development of prediction models for delirium. Inouye and her colleagues have, like none other, fleshed out these concepts into a multifactorial model of delirium (Inouye and Charpentier 1996; Inouye 1998). They first developed a prediction rule for predisposing variables (i.e. frailty, vulnerability) in a cohort of hospitalized elderly which included visual impairment, severe illness, cognitive impairment, and an elevated blood urea nitrogen (BUN)/creatinine ratio (Inouye *et al.* 1993). In a subsequent similar cohort, precipitating variables (i.e. stressors, insults) were also identified and another predictive model was developed which included the use of physical restraints, malnutrition, more than three new medications, the use of a bladder catheter and 'any iatrogenic event'. When these two predictive models were combined, the incremental effects on the relative risk of delirium were found to be additive (Inouye and Charpentier 1996). Such a model provides an excellent framework for the various aetiologies of delirium in old age (Figure 6.2). What is particularly helpful is the concept of an inverse relationship between baseline vulnerability and the severity of the insult necessary to induce delirium.

Specific causes of delirium

Based on the foregoing conceptual framework, the causes of delirium could be summarized very easily. It would seem that given a sufficiently precarious state, any acute insult

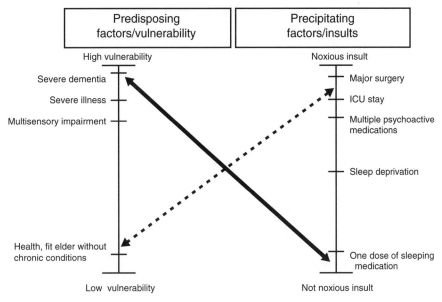

Fig. 6.2 Multifactorial model of delirium.

(illness, substance exposure, or substance intoxication) can precipitate delirium. Any number of predisposing factors may also contribute to the composite state of vulnerability or frailty, especially when the severity of the insult appears to be less intense. The most important predisposing factors for delirium (see Table 6.1) have been discussed in Chapter 3; relevant precipitating variables (see Table 6.2) will now be highlighted.

Precipitating factors

Identification of factors that predispose to delirium is important in its prevention (see Chapter 8). However, in established delirium, the work-up for precipitating variables must proceed urgently. Regardless of the state of vulnerability or frailty, medications top the list of acute insults and must be considered one by one while searching for other acute illness.

Medications

It is at first surprising when reviewing the delirium literature to discover that as a composite endpoint, 'medications' do not always emerge as a strong independent risk factor. This may simply reflect inadequate power, wherein the sheer volume of previous medications used in any cohort obscures the fewer, more hazardous medications, which were more recently prescribed. This effect has been overcome by focusing on the number of new medications or by monitoring only those medications with a high or moderate risk of delirium.

Martin *et al.* (2000) have found an association between the number of medications and delirium. This association was found to be independent of age, cognitive impairment,

Table 6.1 Predisposing Causes of Delirium*

Demographic and Social Factors
  Older Age
  Male gender
  Institutional setting
  Social Isolation
Process of Care
  Iatrogenesis
  Inadequate skills in recognition of delirium
  Negative attitudes toward the care of the elderly
  Rapid pace and technological focus of acute care
  Reductions in skilled nursing staff
Special Sensory Impairment
  Visual Impairment
  Hearing Impairment
Cognitive and Psychiatric Comorbidity
  Dementia
    Degree of stage of dementia
    Late onset Alzheimer's dementia
    Vascular dementia
  Cognitive Impairment
  Depression
Functional Impairments and Disability
  Functional dependence
  Immobility
  Fracture on admission
Malnutrition
  Dehydration
  Alcoholism
Medical Comorbidity
  High burden of illness
  Previous stroke
  Parkinson's disease
  Azotemia

---

* Independent associations are bolded

and the other process of care variables such as surgery, a high number of procedures, and intensive care treatment. Inouye and Charpentier (1996) also found an independent association between delirium and 'more than three medications added' within 24–48 hours prior to its onset.

Medication use in seniors is a topic of great interest in its own right. Common problems include adverse drug reactions, polypharmacy, and non-compliance. Whilst adverse drug reactions may occur as a result of altered pharmacokinetics in the elderly, the pharmacodynamic properties of a large number of medications are at the heart of drug-induced delirium in old age. Large lists of medications, which can cause delirium in the elderly, can be generated. However, in any given patient with delirium, the following variables appear to be crucial.

Table 6.2 Precipitating Causes of Delirium*

Medications	Shock
Substance Withdrawal	**Anemia**
Alcohol	Congestive Heart Failure
Sedative Hypnotics	Chronic Obstructive Pulmonary Disease
Substance Intoxication	Urinary and Fecal Retention
Sedative hypnotics	**Environmental/Psychological Contributors**
Narcotics	Sensory deprivation
Anticholinergics	Sensory overload
Antipsychotics	Psychological stress
Antiparkinsonians	Sleep deprivation
Antidepressants	**Pain**
Severe Acute Illness	**Physical restraint use**
Infections	**Bladder catheter use**
Urinary Tract Infection	**Any iatrogenic event**
Pneumonia	**Intensive care unit treatment**
Metabolic Abnormalities	**Surgery, Anaesthesia and other procedures**
Hyperglycemia/Hypoglycemia	**Orthopedic Surgery**
Hypercalcemia/Hypocalcemia	**Cardiac Surgery**
Thyrotoxicosis/Myxedema	**Duration of cardiopulmonary bypass**
Adrenal Insufficiency	**Non Cardiac Surgery**
Hepatic Failure	**High number of procedures in hospital**
Renal Failure	Neurologic Illness
Hypernatremia/Hyponatremia	Subdural Hematoma
Hyperkalemia/Hypokalemia	Stroke
Hypoperfusion States and Pulmonary	Malignancy
** Compromise**	Cerebral Infection
Hypoxemia	Seizures

* Independent associations are bolded

First, the frailty of the patient combined with their concurrent co-morbidities and medications may set the stage for 'drug–drug' and 'drug–disease' interactions. For example, while a neuroleptic may be helpful in an agitated delirium in a previously healthy senior, the same medication may worsen delirium in a frail senior with Lewy body dementia.

Second, nearly every drug class can cause delirium given the right circumstances. A drug may be commonly observed as a cause of delirium either due to the drug's intrinsic propensity to induce delirium or simply due to the relative frequency with which it is used in clinical practice. Faced with a long list of medications, an important clue when determining which seem to be the 'culprits' is to match recent changes in medications with recent changes in cognition.

The term 'psychoactive medications' is used broadly, referring to medications that have a well-established association with delirium. Independent associations have been found in various populations. In a palliative care population (Lawlor *et al.* 2000), 'psychoactive medication use' conferred an independent relative risk of 6.6. In general medicine in-patients (Francis *et al.* 1990), logistic regression revealed that 'psychoactive medications' increased the risk of delirium by a factor of 3.9. Similar results have been seen in a general surgical (Dai *et al.* 2000) and an orthopaedic population (Rogers *et al.* 1989). Medications that cause delirium have been reviewed extensively and can be classified as 'high risk', 'moderate risk' and 'low risk', based on their individual potential to cause delirium when used (Karlsson 1999). When newly prescribed, the drugs most likely to cause delirium include sedative hypnotics (benzodiazepines), opioids, anticholinergic medications, neuroleptics, dopamine-activating medications, antipsychotics, and antidepressants.

High-risk medications Benzodiazepines are used primarily for their CNS effects, especially sedation. Marcantonio *et al.* (1994a) found a significant association between delirium after non-cardiac surgery and the use of these drugs (odds ratio 3.3). The risk of delirium increased with increasing total dose (odds ratio 3.3) and with the use of long-acting, lipid-soluble medications (odds ratio 5.4) (Marcantonio *et al.* 1994b). An independent association was demonstrated in a group of hospitalized elderly who developed new cognitive impairment in hospital, having had intact cognition previously (Foy *et al.* 1995). As described above, the potential deliriogenic effects of a benzodiazepine must be balanced against the possibility that the sedative will help resolve delirium in the setting of alcohol or sedative withdrawal.

In clinical practice, narcotics are widely recognized to be associated with delirium. Analogous to the push/pull dilemma with benzodiazepine use in alcohol and sedative withdrawal, narcotic use in the context of pain may be either a help or a hindrance. After all, pain itself can contribute to delirium. Fortunately, effective alternative analgesics can often be identified, allowing both the narcotics and the pain syndrome to be addressed concurrently. Independent associations between delirium and narcotic use have been found in some studies (Schor *et al.* 1992; Foy *et al.* 1995), but not others (Marcantonio *et al.* 1994b).

As pointed out by Karlsson, 'all drugs with pure anticholinergic activity will in sufficiently high dose induce delirium, especially in susceptible individuals…' (Karlsson 1999). In the frail elderly, commonly used drugs with anticholinergic effects include oxybutynin and tolteridine, antinauseants and promotility agents. Other drug classes such as antidepressants and antipsychotics also possess anticholinergic properties and must be used cautiously. A classic example from the antidepressant class is amitriptyline, which possesses significant anticholinergic properties, and is best avoided in susceptible individuals such as those with dementia. It is also important to bear in mind that many of the drugs commonly prescribed to elderly patients, such as digoxin, cimetidine, and prednisolone, also have a degree of anticholinergic activity, and the cumulative effect of this may be clinically significant (Tune and Egeli 1999). Despite ample clinical experience and case reports implicating this class of drugs as a cause of delirium (see Chapter 4), it is surprising that this is not always supported by the evidence-based literature (Gustafson *et al.* 1988; Foreman 1989; Francis *et al.* 1990; Schor *et al.*1992; Marcatonio *et al.* 1994b). One study, however, has demonstrated that in delirious patients, exposure to anticholinergic medications is independently associated with an increase in the subsequent severity of the delirium (Han *et al.* 2001).

Any neuroleptic can paradoxically worsen a delirium. Lower potency neuroleptics such as chlorpromazine have anticholinergic properties, whereas higher potency neuroleptics such as haloperidol possess dopaminergic properties, both of which can contribute to delirium. Theoretically, atypical neuroleptics appear to have a lower incidence of parkinsonism. Whether these drugs are less likely to worsen delirium is not known. Delirium which consistently results from a minimal dose of neuroleptics may prompt the clinician to consider Lewy body dementia in the classic clinical setting (features of parkinsonism, visual hallucinations, and a 'picture of delirium').

While the evidence-based literature is scanty, at least one other class of medications must be considered to be high risk: the antiparkinsonians, including dopamine-activating drugs. Hallucinations and inattention in Parkinson's disease are common manifestations of the primary disorder. However, nearly every drug used to treat the physical manifestations of the disease can also cause delirium. These include, in order of risk of delirium, dopamine agonists (including newer agents), levodopa, and anticholinergic medications. Thus, as in other high-risk drugs (sedative hypnotics in alcohol withdrawal, narcotics in pain syndromes, and neuroleptics in Lewy body dementia), yet another clinical backdrop for delirium can exist (dopamine activators in Parkinson's disease), in which it will be unclear whether it is best to taper down or to increase the amount of drug given.

Moderate-risk medications Of the remaining medications, only one has been documented to have an independent association with delirium: the β-receptor antagonists (Rogers *et al.* 1989). This was demonstrated in a relatively young orthopaedic population (average age of 69). Considering the poor β-receptor responsiveness in elderly patients, this effect may be more difficult to demonstrate in an older cohort.

Having first considered the high-risk medications above, other medications that may be the 'generator' of a delirium include steroids, antihistaminergic drugs, anti-arrhythmics, calcium channel blockers, antidepressants and non-steroidal anti-inflammatory drugs (Karlsson 1999). To this list could be added anti-epileptics, H2 blockers, laxatives, antibiotics, diuretics, digitalis, and chemotherapeutic drugs.

Substance withdrawal

Delirium, which occurs in the context of suspected substance dependence, such as alcohol and benzodiazepines, can be particularly vexing. Substance dependence may set the stage for delirium due to substance withdrawal within hours to days of abstinence. Timely treatment with a benzodiazepine is often helpful. However, failure of resolution after such treatment makes the sedative itself suspect. Without a clear record of previous substance usage, the clinician will be left to chart a therapeutic course without a clear direction. In the context of ongoing delirium in a partially treated syndrome of withdrawal, it will often be unclear whether the newly prescribed benzodiazepine should be switched, the dosage increased, the dosage decreased, the frequency increased, or the frequency decreased.

Severe acute illness

Returning to the multifactorial model of delirium (Figure 6.2), but analogous to medications, any insult of sufficient severity can cause delirium, even when the predisposing factors are relatively minimal. Accordingly, there is a solid body of literature supporting the occurrence of a severe acute illness in general medicine populations as an independent cause of delirium (Francis et al. 1990; Levkoff et al. 1992; Inouye et al. 1993; O'Keeffe and Lavan 1996). An independent association between delirium and individuals who were 'unstable on admission' is established (Rockwood 1989). In a systematic review (Elie et al. 1998), this composite variable alone carried a relative risk of 3.8 (2.2–6.6).

Infectious causes

As a composite variable, documentation of 'any symptomatic infection' was significantly and independently associated with delirium in one prospective series. Infection was associated in this mixed medical and surgical population with a relative risk for delirium of 2.96 (1.42–6.15) (Schor et al. 1992). Similarly, 'definite site of infection' was an independent risk factor in another series of 184 consecutive admissions to an acute geriatric floor in a city hospital in London (Jitapunkul et al. 1992). Independent associations with delirium have been observed with 'non-respiratory infections' (Lawlor et al. 2000) and urinary tract infections (Levkoff et al. 1988). Documentation of a fever (Francis et al. 1990) and leukocytosis (Levkoff et al. 1988) also maintain an association with delirium after correction for other variables. In short, any infection superimposed on a sufficiently predisposed individual has the potential to cause delirium. Thus, soft tissue, pulmonary, abdominal, and central nervous system infections must also be considered in older individuals. When a thorough collateral history and physical examination fails to reveal an obvious source, it is prudent to rule out atypical manifestations of common infections such as a urinary tract infection and pneumonia.

A complete blood count, differential, urinalysis, and chest X-ray should be ordered early. These may be supplemented by urine, blood, or sputum cultures. In a persistent, unexplained delirium, and especially in a suspicious clinical setting, a lumbar puncture is an important consideration. Not uncommonly in a frail older adult, fever, meningismus, and leukocytosis are absent in such circumstances.

Metabolic causes

There is a relatively weak evidence basis for the association between delirium and metabolic abnormalities, such as acute endocrinological abnormalities, in the current body of literature. This is also true of renal and hepatic failure. Yet clinical experience begs otherwise. Considering the sometimes bland manifestations of these life-threatening conditions in immobile and delirious seniors, there must be vigilance in the investigations planned in response. In a diabetic, hyperglycaemic non-ketotic coma, ketoacidosis, and hypoglycaemia must be considered, and a simple chemstrip is a sensible early measure. Hypercalcaemia in the setting of malignancy or hyperparathyroidism may manifest as delirium. Myxoedema and thyrotoxicosis are important causes of delirium, which must be identified and treated. Adrenal insufficiency may also evolve slowly and remain unrecognized in a sessile, delirious senior. Hepatic failure and renal failure will cause delirium, primarily when fulminant or acute in evolution.

Disorders of water balance are often reflected in the serum sodium levels. There is an independent association between delirium and 'sodium abnormalities' (Francis *et al.* 1990), hypernatraemia and hypokalaemia (Foreman 1989), and dehydration (Seymour *et al.* 1980). Hyponatraemia is the most common electrolyte abnormality in the hospitalized senior and is associated with a relative risk of delirium of 2.2 (1.3–4.0) (Elie *et al.* 1998). Numerous causes are possible and its work-up and appropriate management are thus crucial in a delirious individual. Hypernatraemia in a confused older person is particularly alarming considering the associated mortality. When renal or extrarenal losses of water are not compensated by increased fluid and salt intake, a vicious spiral of immobility and delirium may further exacerbate the situation. These electrolyte disturbances may also be coupled with endocrinological abnormalities cited above. Hypokalaemia, hyperkalaemia, and acid–base disorders can also cause delirium and death.

Without clinical clues, a basic work-up should include serum electrolytes, glucose, creatinine, calcium, and thyroid stimulating hormone (TSH). If necessary, further probing may also include liver function tests and a serum cortisol followed by the cosyntropin test if there is clinical and biochemical suspicion of adrenal insufficiency.

Hypoperfusion states and pulmonary compromise

Considering the potential for cerebral hypoxaemia, hypoperfusion states and pulmonary compromise would seem to be an obvious consideration in an unwell delirious individual. Yet in the work-up of such an individual, it is surprising how often this category of potential aetiology is neglected. Associations with delirium have been recorded for an 'abnormal pulmonary exam' (Jitapunkul *et al.* 1992), hypoxaemia (Aakerlund and Rosenberg 1994), abdominal aortic aneurysms with elevated blood pressure (So *et al.* 1999), and post-cardiotomy shock requiring inotropic support (Rolfson *et al.* 1999). More importantly, a causal linkage has been demonstrated for hypoxaemia (Foy *et al.* 1995; Lawlor *et al.* 2000) and shock (Foreman 1989).

Cardiac arrhythmias have not been associated with delirium when this has been examined (Elie *et al.* 1998). Similarly, no association has been found between delirium and anaemia based on the literature prior to 1995 (Elie *et al.* 1998). However, since then, an independent association with a postoperative haematocrit less than 30% was demonstrated in a non-cardiac surgical (Marcantonio *et al.* 1998) and in a medical population (Martin *et al.* 2000).

Exacerbations of chronic obstructive lung disease and congestive heart failure undoubtedly can stimulate delirium in a susceptible individual. Delirium is witnessed in the context of myocardial infarction and pulmonary embolism. A careful physical examination may be the only clue that suggests a cardiopulmonary source of the delirium. This should be followed by appropriate radiological or electrocardiographic investigations. The synthesis of the literature provided by Elie *et al.* (1998) did reveal an association with an abnormal electrocardiogram and an abnormal chest X-ray. Non-resolving delirium often can be reversed with scrupulous attention to these underlying precipitants.

Urinary and faecal retention

There is a dearth of empirical evidence that urinary and faecal retention causes delirium, and it is difficult to imagine a pathophysiological linkage. Nevertheless, in the care of frail and dependent seniors who develop delirium, this is observed commonly. Retention syndromes are best viewed as contributing causes, similar to the environmental considerations below. In a non-communicative, delirious individual, a physical examination may be sufficient to demonstrate a distended bladder or abdominal and rectal fullness. 'In and out' catheterization or a bladder scan should be sufficient to rule out an elevated post-void residual. Values consistently higher than 200 ml should be taken seriously. An abdominal flat plate is generally sufficient to confirm faecal impaction when such is not obvious by physical examination.

Environmental/psychological contributors

The experience of hospitalization can be compared to the administration of a medication. While anticipating a benefit from admission to an acute care hospital, a delirious individual will also encounter less desirable 'side effects' of the experience. In fact, a 5% absolute risk reduction for incident delirium has been demonstrated simply by prospectively matching hospital admissions to either usual care or a unit which followed protocols to address environmental contributors (Inouye *et al.* 1999). In this study, each of six protocols targeted specific risk factors for delirium. Cognitive impairment was addressed using orientation and therapeutic activity protocols. Sleep deprivation was prevented using non-pharmacological interventions and noise reduction strategies. Immobility was anticipated and an early mobilization protocol employed. Visual and hearing impairment were discovered from the start, resulting in the use of appropriate visual aids, earwax disimpaction, and amplification devices. A simple dehydration protocol was also used.

Such an innovative approach certainly resulted from the observation that environmental and psychological variables contribute to delirium. Intrinsic variables may include sensory deprivation (visual and hearing impairment), psychological stress, sleep deprivation, and pain. Potential extrinsic variables are numerous, and include immobilization and immobility, physical restraint use, bladder catheter use, sensory overload (noise, frequent room changes, 'iatrogenic events', and intensive care unit treatment), and sensory deprivation (the lack of 'orienting objects', 'low social interactions', lack of windows, unfamiliar environments).

Be it nociceptive, neuropathic, or psychological, sufficient pain can lead to irrational behaviour even in the absence of delirium. Thus, it is surprising that until recently, there was insufficient evidence to conclude that pain was a cause of delirium in susceptible individuals (Elie *et al.* 1998). In a prospective cohort of individuals who had undergone elective non-cardiac surgery, there was an independent association between delirium and pain as measured using a visual analogue scale (Lynch *et al.* 1998). This association was independent of the method of postoperative analgesia, the type of opioid used, and the cumulative opioid dose. Pain was also independent of other known risk factors for delirium such as age, alcohol use, cognitive function, physical function, serum chemistries, and the type of surgery.

Independent associations with delirium have been elucidated in the cases of physical restraint use, bladder catheter use, and 'any iatrogenic event' with relative risks (95% confidence interval) of 4.4 (2.5–7.9), 2.4 (1.2–4.7), and 1.9 (1.1–3.2), respectively (Inouye and Charpentier 1996). This association was independent of intercurrent illness and medications. The intensive care unit (ICU) has the potential to combine most if not all of these noxious environmental stimuli. An association between a period of time in the ICU and delirium which is independent of other significant predictors (age, cognitive impairment, number of procedures, number of medications, and surgery) has been observed (Martin *et al.* 2000). There is also a relationship between delirium and the lack of 'orienting objects' (newspapers, timepieces, radios, televisions, and personal belongings) and 'low social interactions' with significant others (Foreman 1989), suggesting the potential for prevention of delirium simply by enhancing the environment and interactions experienced by the senior.

Surgery, anaesthesia, and other procedures

Without question, surgery introduces a series of noxious insults to an older person. Operative and postoperative insults become the 'knockout punches' that can tip a predisposed individual into a delirious state. On a smaller scale, bedside procedures in the hospital can have a similar effect (Martin *et al.* 2000). The incidence of postoperative delirium was estimated in a large cohort undergoing non-cardiac surgery to be 9% (Marcantonio *et al.* 1994a). The highest incidence of delirium in seniors is found on orthopaedic and cardiothoracic surgical units. While there have been differences in the criteria for delirium used and the populations examined, the incidence of delirium in seniors after cardiac surgery is approximately one-third (Smith and Dimsdale 1989; Van Der Mast and Roest 1996). After repair of a hip fracture, the incidence is up to 61% (Gustafson *et al.* 1988), and after pulmonary thrombendarterectomy it is reported to be as high as 81% (Wragg *et al.* 1988). While preoperative (predisposing) and postoperative (precipitating) variables contribute to the remarkable phenomenon, there is also evidence that aspects of the surgery itself are involved.

Delirium was found to be independently associated with general surgery and a 'high number of procedures in the hospital' (Martin *et al.* 2000). More specifically, there is an independent association with aortic aneurysm surgery and non-cardiac thoracic surgery (Marcantonio *et al.* 1994a). An independent association between delirium and both the aortic cross-clamp time (Wragg *et al.* 1988) and the duration of cardiopulmonary bypass has also been observed in cardiac surgical patients (Rolfson *et al.* 1999). In this latter study, the association remained after correcting for preoperative (past stroke, depression, cardiac dysfunction, burden of co-morbidity, alcoholism) and postoperative factors (new medications, cardiac dysfunction, and electrolyte abnormalities). Less well-established associations also exist for orthopaedic and urological surgery (Dai *et al.* 2000).

Components of the surgery itself have been implicated. In cardiac surgery, the mean arterial pressure during bypass and the hypothermic time are possible risk factors linked to the duration of cardiopulmonary bypass. High-dose inotropic support and excessive blood transfusions are also associated with delirium in cardiac (Gokgoz *et al.* 1997) and non-cardiac surgical populations (Marcantonio *et al.* 1998; Dai *et al.* 2000).

The anaesthetic time for seniors undergoing head and neck surgery has been correlated with the incidence of delirium (Weed *et al.* 1995). Whether spinal compared to general anaesthesia reduces the incidence of delirium in orthopaedic surgery is unclear. One study of elective hip replacement has found a higher rate of delirium with general anaesthesia than with epidural analgesia (Hole *et al.* 1980), but this has not been replicated in subsequent trials (Berggren *et al.* 1987; Haan *et al.* 1991). In two consecutive cohorts undergoing non-cardiac surgery at the same institution, no association was found between delirium and the method of postoperative analgesia (Marcantonio *et al.* 1994b; Lynch *et al.* 1998).

Neurological illness

For a younger individual with no co-morbid illness, neurological illness and psychoactive medications will top the list of causes of a new onset of delirium. In the frail elderly person, acute CNS pathology clearly will also cause delirium, but should be downgraded on the differential diagnosis. In the acute setting, delirium will usually be explained by some combination of medications (intoxication or withdrawal), infection, metabolic abnormalities, cardiopulmonary insufficiency, and other contributors such as sensory deprivation, environmental effects, and retention syndromes.

However, a subdural haematoma or new stroke may also occur in the absence of obvious focal neurological signs. Anticipation of such possibilities should rise if there is a history of confusion and falls. One must also be constantly aware of the potential for a cerebral haemorrhage, a primary tumour, brain metastasis, an abscess, meningitis, encephalitis, and petit mal or partial complex seizures. These, too, may occur in the absence of clues on physical examination. It is for this reason that further investigations for these entities should proceed both in the presence of historical or examination clues and when there is persistence of the delirium after ruling out common causes. Practices will vary depending on the composition of the referral population and the comfort level of the clinician. These investigations may include but not be limited to a full blood count and differential, blood cultures, neuroimaging, an electroencephalogram, and a lumbar puncture.

Prediction models and preoperative risk scores

A prediction model is a list of variables, each independently associated with the outcome of interest, which when viewed in combination allow the overall calculation of the risk of the outcome in any individual. Ideally, a prediction model is first developed in one cohort, and then validated in a subsequent cohort with the same characteristics. Because prediction rules are derived from a specific population and setting, their application, like that of simple risk factor calculation must be limited to individuals drawn from a similar population and setting. Prediction models derived from seven populations will be reviewed from general medicine, from a mixture of medicine and surgery, and from surgery (elective non-cardiac surgery, elective orthopaedics surgery, and hip fracture surgery).

Mixed medicine and surgery

In one of the first delirium prediction models developed for seniors, a mixed surgical and medical population of 1285 seniors were considered retrospectively (Levkoff *et al.* 1988). The key risk factors identified through multivariate analysis were urinary tract infections, low serum albumin on admission, elevated leukocyte count on admission, and proteinuria. A subsequent series validated the model.

General medicine

Both predisposing (Inouye *et al.* 1993) and precipitating (Inouye and Charpentier 1996) characteristics were characterized prospectively. Each prediction model was validated by a subsequent prospective cohort. In the first, visual impairment, severe illness, cognitive impairment, and a high BUN to creatinine ratio were found to be significant. By assigning an equal weight to each of these four factors, risk groups could be significantly distinguished and reliably predicted. The risk of delirium in the low-, intermediate-, and high-risk groups were 3%, 16%, and 32%, respectively. The model also predicted death or nursing home placement.

A risk stratification system for precipitating factors was developed and validated by the same group in precisely the same way. The independent variables included in this model were the use of physical restraints, malnutrition, more than three medications added, the use of a bladder catheter, and 'any iatrogenic event'. Separating members of the validation cohort by the number of these factors allowed prediction of the risk of delirium for the low- (4%), intermediate- (20%) and high-risk (35%) groups. What is even more remarkable is that these two risk models were then cross-stratified, showing the interrelationship of predisposing and precipitating variables (Inouye 1998).

Another medical cohort was observed prospectively, resulting in a similar predictive model for delirium (O'Keeffe and Lavan 1996). A similar point system was used, in which one point was assigned for each of the following independent variables: a history of chronic cognitive impairment, severe illness, elevated serum urea, and elevated serum sodium. In the validation cohort of 84 patients, the risk of delirium escalated for each point added: 0 points (13%), 1 point (32%), 2 points (50%), and 3 points (100%).

Non-cardiac surgery

In a large cohort, 1341 consenting patients over the age of 50 were prospectively followed through general, orthopaedic, and gynecological surgery (Marcantonio *et al.* 1994a). Seven independent preoperative risk factors were identified, leading to the development of a prediction rule that stratified patients into a low-, medium-, and high-risk group. One point each was assigned for age greater than 70, alcohol abuse, cognitive impairment, physical impairment, markedly abnormal sodium, potassium, or glucose, and non-cardiac thoracic surgery. Two points were assigned for aortic aneurysm surgery. Using these criteria, the validation cohort found delirium to be present in 2% of low risk (0 points), 8% and 13% of medium risk (1 and 2 points), and over 50% of high-risk individuals (3 or more points). This same prediction rule was applied to another relatively young (mean age 65) population of 138 candidates for major head and neck cancer surgery (Weed *et al.* 1995). The model performed similarly with 8% (1 point), 17% (2 points), and 47% (3 points) developing delirium.

Williams *et al.* (1985) prospectively followed 170 seniors who were admitted for a hip fracture. Admission characteristics that significantly predicted delirium were age, errors on cognitive testing, and low pre-injury activity. These characteristics combined allowed the prediction of delirium with 66% accuracy. This compared favourably with the recognition rates of physicians and nurses. Risk stratification was not reported and the model was not validated in a subsequent cohort.

In a recent cohort of 701 Chinese seniors who underwent orthopaedic and urological surgery (Dai *et al.* 2000), two baseline (older age, cognitive impairment), and one precipitating variable (the use of a psychoactive drug), remained significant after logistic regression analysis. While the risk of delirium remained low for only one factor present (2% for either age or cognitive impairment and 3% for psychoactive drug use), the combination of both led to an estimated probability of delirium of 28%. This prediction model was not prospectively validated.

Conclusion

Delirium in the older adult is common, under-recognized and associated with significant morbidity. Its occurrence is predictable, based on well-recognized predisposing variables: visual impairment, dementia, functional impairment, malnutrition, and multiple co-morbidities. Such a cluster of vulnerability (or frailty) can be identified even prior to hospital admission. Delirium is precipitated largely by factors that are preventable or treatable. The most common of these are medications, severe illness, infections, metabolic abnormalities, hypoperfusion states, and acute pulmonary compromise. Contributing factors also include the physical environment, iatrogenesis, psychological stressors, and retention syndromes. Neurological illness is an uncommon but important consideration when other precipitants are absent.

A combination of these predisposing and precipitating variables appears to be the rule rather than the exception in the older delirious adult. Further, there is an inverse relationship between the degree of vulnerability and the severity of the insult required to induce a delirium. It has been suggested that delirium is a symptom of the quality of hospital care provided to older adults (Inouye *et al.* 1999). Therefore, to the extent that delirium is prevalent in the hospital, there is a significant window of opportunity to focus on its causes and improve the quality of life of hospitalized older adults.

References

Aakerlund, L. P. and Rosenberg, J. (1994). Postoperative delirium: treatment with supplementary oxygen. *British Journal of Anaesthesia*, **72**, 286–290.

American Psychiatric Association (1994). *Diagnostic and Statistical Manual of Mental Disorders*, 4th edn. American Psychiatric Association, Washington, DC.

Berggren, D., Gustafson, Y., Eriksson, B., *et al.* (1987). Postoperative confusion after anaesthesia in elderly patients with femoral neck fractures. *Anesthesia and Analgesia*, **66**, 497–504.

Brauer, C., Morrison, S., Silberzweig, S. B., and Siu, A. L. (2000). The cause of delirium in patients with hip fracture. *Archives of Internal Medicine*, **160**,1858–1860.

Breitbart, W. and Strout, D. (2000). Delirium in the terminally ill. *Clinics in Geriatric Medicine*, **16**, 357–372.

Brocklehurst, J. C. (ed.) (1985). The day hospital. In *Textbook of geriatric medicine and gerontology*, 3rd edn, pp. 982–995. Churchill, London.

Carlson, J. E., Zocchi, K. A., Bettencourt, D. M., *et al.* (1998). Measuring frailty in hospitalized elderly. *American Journal of Physical Medicine and Rehabilitation*, **77**, 252–257.

Dai, Y. T., Lou, M. F., Yip, P. L., and Huang, G. S. (2000). Risk factors and incidence of postoperative delirium in elderly Chinese patients. *Gerontology*, **46**, 28–35.

Drachman, D. A. (2000). Occam's razor, geriatric syndromes, and the dizzy patient. *Annals of Internal Medicine*, **132**, 403–404.

Elie, M., Cole, M. G., Primeau, F. J., and Bellevance, F. (1998). Delirium risk factors in elderly hospitalized patients. *Journal of General Internal Medicine*, **13**, 204–212.

Foreman, M. D. (1989). Confusion in the hospitalized elderly: incidence, onset and associated factors. *Research in Nursing and Health*, **12**, 21–29.

Foy, A., O'Connell, D., Henry, D., Kelly, J., Cocking, S., and Halliday, J. (1995). Benzodiazepine use as a cause of cognitive impairment in elder hospital inpatients. *Journal of Gerontology*, **50**, M99–M106.

Francis, J., Martin, D., and Kapoor, W. N. (1990). A prospective study of delirium in hospitalized elderly. *Journal of the American Medical Association*, **263**, 1097–1101.

Gokgoz, L., Gunaydin, S., Sinci, V., *et al.* (1997). Psychiatric complications of cardiac surgery postoperative delirium syndrome. *Scandinavian Cardiovascular Journal*, **31**, 217–222.

Gray, S. L., Lai, K. V., and Larson, E. B. (1999). Drug induced cognition disorders in the elderly: incidence, prevention and management. *Drug Safety*, **21**, 101–122.

Gustafson, Y., Berggren, D., Brannstrom, B., *et al.* (1988). Acute confusional states in elderly patients treated for femoral neck fractures. *Journal of the American Geriatrics Society*, **36**, 525–530.

Haan, J., van Kleef, J. W., Bloem, B. R., *et al.* (1991). Cognitive function after spinal or general anesthesia for transurethral prostatectomy in elderly men. *Journal of the American Geriatrics Society*, **39**, 596–600.

Han, L., McCusker, J., Cole, M., Abrahamowicz, M., Primeau, F., and Elie, M. (2001). Use of medications with anticholinergic effect predicts clinical severity of delirium symptoms in older medical inpatients. *Archives of Internal Medicine*, **23**, 1099–1105.

Hole, A., Terjesen, T., and Breivik, H. (1980). Epidural versus general anaesthesia for total hip arthroplasty in elderly patients. *Acta Anaethesiologica Scandinavica*, **24**, 279–287.

Inouye, S. K. (1998). Delirium in hospitalized older patients: recognition and risk factors. *Journal of Geriatric Psychiatry and Neurology*, **11**, 118–125.

Inouye, S. K. and Charpentier, P. A. (1996). Precipitating factors for delirium in hospitalized elderly persons: predictive model and interrelationship with baseline vulnerability. *Journal of the American Medical Association*, **275**, 852–857.

Inouye, S. K., Viscoli, C. M., Horwitz, R. I., *et al.* (1993). A predictive model for delirium in hospitalized medical patients based on admission characteristics. *Annals of Internal Medicine*, **119**, 474–481.

Inouye, S. K., Bogardus, S. T., Charpentier, P. A., *et al.* (1999). A multicomponent intervention to prevent delirium in hospitalized older patients. *New England Journal of Medicine*, **340**, 669–676.

Jarrett, P. G., Rockwood, K., Carver, D., Stolee, P., and Cosway, S. (1995). Illness presentation in elderly patients. *Archives of Internal Medicine*, **155**, 1060–1064.

Jitapunkul, S., Pillay, I., and Ebrahim, S. (1992). Delirium in newly admitted elderly patients: a prospective study. *Quarterly Journal of Medicine*, **83**, 307–314.

Karlsson, I. (1999). Drugs that induce delirium. *Dementia and Geriatric Cognitive Disorders*, **10**, 412–415.

Lawlor, P. G., Gognon, B., Mancini, I. L., *et al.* (2000). Occurrence, causes and outcome of delirium in patients with advanced cancer. *Archives of Internal Medicine*, **160**, 786–794.

Levkoff, S. E., Safran, C., Cleary, P. D., *et al.* (1988). Identification of factors associated with the diagnosis of delirium in elderly hospitalized patients. *Journal of the American Geriatrics Society*, **36**, 1099–1104.

Levkoff, S. E., Evans, D. A., Liptzin, B., *et al.* (1992). Delirium: the occurrence and persistence of symptoms among elderly hospitalized patients. *Archives of Internal Medicine*, **152**, 334–340.

Lynch, E. P., Lazor, M. A., Gellis, J. E., Orav, J., Goldman, L., and Marcantonio, E. R. (1998). The impact of postoperative pain on the development of postoperative delirium. *Anesthesia and Analgesia*, **86**, 781–785.

Marcantonio, E. R., Goldman., L., Mangione, C. M., *et al.* (1994a). A clinical prediction rule for delirium after elective noncardiac surgery. *Journal of the American Medical Association*, **271**, 134–139.

Marcantonio, E. R., Juarez, G., Goldman, L., *et al.* (1994b). The relationship of postoperative delirium with psychoactive medications. *Journal of the American Medical Association*, **272**, 1518–1522.

Marcantonio, E. R., Goldman, L., Orav, E. J., Cook, E. F., and Lee, T. H. (1998). The association of intra-operative factors with the development of postoperative delirium. *American Journal of Medicine*, **105**, 380–384.

Martin, N. J., Stones, M. J., Young, J. E., and Bedard, M. (2000). Development of delirium: a prospective cohort study in a community hospital. *International Psychogeriatrics*, **12**, 117–127.

McGuire, B. E., Basten, C. J., Ryan, C. J., and Gallagher, J. (2000). Intensive care unit syndrome: a dangerous misnomer. *Archives of Internal Medicine*, **160**, 906–909.

Meagher, D. J. and Trzepacz, P. T. (1998). Delirium phenomenology illuminates pathophysiology, management and course. *Journal of Geriatric Psychiatry and Neurology*, 11, 150–156.

Meagher, D. J., O'Hanlon, D., O'Mahony, E., Casey, P. R., and Trzepacz, P. T. (1998). Relationship between etiology and phenomenologic profile in delirium. *Journal of Geriatric Psychiatry and Neurology*, 11, 146–149.

O'Keeffe, S. T. and Lavan, J. N. (1996). Predicting delirium in elderly patients: development and validation of a risk stratification model. *Age and Ageing*, 25, 317–321.

O'Keeffe, S. T. and Lavan, J. (1999). Clinical significance of delirium subtypes in older people. *Age and Ageing*, 28, 115–119.

Rockwood, K. (1989). Acute confusion in elderly medical patients. *Journal of the American Geriatrics Society*, 37, 150–154.

Rockwood, K., Fox, R. A., Stolee, P., Robertson, D., and Beattie, B. L. (1994). Frailty in elderly people: an evolving concept. *Canadian Medical Association Journal*, 150, 489–495.

Rockwood, K., Hogan, D. B., and MacKnight, C. (2000). Conceptualization and measurement of frailty in elderly people. *Drugs and Aging*, 17, 295–302.

Rogers, M. P., Liang, M. H., Daltroy, L. H., *et al.* (1989). Delirium after elective orthopedic surgery: risk factors and natural history. *International Journal of Psychiatry and Medicine*, 19, 109–121.

Rolfson, D. B., McElhaney, J. E., Rockwood, K., *et al.* (1999). Incidence and risk factors for delirium and other adverse outcomes in older adults after coronary artery bypass graft surgery. *Canadian Journal of Cardiology*, 15, 771–776.

Ross, C. A., Peyser, C. E., Shapiro, I., *et al.* (1991). Delirium: phenomenology and etiologic subtypes. *International Psychogeriatrics*, 3, 135–147.

Sandberg, O., Gustafson, Y., Brannstrom, B., and Buch, G. (1999). Clinical profile of delirium in older patients. *Journal of the American Geriatrics Society*, 47, 1300–1306.

Sarkisian, C. A. and Lachs, M. S. (1996). 'Failure to thrive' in older adults. *Annals of Internal Medicine*, 124, 1072–1078.

Schor, J. D., Levkoff, S. E., Lipsitz, L. A., *et al.* (1992). Risk factors for delirium in hospitalized elderly. *Journal of the American Medical Association*, 267, 827–831.

Seymour, D. G., Henschke, R. D., Cape, T., *et al.* (1980). Acute confusional states and dementia in the elderly: the role of dehydration/ volume depletion, physical illness and age. *Age and Ageing*, 8, 137.

Smith, L. W. and Dimsdale, J. E. (1989). Postcardiotomy delirium: conclusions after 25 years? *American Journal of Psychiatry*, 146, 452–458.

So, T., Tanaka, H., Tsuchiya, K, *et al.* (1999). Influence of cardiovascular factors on the development of delirium after acute aortic dissection. *International Medical Journal*, 6, 113–117.

Stuck, A. E., Walthert, J. M., Nikolaus, T., Bula, C. J., Hohmann, C., and Beck, J. C. (1999). Risk factors for functional status decline in community-living elderly people: a systematic literature review. *Social Science and Medicine*, 48, 445–469

Tinetti, M. E., Inouye, S. K., Gill, T. M., and Doucette, J. T. (1995). Shared risk factors for falls, incontinence, and functional dependence. Unifying the approach to geriatric syndromes. *Journal of the American Medical Association*, 273, 1348–1353.

Trzepacz, P. T. (1999). Update on the neuropathogenesis of delirium. *Dementia and Geriatric Cognitive Disorders*, 10, 330–334.

Trzepacz, P. T., Baker, R. W., and Greenhouse, J. (1988). A symptom rating scale for delirium. *Psychiatry Research*, 23, 89–97.

Tune, L. and Egeli, S. (1999) Acetylcholine and delirium. *Dementia and Geriatric Cognitive Disorders*, 10, 342–344.

Van der Mast, R. C. and Roest, F. H. (1996). Delirium after cardiac surgery: a critical review. *Journal of Psychosomatic Research*, 41, 13–30.

Weed, H. G. Lutman, C. V., Young, D. C., and Schuller, D. E. (1995). Preoperative identification of patients at risk for delirium after major head and neck cancer surgery. *Laryngoscope*, **105**, 1066–1068.

Williams, M. A., Campbell, E. B., Raynor, W. J., *et al.* (1985). Predictors of acute confusional states in hospitalized elderly patients. *Research in Nursing and Health*, **8**, 31–40.

Wragg, R. E., Dimsdale, J. E., Moser, K. M., *et al.* (1988). Operative predictors of delirium after pulmonary thrombendarterectomy. A model for postcardiotomy delirium? *Journal of Thoracic and Cardiovascular Surgery*, **96**, 524–529.

Chapter 7

The management of delirium

Edward Marcantonio

Delirium is common, morbid, and costly, especially among hospitalized older patients. Nonetheless, it remains under-recognized and often poorly managed. The goals of this chapter are to review the principles of non-pharmacological and pharmacological management of delirium. The medico-legal ramifications of caring for delirious patients are also discussed. Before beginning this discussion, several key management principles that are covered in other chapters of this book should be highlighted. First and foremost, the appropriate management of delirium requires timely recognition. Failure to detect delirium entirely, misdiagnosis of delirium as dementia or a psychiatric disorder, or diagnosis too late after significant complications have supervened, are the most common errors in its management. Therefore, systematic case-finding efforts involving regular assessment of mental status and use of a standardized diagnostic algorithm such as the Confusion Assessment Method (Inouye *et al.* 1990), are key in identifying patients with delirium as early as possible in their course. Second, a thorough diagnostic evaluation of the delirious patient is a key step in management. This may involve a significant degree of 'detective' work. Often, a single clear-cut aetiology cannot be found. In older patients, delirium typically results from an interaction between predisposing and precipitating factors (Inouye and Charpentier 1996). Therefore, all potentially reversible contributing factors must be addressed. Finally, as with other geriatric syndromes, the prevention of delirium is easier and more effective than treatment and restoration of the patient after the syndrome has developed. A growing body of literature documents the effectiveness of interventions designed to prevent delirium before it begins (Cole *et al.* 1996; Inouye *et al.* 1999a, Marcantonio *et al.* 2001). Therefore, systematic risk assessment and proactive multifactorial preventive strategies should be implemented for all high-risk patients.

This chapter describes the key steps in managing the delirious patient. These include:

- addressing the underlying cause or causes of delirium;
- maintaining behavioural control through non-pharmacological and, if necessary, pharmacological interventions;
- anticipating and preventing common complications of delirium;
- supporting functional needs and restoring function, including family education and support.

Also discussed are: delirium in terminal care and the medico-legal aspects of delirium, including informed consent, emergency treatment, failure to diagnose, and mismanagement.

Key steps in managing the delirious patient

Step 1: address underlying causes

Treatment of the underlying cause or causes of delirium may lead to its resolution, and should be attempted whenever possible. As stated above, a prerequisite to this crucial step is a thorough diagnostic evaluation. In the right situation, almost any medication or any acute medical problem can cause delirium. Therefore, it is beyond the scope of this chapter to review the treatment of all problems that might cause delirium. The management of the most common reversible causes of delirium in elderly patients are highlighted:

- medications
- infections
- fluid balance and metabolic disorders
- impaired CNS oxygenation
- severe pain
- sensory deprivation
- elimination problems.

Medications are the most common reversible causes of delirium. Therefore, all delirious patients require a careful medication review. In the hospital or institutional setting, this involves careful review of the nursing drug administration record to determine exactly what the patient has received. In out-patients, this must also include non-prescription medications and alcohol. Any medication newly prescribed, newly discontinued (whether on purpose or inadvertently), or with its dosage changed is particularly suspect. Drug–drug interactions are another common cause of delirium. Prescription of a new medication without psychoactive properties may alter the metabolism of a psychoactive drug, leading to increased serum levels and new mental status changes. The prescription of any new medicine in an elderly patient with a complex medication regimen requires a thorough review for drug–drug interactions. Sometimes, the medication regimen does not change but the patient's metabolism does, leading to drug toxicity. For example, a patient with acute renal failure will build up toxic levels of all renally excreted medications unless their dosage is appropriately adjusted. A subtler scenario involves the patient on long-standing psychoactive medications (such as a hypnotic), who with gradual changes in body composition and metabolism, and age-associated increased drug sensitivity, becomes increasingly susceptible to side effects, including confusion.

If a medication is suspected to be causing or contributing to delirium, it should be discontinued if at all possible. If this is not possible, reduction to the lowest possible dose, or substitution of a similar but lower risk drug should be attempted. Table 7.1 lists some of the most common drugs implicated in delirium, and recommendations for alternative treatments if discontinuation is necessary. Of course, drugs have different elimination half-lives, so the time interval between when the drug is discontinued and when serum levels have dropped sufficiently is highly variable. Drugs with significant fat absorption (the fat compartment increases as a percentage of total body weight in elders), and those that require phase I oxidative metabolism in the liver have particularly long and unpredictable half-lives in elders (Avorn *et al.* 1997). Drugs with known psychoactive properties and prolonged half-lives should be avoided in older patients in favour of similar drugs with shorter half-lives.

There are a few situations in which treatment with drugs may actually help to reverse delirium. The most common situation is delirium due to sedative withdrawal, in which reinstitution of a sedative may help to terminate the delirium. The most common drugs that cause sedative withdrawal are the benzodiazepines, barbiturates, and, of course, alcohol. For treatment of withdrawal, the benzodiazepines have the best pharmacokinetic and side effect profile, and are usually the agents of choice, not only for benzodiazepine withdrawal, but also for alcohol and barbiturate withdrawal (Mayo-Smith 1997). Even the benzodiazepines run the risk of oversedation and paradoxical excitatory responses, so the lowest effective dose of a short-to-intermediate duration agent (such as lorazepam or oxazepam) is preferred. The most severe manifestation of alcohol withdrawal is delirium tremens. In addition to severe agitated delirium, this entity is manifested by autonomic instability such as blood pressure lability, tachycardia, fever, and diaphoresis. Treatment includes benzodiazepines for withdrawal and excellent supportive care. Despite this, delirium tremens still has a mortality of greater than 10%.

In other cases of drug-induced delirium, a direct antidote or antagonist exists that can be administered. Examples include use of naloxone for treatment of opioid overdose and flumazenil for treatment of benzodiazepine overdose (Weinbroum *et al.* 1996). Unfortunately, these antagonists have very short half-lives, so in practice they are more useful in the diagnosis of an overly sedated patient than the true reversal of delirium. In severe delirium due to anticholinergic agents, the central acetylcholinesterase inhibitor physostigmine may be tried, provided that careful attention is paid to peripheral cholinergic toxicity (Burns *et al.* 2000). The efficacy of the less toxic cholinesterase inhibitors such as donepezil and rivastigmine has not yet been demonstrated in the setting of anticholinergic delirium. Similarly, it is not yet known if these drugs have a more general contribution to make to the treatment and prevention of delirium. The theoretical basis of possible drug treatments for delirium is discussed more fully in Chapter 4.

Infections are another important, readily treatable cause of delirium. It is important to remember that in elderly individuals, delirium is usually the atypical presentation of

Table 7.1 Drugs to reduce or eliminate in the management of delirium

Agent	Mechanism of action	Possible substitute	Notes
Benzodiazepines: especially long-acting, including diazepam, flurazepam, chlordiazepoxide	CNS sedation	Non-pharmacological sleep management (McDowell et al. 1998), intermediate agents (lorazepam, temazepam)	Associated with delirium in medical and surgical patients (Schor et al. 1992; Marcantonio et al. 1994)
Benzodiazepines: ultra short-acting, including triazolam, alprazolam	CNS sedation and withdrawal	Non-pharmacologic sleep management (McDowell et al. 1998), intermediate agents (lorazepam, temazepam)	Associated with delirium in case reports and series (Rothschild 1992)
Barbiturates	Severe withdrawal syndrome	Avoid inadvertent abrupt discontinuation, or substitute benzodiazepine	
Choral hydrate	CNS sedation	Non-pharmacologic sleep protocol (McDowell et al. 1998)	No better for delirium than benzodiazepines
Alcohol	CNS sedation Withdrawal syndrome	If history of heavy intake, careful monitoring and benzodiazepines if withdrawal symptoms	Alcohol history is imperative
Antidepressants, esp. the tertiary amine tricyclic agents: amitriptyline, imipramine, doxepin	Anticholinergic toxicity	Secondary amine tricyclics: nortriptyline, desipramine. SSRI or other agents	Secondary amines as good as tertiary for adjuvant treatment of chronic pain (Max et al. 1992)
Antihistamines, including diphenhydramine	Anticholinergic toxicity	Non-pharmacological protocol for sleep (McDowell et al. 1998) Pseudoephedrine for colds	Must take over-the-counter medication history

Medication	Effect	Recommendation	Comments
Anticholinergics: oxybutynin, benzotropine	Anticholinergic toxicity	Lower dose, behavioural measures	Rare at low doses (Donnellan et al. 1997)
Opioid analgesics: especially meperidine (Richardson and Bresland 1998)	Anticholinergic toxicity CNS sedation Faecal impaction	Use local measures and non-psychoactive pain medications round-the-clock. (Abrahm 2000) Save opioids for breakthrough and severe pain	Higher risk in patients with renal insufficiency Must titrate risks from drugs vs. risks from pain
Antipsychotics: esp. low potency, anticholinergic agents and atypical agents (clozapine)	Anticholinergic toxicity CNS sedation	Eliminate, or if necessary use low dose high potency agents	
Anticonvulsants, esp. mysoline, phenobarbitone, phenytoin	Mysoline is converted to pheno-barbitone, which is a sedating long-acting barbiturate	Consider need for agent. Alternative agent	Toxic reactions can occur despite 'therapeutic' drug levels
Histamine-2 blocking agents	?Anticholinergic toxicity	Lower dosage Consider antacids or proton pump inhibitors	
Antiparkinsonian agents: levodopa-carbidopa, dopamine agonists, amantidine	Dopaminergic toxicity	Lower dose Adjust dosing schedule	Usually with end-stage disease and high doses
Almost any medication if time course is appropriate	Consider risks/benefits of all medications in the elderly		

Reproduced from: Marcantonio, ER. PIER Module: Delirium. American College of Physicians. 2002.

a non-central nervous system disorder (Resnick and Marcantonio 1997). Therefore, while presentation of high fever and confusion in a young patient leads to the almost reflex diagnosis of meningitis or other CNS catastrophe, in older patients it is most likely due to a common extra-CNS infection. The urinary tract, upper or lower respiratory tract, skin/soft tissue, and abdomen are the most likely sites of infection presenting with acute mental status changes in older patients. In each case, prompt and appropriate antibiotic treatment of the underlying infection as well as supportive care of the patient should help to ameliorate and reverse the delirium.

At times, diagnosis of an infection in elderly patients can be challenging. It is also important to remember that as people age, they are less able to mount a febrile response. Therefore, the absence of fever does not rule out infection in elderly patients. Even the white blood cell count may not be elevated, or could be chronically elevated due to another condition. There is really no substitute for a careful physical examination, supplemented by appropriate cultures or radiology studies as necessary.

One potential pitfall requires further elaboration. In many settings, particularly nursing homes, the nursing staff have a strong belief that delirium is caused by urinary tract infection (UTI). Therefore, any patient presenting with acute confusion results in an almost automatic order for urinalysis and culture. The problem is that it is also known that older patients, particularly frail ones in an institutional setting, have a very high incidence of asymptomatic bacteriuria and pyuria. Therefore, the finding of bacteria and white cells in the urine is no guarantee that UTI is the cause of the patient's mental status changes. The error is not in checking the urine, but doing so to the exclusion of evaluating medications, other sources of infection, and the other reversible factors discussed below.

Fluid and electrolyte disorders represent another common class of reversible causes of delirium. Included in this class are dehydration, congestive heart failure, and disorders of sodium, glucose, and calcium. Dehydration may be one of the most common causes of delirium in the institutional setting, where frail and/or demented elders have difficulty maintaining adequate oral intake. Of course, once delirium develops, these patients become progressively less able to take adequate amounts of fluid, which leads to a vicious cycle of worsening dehydration and worsening mental status. Optimal management involves timely recognition, confirmatory laboratory testing, and prompt treatment with intravenous fluids, or if very mild, monitored oral rehydration. Some nursing facilities also utilize 'clysis', in which fluids are introduced subcutaneously, and then absorbed systemically. Approximately 1–1.5 litres of fluid per day can be introduced via clysis, which makes it a useful adjunct in the management of the mildly to moderately dehydrated patient in the institutional setting (Hussain and Warshaw 1996). Dehydration is often accompanied by hypernatraemia, or less commonly, hyponatraemia, which may in turn further exacerbate delirium. Appropriate adjustment of fluid replacement can correct these disorders concomitantly with treatment of dehydration.

Congestive heart failure (CHF) of any aetiology may also contribute to delirium. The actual cause of delirium may be hypoxia, poor cerebral blood flow, or excess catecholamines. Delirium due to CHF is usually accompanied by shortness of breath and characteristic physical and X-ray findings. Treatment is geared to the underlying cause of the CHF, but oxygen and diuretics remain the cornerstone of acute treatment. Patients with CHF due to certain aetiologies are an increased risk for cerebral embolic phenomenon. If delirium is accompanied by new focal findings in these patients, work-up should include cerebral imaging.

There are several less common metabolic causes of delirium that are seen primarily in specific circumstances. In diabetics, hypoglycaemia, or severe hyperglycaemia with or without hyperosmolar state should be considered. A glucose obtained by fingerstick should be obtained on any acutely confused diabetic patient. Of note, some frail elderly individuals may present with a hyperosmolar state even without a prior history of diabetes. Patients with cancer, Paget's disease, hyperparathyroidism, and vitamin D toxicity may present with delirium due to hypercalcaemia. Treatment involves correcting the calcium and addressing the underlying condition. Finally, both hyper- and hypothyroidism may present with delirium in elderly individuals. The onset of these disorders can be insidious, so subacute to chronic worsening of cognition is more common than an acute change. A serum TSH level should be checked as part of a work-up for reversible cognitive impairment, whether acute or chronic.

Inadequate delivery of oxygen to the CNS is another broad category of causes of delirium in elderly individuals. Hypotension and hypoxaemia should be treated based on their underlying aetiology. Another common cause is severe anaemia. Elderly persons have a limited ability to increase cardiac output with increased demand, so tissue oxygen delivery begins to become compromised when the haematocrit falls below 30%. Low haematocrit has been found to be a risk factor for postoperative delirium, and transfusion should be considered for any delirious patient with a haematocrit <30% (Marcantonio *et al.* 1998). Closely related to poor tissue oxygenation is inadequate ventilation. Hypercapnoea must always be considered in a patient with chronic obstructive pulmonary disease and severe hypoactive delirium. Often, treatment requires temporary intubation and artificial ventilation.

Severe pain is another common, readily treatable cause of delirium. Increased pain at rest has been associated with delirium after elective non-cardiac procedures (Lynch *et al.* 1998), and in several mixed medical/surgical delirium cohorts (Schor *et al.* 1992). Unfortunately, many of the medicines used to treat pain can also cause delirium, so the goal is to treat pain effectively with the minimum dose of the least psychoactive drugs possible. Several principles guide this strategy. First, non-pharmacological analgesic strategies, such as use of heat and cold, immobilization, or repositioning, should be considered and implemented when useful. Second, when medication must be used, local or regional treatments to reduce pain with a minimum of systemic drug absorption (local blocks, epidural catheters) are usually preferable to systemic medications.

Third, use of scheduled, round-the-clock analgesia is preferable to as-needed (PRN) dosing. Studies have demonstrated that scheduled analgesics result in better pain control with less total dose administered (Agency for Health Care Policy and Research 1992; Abrahm 2000). Patient-controlled analgesia has also been associated with improved analgesia and decreased total analgesic doses, and is preferable to physician/nurse-controlled analgesia if the patient has adequate cognitive function (Egbert *et al.* 1990). The fourth principle of pain management is the use of adjunctive, non-psychoactive medications. Several studies have shown that round-the-clock paracetamol (acetaminophen), aspirin, or non-steroidal agents reduce the total dose of opioid analgesic required, and should be considered in most elderly patients without contraindications (Richardson and Bresland 1998). Finally, not all opioids are equal with respect to delirium. Meperidine, with its highly anticholinergic properties, idiosyncratic metabolism, and psychoactive metabolic products, has been associated with a more than 2.5× increased risk of delirium compared to other opioids and should be avoided in most elderly patients (Marcantonio *et al.* 1994). Morphine, which is inexpensive, effective, and available in a variety of routes, is a good first choice.

Sensory deprivation, whilst rarely the sole cause of delirium, is a frequent contributor, especially in the hospital setting, and is also usually readily treatable (Inouye *et al.* 1993). Glasses and hearing aids should be brought to the hospital and used. For very hard of hearing patients with no aids, a pocket amplifier may help with interactions with the hospital staff. Adequate lighting should be provided, but incandescent lamps, which provide a more home-like environment, are preferable to institutional overhead bright fluorescent lights, especially during the evening hours. The appropriate level of external sensory stimulation varies from patient to patient, so sweeping generalizations about private rooms, rooms near the nursing station, etc., cannot be made. In general, agitated delirious patients need a more calming environment, whereas hypoactive patients need a more stimulating environment. The environment is discussed further below.

Finally, elimination problems, in particular urinary retention and faecal impaction, are common reversible contributors to delirium in elderly patients. Moreover, the two are often related, with faecal impaction precipitating urinary retention, particularly in postoperative patients. Case reports have documented the resolution of delirium after treatment of these conditions (Blackburn and Dunn 1990), although more often they are one of several interacting aetiological factors. Careful intake and output records, and recording of bowel movements, are crucial in the assessment for these conditions. If these suggest a problem, suprapubic palpation for bladder fullness and/or rectal examination for impaction should be performed. An abdominal plain film may be helpful in ruling out impaction higher than the rectum. For treatment of urinary retention, intermittent catheterization is preferable to an indwelling bladder catheter in delirious patients. Discontinuation of offending medications, mobilization out of bed, and treatment of faecal impaction may also help. Treatment of faecal impaction may involve manual disimpaction and use of suppositories or enemas. Laxatives should be started to prevent a recurrence, but should not be the primary treatment in most instances.

As stated above, treatment of all potentially correctable contributing causes for delirium is the first and most critical step in its management. In some cases, particularly in younger individuals, the delirium will clear rapidly and little further intervention will be required. Unfortunately, in most elderly individuals, the delirium may persist for a significant time period after medications and medical status are optimized. This represents a vulnerable period during which additional problems may develop, so a vigilant eye for new problems is required until the delirium resolves. Periodic and careful reassessments are necessary to rule out the development of new aggravating or perpetuating factors. In addition, a variety of supportive and restorative measures may be necessary. These will be the next topics of discussion.

Step 2: maintain behavioural control

For the harried, sleep-deprived medical house officer called in the middle of the night by the nursing staff to order something to 'quiet down' the acutely agitated delirious patient, behavioural control may be the *sine qua non* of delirium management. However, management of agitation is best understood as a side issue for delirium, much as it is for dementia. The treatment of agitation is more an issue imposed by our health-care system than an integral part of delirium management. Moreover, there is as yet little evidence that the currently available pharmacological treatments for agitation address the underlying pathophysiology leading to delirium (see Chapter 4). In fact, in many cases these drugs, which are best viewed as chemical restraints, worsen and prolong delirium, albeit converting it from a hyperactive to hypoactive variant (Flacker and Marcantonio 1998; Meagher 2001).

As with dementia, agitation in delirium is best viewed as a behavioural disorder treated (or prevented) through behavioural means. Behavioural disorders often result from the difficulty delirious patients have with attending to, perceiving, and interpreting their environment. Additional contributors to agitation are:

- the loss of familiar surroundings and persons,
- the sterile, unfamiliar, and frenetic hospital environment and routine, and
- the delirious patient's difficulty communicating and attending to their needs.

Effective prevention and treatment strategies must address each of these issues.

There is a growing trend toward liberalizing visiting policies for immediate family members of elders with delirium or at high risk for developing delirium. In some hospitals, cots are provided to allow family members to sleep beside the patient. Whilst such duties can be exhausting for family members (it is best if several can take 'shifts'), it is clear that family members can advocate for and support delirious elders far better than today's overworked and harried hospital staff. The presence of a reassuring family member in the middle of the night may save the patient from getting an intolerably high dose of a psychoactive substance to 'calm him down'. In the absence of family members, sitters can be ordered to supervise delirious patients. Sitters were originally implemented for unstable psychiatric patients who required management on the medical service. There has been little written about the use of sitters in the management of delirium, but most observers feel they are clearly inferior to motivated family members, except perhaps for the prevention of gross physical injury. Alternative arrangements for patients with no families, such as the use of volunteers, must be explored.

The hospital staff's interaction with the delirious patient can escalate or ameliorate behavioural disturbances. Every effort should be made to provide delirious patients with a consistent nursing staff. Staff should approach these patients in a calm, non-confrontational manner. Sitting at the bedside is preferred to standing and hovering over the patient. The patient should be reoriented to their surroundings as often as possible in a non-threatening manner that does not 'test' the patient's cognition. It would seem obvious, but the hospital staff should always explain what they are doing and why, even if the patient seems profoundly impaired. There is no excuse for moving the patient in and out of bed, adjusting intravenous lines, etc., without talking to the patient. The staff should avoid using medical jargon, which can contribute to misunderstanding and lack of control. Providers who speak other languages should also avoid using these in the presence of the patient. If the patient is actively hallucinating or delusional, it is best to take an empathic approach, acknowledging the person's distress while neither accepting nor refuting the content of the perceptual disturbance or thought disorder. The use of touch can be effective, but also can exacerbate agitation and needs to be individualized. In addition to these interpersonal approaches, modifications of the hospital environment may serve to ameliorate behavioural disturbances in delirium. These will be discussed in detail under *Step 4: supporting functional needs and restoration of function.*

Should behavioural measures fail to control agitation, physical and chemical restraints may be necessary. Physical restraints, while objectionable, may be required because of violent behaviour, or to prevent the removal of important devices such as endotracheal tubes, intra-arterial lines and catheters. In such cases, it is important to reassess continually the indication for the indwelling devices, and remove them (and thus the indication for the restraints) as soon as possible. It is also important to carefully monitor the patient for signs of injury (e.g. bruising) related to the restraints. Because of the frenetic hospital environment in which nurses are unable to monitor confused patients continuously, restraints may be applied as an insurance policy against falls. Although this practice has not been well studied in the acute hospital setting, evidence from nursing homes suggests that restraints probably do not decrease the rate of falls in confused ambulatory individuals, and may actually increase the risk of injury (Tinetti *et al.* 1992; Capezuti *et al.* 1996). In this situation, the use of a sitter is preferable to the application of restraints.

Pharmacological restraints are also often used as 'time-savers', but they extract a particularly costly toll in terms of adverse effects, prolonged delirium, and loss of mobility, and should be avoided if possible. Chemical intervention may be necessary and effective for true psychotic symptoms, such as delusions or hallucinations that are frightening to the patient when verbal comfort and reassurance are not successful. Some delirious patients display behaviour that is dangerous to themselves or others, and providing a sitter or family companionship is ineffective or impossible. However, the mere presence of delirium is *not* an indication for pharmacological intervention. The indications for such intervention should be clearly identified, documented, and constantly reassessed.

The literature investigating the optimal pharmacological treatment of agitated delirium in elderly individuals is remarkably scant and consists primarily of case series rather than randomized controlled clinical trials (Cole *et al.* 1996). However, the data that do exist suggest that high potency antipsychotics are the drugs of choice because of their low anticholinergic activity and minimal hypotensive effects (Breitbart *et al.* 1996; Flacker and Marcantonio 1998; Meagher 2001). However, these medications must be used cautiously as they may actually prolong delirium and may increase the risk of complications by converting a hyperactive, confused patient into a stuporous one whose risk of falling or aspiration may be increased. In elderly patients with mild hyperactivity, low doses of haloperidol (0.5–1 mg orally) should be used initially, with careful reassessment before giving additional doses. Keeping the total daily dose of haloperidol below 3 mg may reduce the risk of extrapyramidal side effects (Hassan *et al.* 1998). In more severe delirium, somewhat higher initial doses may be used (0.5–2 mg parenterally), with additional doses every 30–60 minutes as required. Data suggest that parenteral haloperidol may be less likely to cause extrapyramdial side effects (Menza *et al.* 1987).

Case series have documented the successful use of the newer atypical antipsychotic compounds, olanzepine and risperidone, in the management of delirium (Sipahimalani and Masand 1997, 1998). Although these compounds have clear advantages over haloperidol for long-term management of agitation in dementia, their advantage for the short-term treatment of delirium is less clear. The atypical antipsychotic agent risperidone is also available in oral and parenteral forms, and may be effective in agitated delirium in doses similar to those described above for haloperidol (Sipahimalani and Masand 1997). Although marketed as having less extrapyramidal effects (EPS) than haloperidol, in higher doses it does have substantial EPS. Olanzepine may have less risk of EPS than either haloperidol or risperidone, but has increased anticholinergic effects that may make it less desirable for treatment in delirium. One small open trial did not find these to be problematic, however (Kim *et al.* 2001). Olanzepine is currently available only orally, which may limit its utility in critically ill or uncooperative patients (Sipahimalani and Masand 1998; Meagher 2001).

Care must be taken to assess the patient for akathisia (motor restlessness), which may be an adverse effect of high potency antipsychotics, and can be confused with worsening hyperactive delirium. The treatment of akathisia is less, not more, antipsychotic medication. Haloperidol should be avoided in elderly persons with parkinsonism (including those with true Parkinson's disease, the 'Parkinson's-plus' syndromes, and diffuse Lewy body dementia) because of its extrapyramidal side effects. In these cases, a benzodiazepine such as lorazepam may be substituted. Among benzodiazepines, lorazepam is a good choice because of its short-to-intermediate duration of action, absence of active metabolites, and its availability in both oral and parenteral forms (Meagher 2001). However, in general, benzodiazpines have a less favourable side effect profile in delirious patients, including an increased risk of oversedation, paradoxical excitation, and respiratory depression (Flacker and Marcantonio 1998; Meagher 2001). The agents used in the pharmacological management of agitated delirium are summarized in Table 7.2.

High-dose intravenous haloperidol may be the treatment of choice in critically ill intensive care unit patients (Seneff and Matthews 1995; Shapiro *et al.* 1995). In such patients, the risk/benefit ratio of adverse drug reactions versus the removal of lines and devices often favours pharmacological treatment. Such therapy must be used with special caution in older patients. In addition to EPS, the potential for QT interval prolongation and *torsades de pointes*, neuroleptic malignant syndrome, and withdrawal dyskinesias remain important concerns (Metzger and Friedman 1993). As with mechanical restraints, in all cases where pharmacological restraints are used the health-care team must clearly identify the target symptoms necessitating their use, frequently review the efficacy of the agent in controlling the target symptoms, and assess the patient for adverse effects and complications. Use of the lowest dose of the least toxic agent for the shortest duration of time is the best rule of thumb.

There are relatively new data supporting the use of alternative agents in the management of agitated delirium. Trazodone and mianserin are atypical antidepressants that are serotonin reuptake inhibitors. Studies have suggested that these drugs are very effective in treating non-specific agitation in dementia (Sultzer *et al.* 1997), independent of their antidepressant effects. They are also used quite effectively as sedative-hypnotics in elders and may have a better side effect profile than benzodiazepines. Two case series have shown some benefit of these agents in treating agitation in delirium (Nakamura *et al.* 1997; Okamoto *et al.* 1999). However, because these drugs are highly sedating, they are probably not the agents of choice.

Discussions of drug use to maintain behavioural control in delirium usually focus on hyperactive delirium, and have little or nothing to say about management of the hypoactive variant. This is probably because hypoactive delirium does not obviously distress the patient or cause problems with ward routines. However, it impairs effective communication with others, and is associated with significant adverse consequences, such as pressure sores and chest infections (see below). Given that sedative drugs often cause hypoactive delirium, the most effective intervention in such cases is probably to

Table 7.2 Pharmacological therapy of agitated delirium

Agent	Mechanism of action	Dosage	Benefits	Side effects	Comments	Notes
Haloperidol	Antipsychotic	0.5–1.0 mg PO/IV Q4h. PRN agitation	Relatively non-sedating. Few haemodynamic effects	Extrapyramidal symptoms (EPS), esp. if >3 mg/day	Usually agent of choice	In a randomized trial comparing haloperidol, chlorpromazine, and lorazepam in the treatment of agitated delirium in young patients with AIDS, all were equally effective, but haloperidol had the least side effects or adverse sequelae (Breitbart et al. 1996)
Risperidone	Antipsychotic	0.5–1.0 mg PO/IV Q4h. PRN agitation	Similar to haloperidol	Might have slightly less EPS		A case series demonstrated that risperidone was effective and reasonably safe in treating agitated delirium (Sipahimalani and Masand 1997)
Lorazepam	Sedative	0.5–1.0 mg PO/IV Q4h. PRN agitation	Use in sedative and alcohol withdrawal, Parkinson's, and patients with h/o neuroleptic malignant syndrome	More paradoxical excitation, respiratory depression than haloperidol	Second-line agent, except in specific cases noted	

Reproduced from: Marcantonio, E.R. *PIER Module: Delirium*. American College of Physicians, 2002.

reduce or withdraw these. There are case reports supporting the use of psychostimulant drugs such as methylphenidate to improve functioning in hypoactive delirium due
to other causes (e.g. Morita *et al.* 2000), but no trials as yet.

Step 3: anticipating and preventing common complications of delirium

Delirious patients are vulnerable to complications that may further compound and
complicate their problems. In fact, delirium has been postulated to play a central role
in the cascade of adverse events that befalls many hospitalized elderly patients, ultimately leading to long-term functional decline and loss of independence (Creditor
1993). Like the causes of delirium, the complications are so numerous that a comprehensive discussion is beyond the scope of this chapter. However, several complications
are so predictably frequent that the diagnosis of delirium should trigger immediate
implementation of a proactive strategy to prevent or manage them. These will be discussed below and include urinary incontinence, immobility, and falls, pressure ulcers,
sleep disturbance, and feeding disorders.

Delirium is cited as one of the most common causes of transient urinary incontinence (Resnick 1995). Up to one half of hospitalized elders have transient urinary
incontinence, and most of this is attributed to delirium. The major reasons for incontinence in delirious patients are their inability to appropriately attend to the sensation of
needing to urinate, their inability to effectively communicate the need to urinate, and,
most unfortunately, the shortage of hospital personnel to provide a bedpan or assistance to get to the bathroom. Urinary incontinence, when it occurs, may contribute to
several other problems below, including falls, which occur when the delirious patient
tries to get up by him/herself and go to the bathroom, and pressure ulcers, which result
from moist and macerated perineal skin. The best treatment for incontinence is a
scheduled toiletting regimen, in which the delirious patient is offered a bedpan or,
preferably, assisted to the bathroom, every 2–3 hours. Unfortunately, the worst treatment is the one most commonly employed, namely, an indwelling urinary catheter.
Indwelling catheters, in addition to predisposing to urinary tract infection (which in
turn may prolong delirium), may also result in significant urinary tract trauma if the
delirious patient tries to remove the catheter, or the need for physical restraints to
avoid inadvertent removal. If catheterization is absolutely required, intermittent is
preferable to indwelling. Antispasmodic bladder medications (such as oxybutynin) are
also occasionally prescribed to reduce bladder urgency. These are best reserved for stable out-patients with established urinary incontinence due to detrusor overactivity.
In delirious patients, the anticholinergic properties of these drugs run the risk of
worsening the delirium and predisposing patients to numerous other complications,
including urinary retention and faecal impaction (Donnellan *et al.* 1997).

Delirious patients are frequently immobilized, and yet also frequently fall. This
seeming paradox is explained by the finding that physical restraints do not prevent

falls; in fact, they have been shown to increase fall-related injuries (Tinetti *et al.* 1992; Capezuti *et al.* 1996). Immobility and bedrest are not benign conditions for hospitalized elders. Studies have shown that elderly patients lose up to 5% of their muscle mass for every day at bedrest, compared to 1.5% in younger persons (Creditor 1993). Bone mineral density declines at an equally rapid rate. Many delirious patients lack judgement, and may attempt to do inappropriate things, such as get out of bed and go to the bathroom, despite a recent orthopedic procedure or an indwelling bladder catheter. The solution is not to untie delirious elders and allow them free, unsupervised activity around the hospital ward. Delirious patients need carefully supervised mobilization, provided by therapists, nurses, or aides. Delirious patients with mobility problems should be evaluated and treated by a physical therapist, even in the absence of a traditional 'rehab' diagnosis (stroke, hip fracture, etc.). One recent study found that delirium was a strong risk factor for in-hospital falls and fall-related injuries (Bates *et al.* 1995). Again, the solution is neither physical nor chemical restraints. Instead, it is careful supervision and structured mobilization programmes.

One of the adverse sequelae of the immobilization of delirious patients is the development of pressure ulcers (Allman 1989; O'Keeffe and Lavan 1999). Again, the best management is prevention, through early and judicious mobilization. For patients who must be immobilized, a careful turning and repositioning programme is necessary, along with vigilant monitoring of pressure points. Delirious patients cannot be expected to shift and turn themselves, and in some cases may exacerbate their condition by constantly rubbing at bedsheets. The development of pressure ulcers in a delirious patient is a truly unfortunate occurrence, because its management requires yet another set of medical interventions that may serve to agitate, tether, or otherwise impede rehabilitation. Moreover, the incontinence and malnutrition that are often associated with delirium may serve to exacerbate the pressure ulcer. Although the detailed management of pressure ulcers is beyond the scope of this chapter, when options are available, it is best to choose the one that requires the least medical intervention (fewest dressing changes, medications, etc.) and is still consistent with a favourable outcome.

The sleep–wake cycle is frequently disordered in delirious patients, and this leads to a host of complications. Delirious patients may sleep much of the day, and then be awake (and agitated) much of the night. This in itself is not a cause for too much concern, except that hospitals are staffed expecting that patients will be relatively active during the day, and sleeping at night. Moreover, the agitated patient in the middle of the night is likely to disturb others. Unfortunately, the most commonly used intervention for disordered sleep–wake cycle in hospitals is sedative-hypnotic medication (O'Reilly and Rusnak 1990). These medications are likely to exacerbate the patient's confusion and agitation, and may even worsen the sleep problem for which they were prescribed (Zisselman *et al.* 1996). Much more appropriate is a programme of non-pharmacological sleep hygiene, which can be applied to all hospitalized patients, but most particularly the delirious. Elements of this programme include exposure to light and activities during the day in an attempt to minimize the all too frequent mid-day napping. Avoidance of caffeine and diuretics after noon, which may increase urinary output in the evening, is also helpful. Patients should be allowed to go to sleep at their usual hour, rather than the often enforced 'in bed by 7, asleep by 8' rule, which almost ensures awakening in the middle of the night. Also helpful are modifications of the hospital environment in the evening and night-time hours, such as soft lighting and minimizing noise.

Perhaps most important is elimination of the ubiquitous use of sedative-hypnotics at bedtime, and substitution of a non-pharmacological sleep protocol. One such protocol, developed by Inouye and colleagues at Yale University, has been proved effective and was perhaps the most important component of a multifactorial protocol that reduced the incidence of delirium in the acute hospital setting (Inouye *et al.* 1999a). This involved use of soft lighting, playing relaxation tapes, provision of a warm non-caffeinated beverage (such as milk or herbal tea), and giving the patient a short but relaxing back rub (Fakouri and Jones 1987). This protocol was successful in inducing sleep and obviating the need for sedatives in over 85% of patients (McDowell *et al.* 1998). More importantly, the patients who received this protocol slept longer and better than those who received sleeping pills. Obviously, provision of this protocol is more time-consuming for the staff than distribution of sleeping pills: Inouye's team utilized a cadre of trained volunteers. Alternatives include using trained nursing aides, or family members who might be 'sleeping over' with the patients. It is a challenge for modern hospitals to develop creative ways of delivering low-technology, high-caring services needed by elders in the face of growing financial difficulties.

Finally, delirious patients are at risk for malnutrition. The basic problem is simple: because of their attentional deficits, delirious patients have difficulty attending to food and feeding themselves properly. Further complicating the problem is that institutional food often arrives in a hermetically sealed container. Plastic lids and cellophane wrap that might present no problem for most patients represent insurmountable barriers for delirious individuals. Therefore, delirious elders need help with feeding, including set-up, monitoring, and possibly, hand feeding. Delirious elders are also at risk for aspiration, so they should be fed out of bed, or if unable, sitting up at 90 degrees. Because of the aspiration risk, patients who are stuporous or very drowsy should not be orally fed. Often, the cause of this state is oversedation for agitation. If chewing and swallowing difficulties persist despite appropriate use of dentures and a normal level of consciousness, referral to speech therapy for a swallowing evaluation may be indicated.

Oral intake needs to be monitored very closely. Acutely ill medical patients, or postoperative surgical patients, have increased protein and calorie requirements to help reverse the catabolism that is associated with these conditions (Mizcock and Troglia 1997). It is often difficult for the delirious patient to eat adequately to meet these increased needs. Obviously, the best solution is to reverse the delirium as quickly as possible so that the patient's eating can improve. In cases where the delirium is slow to improve, alternative means to increase intake should be considered. Sometimes, temporarily liberalizing the patient's dietary restrictions, or asking the family to bring in the patient's favourite foods, may be enough to improve intake. Oral nutritional supplements in the form of calorie and protein-fortified milk shakes are another option (McWhirter and Pennington 1996). These should be given between meals rather than at mealtime, so they can truly be supplements rather than substitutes for regular food. In some cases, oral intake cannot be maintained despite supplements. In this case, short-term feeding via a nasogastric tube, or parenteral feeding via an intravenous line, needs to be considered (McWhirter and Pennington 1996). Unfortunately, these create another irritant or tether that is likely to agitate the patient and may require restraints, so these should only be used as a last resort when oral options have been exhausted. Except for situations when the impaired mental status is expected to continue for a very long time, surgically or endoscopically placed feeding tubes have no role in the management of delirious patients.

Step 4: supporting functional needs and restoring function; family education and support

As discussed above, delirious patients are at risk of sustaining permanent and significant functional decline. Therefore, concomitant with the diagnosis of delirium, a rehabilitation plan should be put into place with the goal of restoring the patient to his/her pre-morbid functional state. To this end, each of the steps described above are critical. First and foremost, the causes and contributors to delirium must be identified and corrected as promptly as possible. Behavioural disturbances, if present, must be managed in a fashion least likely to cause additional complications and functional decline. Common complications, which for the most part bear a direct correspondence to the patient's basic activities of daily living (ADL) needs (toileting, mobility, sleep, and feeding), must be anticipated and averted or managed in a way least likely to contribute to additional problems. Indeed, without each of the steps noted above, restoration of function will be fruitless because delirium and its complications will continue to ravage the patient. In addition, a systematic rehabilitation plan for delirious patients should be implemented with the following key steps:

- modification of the hospital environment;
- implementation of a systematic cognitive reconditioning programme;
- frequent reassessment of ADL capacity, and matching performance to capacity;
- family education, support, and participation in the rehabilitation plan; and
- discussion of delirium in the context of discharge.

Modifications to the environment may be helpful in the management of delirium (Meagher *et al.* 1996; McCusker *et al.* 2001). Family members should be encouraged to bring in familiar objects and pictures of family members from home. More importantly, hospitals can provide simple modifications to the environment that can make a big difference. Large clocks, calendars, and an orientation board should be provided at the bedside and used as part of a cognitive reconditioning programme. This is discussed further below. Both visual and hearing impairment have been shown to be risk factors for delirium, so glasses and hearing aids should be provided and worn properly. Incandescent lighting should be provided at the bedside and used, especially during evening hours. A portable tape recorder to play relaxing music may be helpful in the management of agitation for some patients and can be used as part of the non-pharmacological sleep protocol described above (Mornhinweg and Voignier 1995; McDowell *et al.* 1998).

In addition to these simple bedside devices, systematic changes in hospital practices may also be important in delirium management. In particular, delirious patients benefit from familiar routine, so consistent nursing staff should be assigned whenever possible. Reducing noise and light levels at night may help to facilitate a good night's sleep. Hospital staff should always explain who they are and what they are doing. Further description of how to interact with the delirious patient can be found in the section above on behavioural disturbances. Reduction of the general clutter of the hospital environment can also be helpful (Meagher *et al.* 1996). Any unfamiliar objects in the delirious patient's room may serve as a basis for misperceptions or distortions that may further agitate the patient. Moreover, they serve as obstacles that increase risk of falls and injury. Frequent room changes should be avoided, as this increases the risk of delirium (McCusker *et al.* 2001).

Delirious patients should receive a cognitive reconditioning programme (Inouye 2000). All hospital staff who come into contact with the patient can participate, as can the family once properly educated. At least three times daily, the patient should be reminded of the date, day, time, and location in the hospital. Appropriate times include first thing in the morning when the nurse comes in to do morning vital signs and care, last thing in evening prior to the non-pharmacological sleep protocol, and at the beginning of any therapy sessions or nursing treatments. Any upcoming testing, treatments, surgery, and discharge should be described. This should be done in a gentle, non-confrontational manner rather than as a test of orientation.

The hospital staff should also frequently reassess the delirious patient's ADL capacity. Many of these patients may be severely delirious at the time of admission or shortly thereafter and therefore require total care for ADL needs. In such cases, the hospital staff must perform all basic functions for them. However, as the patient's delirium clears, he/she may be able to begin to participate in ADL activities. If the staff continues to provide total care, this may reinforce a cycle of dependence that prevents functional recovery. In the hospital environment, large changes can happen rapidly, so it is probably worthwhile to reassess ADL capacity on a daily basis, at least for the first several days. ADL capacity can be assessed by encouraging the patient to perform his/her

ADLs before performing them for him/her. The goal is to match ADL performance with ADL capacity, in other words, to maximize functional independence.

Family education and support are also crucial to management and restoration of the delirious patient (Chatham 1978) (see Chapter 9). The family is often the best source of information about the patient's baseline mental status, which can be crucial in differentiating delirium from dementia. Family members are usually overwhelmed by the acute onset or worsening of confusion in a loved one. In previously intact patients, the family may mistakenly attribute the changes to dementia. Alternatively, a patient may have preexisting dementia, but have had an acute decompensation or exacerbation of confusion. In either case, the onset of delirium may raise family concerns about long-term prognosis and living situation. It is extremely relieving to these family members to explain the syndrome of delirium, that it is usually caused by medicines and medical problems, and that it is usually reversible. However, it is also important to share concerns about prognosis and engage the family to help manage the patient. As described above, the presence of a familiar face can often prevent the need for physical or chemical restraints. Family members can also advocate for their delirious relatives' functional needs, and with training, even provide functional assistance (such as feeding). However, just because someone is a relative or friend does not mean that they will be a calming influence. It is important to assess each relative's motivation to participate in the delirium abatement team, and also to provide the proper training as to how to interact with the delirious patient. In some cases, this may require a major shift from their usual way of interacting with the family member, and the relative may not be able to help.

Part of family education includes the management of delirium at discharge. It is known that delirium symptoms may persist in a significant portion of patients for weeks to months after the acute illness (Levkoff *et al.* 1992). If the patient is to be discharged home during this period of time, he/she will need increased supervision and ADL support during the period. In today's environment, very little of this is provided by skilled home care agencies, so most of the burden falls on family members. Alternatively, the patient may be discharged to a rehabilitation hospital or skilled nursing facility. Family members can play a crucial role in these facilities by explaining to the medical and nursing staff that the patient is in fact not at his/her baseline mental state and needs additional cognitive and functional rehabilitation. The family member should also realize that delirium or mental functioning may be a crucial barometer of the patient's overall medical status. In particular, if the patient suddenly becomes much more confused, this suggests a new medical problem or an adverse reaction to a medicine has supervened and requires an urgent and thorough medical reinvestigation.

Some patients, despite what seems to be optimal medical management and functional support, fail to recover completely (Francis and Kapoor 1992; Murray *et al.* 1993). One reason is that delirium may have been a manifestation of a serious medical problem in another organ system that is not reversible (for instance, a major myocardial infarction). However, in some cases, the primary problem is readily reversible (for instance, hip fracture), but the patient still sustains a permanent decline in cognitive and functional status. The reasons for this remain unclear, but it is possible that the process of delirium itself exerts a direct toxic effect on the brain, leading to irreversible damage. Although family members should be encouraged to remain optimistic for a complete recovery, this can never be guaranteed. A good rule of thumb is that the longer delirium and its sequelae persist, the less likelihood of a complete recovery. Thus, one can be much more optimistic one or two days into delirium than one or two months. Research into how delirium exerts its influence on permanent cognitive and functional decline is a priority for the future. Because of the uncertain prognosis of prolonged delirium, careful reassessment of mental status is indicated over several months following the acute illness.

There has been virtually no research into the effects of rehabilitation and other forms of community support for patients with delirium following hospital discharge. One recent study by Rahkonen *et al.* (2001) has examined the effect of a programme involving case management by a nurse specialist and annual rehabilitation periods of 1 week for up to 3 years following discharge from hospital. When compared with a group of controls receiving usual after-care, the intervention group spent significantly less time in long-term institutional care (19 person-years overall), without requiring any more acute hospital admissions. This was a relatively small study, and there was no formal randomization into the intervention and control groups; however, their findings suggest that formal community support strategies may have an important role in the after-care of the delirious patient. Indeed, delirium as an in-patient may be an indicator of the need for more intensive community support than is usually the case following hospital discharge. Further research in this area is necessary.

Delirium and terminal care

There is one group of patients for whom the discussion above is largely irrelevant, that is, patients who are dying. Delirium may be the manifestation of the terminal phases of illness (Breitbart and Strout 2000; Casarett and Inouye 2001), and in fact may have evolved as the body's protective mechanism against the pain and anguish of death. In dying patients, medication adjustment and other straightfoward interventions to improve mental status should be considered. However, a vigorous diagnostic work-up to identify causes of delirium, and multifaceted interventions to reverse delirium and restore function may not be appropriate. Instead, the main focus should be to provide comfort for both the patient and family. This should include family education about delirium and its natural role in the dying process. Whilst many patients would like to remain lucid until the end, this is often not compatible with maintaining comfort. Discussions about priorities for the dying process should be discussed in advance of the actual events to allow the treatment team to deliver care in the manner most consistent with patient and family wishes.

Medico-legal aspects of delirium

Whilst the appropriate medical care for delirium transcends national boundaries, laws vary from country to country, and in some cases from state to state within countries. Rather than focusing on specific legislation, this discussion emphasizes general principles that must be considered in managing delirious patients. How the doctrine of informed consent applies to patients is discussed first, followed by discussion of how a country's mental health legislation may be used in their management. Third, how delirium is a syndrome of increasing interest among malpractice attorneys is discussed, together with the situations most likely to result in legal action.

Informed consent implies that the patient agrees to a given treatment course after being fully informed of the risks and benefits, as well as alternatives. Although informed consent is implied in all medical interactions, the degree to which the informed consent is documented and required is proportionate to the risks involved. Thus, there is rarely a formal written consent for the initiation of a new drug in the ambulatory setting, whereas there is almost always a signed informed consent prior to a major surgical procedure. A prerequisite of informed consent is that the patient be capable of being informed, that is, understand the consequences of the proposed medical actions, as well as the alternatives. In practice, the informed consent process often fails. First, hurried and harried clinicians may not provide adequate explanations of medical treatments. Second, these same clinicians almost never ask the patient questions to assess whether, in fact, the necessary information has been transmitted and processed. Thus, even with an entirely mentally intact patient, informed consent may not truly be 'informed'.

Delirious patients, because of their impaired attention and thought organization, are rarely able to provide truly informed consent. Therefore, the doctrine of substituted judgement pertains, in which informed consent must be obtained from a substituted decision-maker. In some countries, such as the USA, this may take the form of a predesignated health-care proxy. In this case, the patient has signed a legal document (termed an advance directive) designating that the health-care proxy has full decision-making authority related to health care if he/she were mentally or physically unable to provide informed consent. The health-care proxy is supposed to make medical decisions in the way the patient would have wanted them made, if he or she were able to do so. Whilst a legally appointed health-care proxy can be extremely helpful, many persons have not filled out an advance directive. In this case, the next of kin can provide substituted judgement. However, if multiple next of kin (such as children) are unable to reach a consensus and there is no designated proxy, the situation can become quite problematic.

Different approaches to informed consent may be required depending on the severity of the delirium. In severe delirium (such as stupor), the patient is clearly unable to provide informed consent and the substitute decision-maker, if there is one, must be utilized. In cases of mild delirium, the patient may be able to understand some medical discussions and give some opinions as to his or her care, particularly during lucid intervals. One case series documents the use of flumazenil, a competitive benzodiazepine antagonist, to temporarily restore mental capacity in patients with delirium and allow participation in medical decisions (Bostwick and Masterson 1998). In cases when mental status is questionable or fluctuating rapidly, it is often wise to involve both the patient and the substituted decision-maker. Unfortunately, the approach described above rarely happens. A recent study examined informed consent in a cohort of patients who were known to be delirious. In over half, the patient's signature was the only one on the informed consent document (Auerswald *et al.* 1997). If adverse consequences resulted from the treatment and led to legal action, the physicians obtaining informed consent in these cases would be in a rather tenuous situation.

Another approach to substituted decision-making is mental health legislation. Most countries have some form of legislation which makes provisions for the management and care of those with a mental disorder who are unable by virtue of their disorder to give valid consent. Such legislation defines the circumstances in which patients may be admitted involuntarily to hospital, and receive treatment against their wishes. There are usually safeguards in place, such as consent from next of kin, independent second opinions, etc., to ensure that these powers are not abused. Delirium is classified as a mental disorder, so this legislation can and should be used to enable incompetent and resistive patients to receive the assessment and treatment they need. Unfortunately, non-psychiatrists are often unaware of the status of delirium as a mental disorder, they have limited knowledge of their national mental health law, and most non-psychiatric hospitals do not have the experience or the capacity to administer it.

A life-threatening emergency is a special situation that deserves mention. In this case, the physician has the authority to initiate life-saving or sustaining treatment, even in the absence of informed consent (Meagher 2001). This could include administration of medicines and invasive procedures, including intubation and surgery. The general rule of thumb is that treatment may be given without consent if medical colleagues would generally consider it to be appropriate, and a reasonable person would want it. This is important, because many critically ill patients are delirious and unable to give informed consent, and a substitute decision-maker may not exist, or be readily available. The physician should obtain consent from any substitute decision-maker (or, rarely, the patient) as soon as possible after the situation has stabilized. In an acutely agitated delirious patient who is a danger to him/herself, the use of physical restraints and administration of sedatives can also be performed in the acute setting without informed consent. Of course, as described above in the section on behavioural management, these measures should only be used when absolutely necessary, and should be discontinued as soon as possible.

Finally, there is growing interest in delirium by attorneys who specialize in suing doctors. Because it is so frequently missed or mismanaged by physicians, delirium is a potentially happy hunting ground for these attorneys. The major grounds for suit are either failure to diagnose, or mismanagement. Among the most concerning errors are the following:

- misdiagnosis as an acute psychiatric condition, treated primarily with chemical or physical restraints, with little or no attention to underlying medical problems, with resultant life-threatening sequelae;

- appropriate diagnosis of delirium, but administration of excessive doses of sedative medication, which result in adverse sequelae;

- mismanagement of the delirious patient with prolonged restraints and immobility, leading to complications such as injuries from restraints and pressure ulcers.

While there is increasing interest in delirium among malpractice attorneys, fear of litigation should not be the primary motivation for the appropriate management of delirium. Errors in diagnosis and management are extremely common, and few result in legal action. There may also be grounds for suit if the patient is unlawfully detained or treated without their consent; doctors should be aware of their national legal framework determining how such decisions should be made.

Summary

This chapter reviews the key steps in the management of delirium (Table 7.3). First, timely diagnosis is key. Systematic case-finding efforts, including regular assessment of mental status as a 'vital sign' and application of a standardized algorithm such as the Confusion Assessment Method, should be considered for all high-risk hospitalized elders. Once delirium is detected, the first and key step in its management is a thorough evaluation for potential causes and contributors, and the prompt treatment of all correctable factors. Common factors amenable to intervention include: medications, infections, fluid and electrolyte disorders, severe pain, sensory deprivation, and elimination problems. Another key step in delirium management is the control of problematic behaviour. For the most part, this should be achieved by non-pharmacological means, including appropriate interactions with the hospital staff and the involvement of family members. In some cases, physical or chemical restraints are required for patient safety. In general, low doses of high potency neuroleptics (such as haloperidol) are the drugs of choice. Once reversible factors and behavioural problems have been addressed, the physician should anticipate, prevent, and manage common complications of delirium. These include urinary incontinence, immobility and falls, pressure ulcers, sleep disorders, and feeding problems. In each case, a programme should be implemented to meet the patient's functional needs and to prevent adverse consequences that might perpetuate the cascade of adverse events often precipitated by delirium. Finally, the need to implement a systematic plan to restore function in delirious patients is discussed. The family can play a critical role in the restorative plan, after having been appropriately educated and engaged.

Table 7.3 Summary of management of delirium

Step	Key issues	Proposed treatment
Identify and treat reversible contributors	Medications	Reduce or eliminate offending medications, or substitute less psychoactive medications (see Table 7.1)
	Infections	Treat common infections: urinary, respiratory, soft-tissue
	Fluid balance disorders	Assess and treat dehydration, CHF, electrolyte disorders
	Impaired CNS oxygenation	Treat severe anaemia (transfusion), hypoxia, hypotension
	Severe pain	Assess and treat, using local measures, scheduled pain regimens that minimize opioids. Avoid meperidine
	Sensory deprivation	Use glasses, hearing aids, portable amplifiers
	Elimination problems	Assess and treat urinary retention and faecal impaction
Maintain behavioural control	Behavioural interventions	Teach hospital staff appropriate interaction with delirious. Encourage family visitation
	Pharmacological interventions	If necessary, low-dose high potency neuroleptics are usually agents of choice (haloperidol 0.5–1 mg) (see Table 7.2)
Anticipate and prevent or manage complications	Urinary incontinence	Implement scheduled toiletting programme
	Immobility and falls	Avoid physical restraints. Mobilize with assistance. Physical therapy
	Pressure ulcers	Mobilize. If immobile, reposition frequently and monitor pressure points
	Sleep disturbance	Implement a non-pharmacological sleep hygiene program, including a night-time sleep protocol. Avoid sedatives
	Feeding disorders	Assist with feeding. Aspiration precautions. Nutritional supplementation as necessary

Restore function in delirious patients	
Modify hospital environment	Reduce clutter and noise (esp. at night). Adequate lighting. Bring in familiar objects from home
Implement cognitive reconditioning programme	Staff reorients to time, place, person at least 3 times daily
Reassessment of ADL capacity	As delirium clears, match performance to capacity to break 'circle of dependence'
Family education, support, and participation	Education about delirium, its causes, its reversibility, how to interact, and family's role in restoration of function
Delirium and discharge	Delirium may persist – need for increased ADL supports, mental status changes as 'barometer' for recovery

The proper management of the delirious patient can be a very time-intensive process. However, failure to invest the appropriate effort can result in severe adverse consequences, ranging from permanent functional decline to death. New models of acute care delivery must be developed to bring the recognition and management of delirium to the forefront (Inouye *et al.* 1999a, 1999b), such as specialized hospital units. Environmental modifications, altered routines of care, trained professional staff with expertise in delirium, and the use of non-professional staff or volunteers for functional support may be some of the key components in such units. The hospitals of the future will need to be friendlier for older patients (Landefeld *et al.* 1995). If so, the incidence of delirium and its adverse sequelae will be reduced. Much as the public health advances of the early twentieth century reduced infectious diseases before antibiotics came into use, changes in how we care for older patients have the potential to have a positive impact on delirium before advances in our understanding of its pathophysiology result in pharmacological treatments. Developing, implementing, and testing new models of care for delirium are important priorities for clinicians and researchers.

Acknowledgement

I would like to thank Margaret Bergmann, RN, MS, GNP for her careful review and helpful comments on this manuscript.

Further reading

American Psychiatric Association (1999). *Practical guidelines for the treatment of patients with delirium.* American Psychiatric Association, Washington, DC.

References

Abrahm, J. L. (2000). Advances in pain management for older patients. *Clinical Geriatric Medicine,* **16**, 269–311.

Agency for Health Care Policy and Research. (1992). *Acute pain management in adults: Quick reference guide for clinicians.* Publication 92-0019.

Allman, R. M. (1989). Pressure ulcers among the elderly. *New England Journal of Medicine,* **320**, 150–153.

Auerswald, K. B., Charpentier, P. A., and Inouye, S. K. (1997). The informed consent process in older patients who developed delirium: a clinical epidemiologic study. *American Journal of Medicine,* **103**, 410–418.

Avorn, J. and Gurwitz, J. H. (1997). Principles of pharmacology. In: *Geriatric medicine* (eds C. K. Cassel, *et al.*), 3rd edn. Springer-Verlag, New York.

Bates, D. W., Pruess, K., Souney, P., and Platt, R. (1995). Serious falls in hospitalized patients: correlates and resource utilization. *American Journal of Medicine,* **99**, 137–143.

Blackburn, T. and Dunn, M. (1990). Cystocerebral syndrome: acute urinary retention presenting as confusion in elderly patients. *Archives of Internal Medicine,* **150**, 2577–2578.

Bostwick, J. M. and Masterson, B. J. (1998). Psychopharmacological treatment of delirium to restore mental capacity. *Psychosomatics,* **39**, 112–117.

Breitbart, W., Marotta, R., Platt, M. M., *et al.* (1996). A double-blind trial of haloperidol, chlorpromazine, and lorazepam in the treatment of delirium in hospitalized AIDS patients. *American Journal of Psychiatry*, **153**, 231–237.

Breitbart, W. and Strout, D. (2000). Delirium in the terminally ill. *Clinical Geriatric Medicine*, **16**, 357–372.

Burns, M. J., Linden, C. H., Graudins, A., Brown, R. M., and Fletcher, K. E. (2000). A comparison of physostigmine and benzodiazepines for treatment of anticholinergic poisoning. *Annals of Emergency Medicine*, **35**, 374–381.

Capezuti, E., Evans, L., Strumpf, N., *et al.* (1996). Physical restraint use and falls in nursing home residents. *Journal of the American Geriatrics Society*, **44**, 627–633.

Casarett, D. J. and Inouye, S. K. (2001). Diagnosis and management of delirium near the end of life. *Annals of Internal Medicine*, **135**, 32–40.

Chatham, M. A. (1978). The effect of family involvement on patients' manifestations of postcardiotomy psychosis. *Heart and Lung*, **7**, 995–999.

Cole, M. G., Primeau, F., and McCusker, J. (1996). Effectiveness of interventions to prevent delirium: a systematic review. *Canadian Medical Association Journal*, **155**, 1263–1268.

Creditor, M. C. (1993). Hazards of hospitalization in the elderly. *Annals of Internal Medicine*, **118**, 219–223.

Donnellan, C. A., Fook, L., McDonald, P., and Playfer, J. R. (1997). Oxybutynin and cognitive dysfunction. *British Medical Journal*, **315**, 1363–1364.

Egbert, A. M., Parks, L. H., and Short, L. M. (1990). Randomized trial of postoperative patient controlled analgesia vs. intramuscular narcotics in frail elderly men. *Archives of Internal Medicine*, **150**,1897–1903.

Fakouri, C. and Jones, P. (1987). Relaxation Rx: slow stroke back rub. *Journal of Gerontological Nursing*, **13**, 32–35.

Flacker, J. M. and Marcantonio, E. R. (1998). Delirium in the elderly: optimal management. *Drugs and Aging*, **13**, 119–130.

Francis, J. and Kapoor, W. N. (1992). Prognosis after hospital discharge of older medical patients with delirium. *Journal of the American Geriatrics Society*, **40**, 601–606.

Hassan, E., Fontaine, D. K., and Nearman, H. S. (1998). Therapeutic considerations in the management of agitated or delirious critically ill patients. *Pharmacotherapy*, **18**, 113–129.

Hussain, N. A. and Warshaw, G. (1996). Utility of clysis for hydration of nursing home residents. *Journal of the American Geriatrics Society*, **44**, 969–973.

Inouye, S. K. (2000). Assessment and management of delirium in hospitalized older patients. *Annals of Long Term Care*, **8**, 53–59.

Inouye, S. K. and Charpentier, P. A. (1996) Precipitating factors for delirium in hospitalized elderly persons. Predictive model and interrelationship with baseline vulnerability. *Journal of the American Medical Association*, **275**, 852–857.

Inouye, S. K., van Dyck, C. H., Aless, C. A., Balkin, S., Siegal, A. P., and Horwitz, R. I. (1990). Clarifying confusion: the confusion assessment method. A new method for detection of delirium. *Annals of Internal Medicine*, **113**, 941–948.

Inouye, S. K., Viscoli, C. M., Horwitz, R. I., Hurst, L. D., and Tinetti, M. E. (1993). A predictive model for delirium in hospitalized elderly medical patients based on admission characteristics. *Annals of Internal Medicine*, **119**, 474–481.

Inouye SK, Bogardus, S. T., Charpentier, P. A., *et al.* (1999a). A multicomponent intervention to prevent delirium in hospitalized older patients. *New England Journal of Medicine*, **340**, 699–676.

Inouye, S. K., Schlesinger, M. J., and Lydon, T. J. (1999b). Delirium: a symptom of how hospital care is failing older persons and a window to improve quality of hospital care. *American Journal of Medicine*, **106**, 565–573.

Kim, K. S., Pae, C. U., Chae, J. H., Bahk, W. M., and Jun, T. (2001). An open pilot trial of olanzapine for delirium in the Korean population. *Psychiatry and Clinical Neurosciences*, **55**, 515–519.

Landefeld, C. S., Palmer, R. M., Kresevic, D. M., Fortinsky, R. H., and Kowal, J. (1995). A randomized trial of care in a hospital medical unit especially designed to improve the functional outcomes of acutely ill older persons. *New England Journal of Medicine*, **332**, 1338–1344.

Levkoff, S. E., Evans, D. A., Liptzin, B., *et al.* (1992). Delirium. The occurrence and persistence of symptoms among elderly hospitalized patients. *Archives of Internal Medicine*, **152**, 334–340.

Lynch, E. P., Lazor, M. A., Gellis, J. E., Orav, J., Goldman, L., and Marcantonio, E. R. (1998). The impact of postoperative pain on the development of postoperative delirium. *Anesthesia and Analgesia*, **86**, 781–785.

McCusker, J., Cole, M., Abrahamowicz, M., Han, L., Poboda, J. E., and Ramman-Haddad, L. (2001). Environmental risk factors for delirium in hospitalized older people. *Journal of the American Geriatrics Society*, **49**, 1327–1334.

McDowell, J. A., Mion, L. C., Lydon, T. J., and Inouye, S. K. (1998). A nonpharmacologic sleep protocol for hospitalized older patients *Journal of the American Geriatrics Society*, **46**, 700–705.

McWhirter, J. P. and Pennington, C. R. (1996). A comparison between oral and nasogastric nutritional supplements in malnourished patients. *Nutrition*, 12, 502–506.

Marcantonio, E. R., Juarez, G., Goldman, L., *et al.* (1994). The relationship of postoperative delirium with psychoactive medications. *Journal of the American Medical Association*, **272**, 1518–1522.

Marcantonio, E. R., Goldman, L., Orav, E. J., Cook, E. F., and Lee, T. H. (1998). The association of intraoperative factors with the development of postoperative delirium. *American Journal of Medicine*, **105**, 380–384.

Marcantonio, E. R., Flacker, J. N., Wright, J., and Resnick, N. M. (2001). Reducing delirium after hip fracture: a randomized trial. *Journal of the American Geriatrics Society*, **49**, 516–522.

Mayo-Smith, MR. (1997). Pharmacological management of alcohol withdrawal: a meta-analysis and evidence-based practice guideline. *Journal of the American Medical Association*, **278**, 144–151.

Max, M. B., Lynch, S. A., Muir, J., Shoaf, S. E., Smoller, B., and Dubner, R. (1992). Effects of desipramine, amitriptyline, and fluoxetine on pain in diabetic neuropathy. *New England Journal of Medicine*, **326**, 1250–1256.

Meagher, D. J. (2001). Delirium: optimising management. *British Medical Journal*, **322**, 144–149.

Meagher, D. J., O'Hanlon, D., O'Mahony, E., and Casey, P. R. (1996). Use of environmental strategies and psychotropic medical in the management of delirium. *British Journal of Psychiatry*, **168**, 512–515.

Menza, M. A., Murray, G. B., Holmes, V. F., and Rafulis, W. A. (1987). Decreased extrapyramidal symptoms with intravenous haloperidol. *Journal of Clinical Psychiatry*, **48**, 278–280.

Metzger, E. and Friedman, R. (1993). Prolongation of the corrected QT and torsades de pointes cardiac arrhythmia associated with intravenous haloperidol in the medically ill. *Journal of Clinical Psychopharmacology*, **13**, 128–132.

Mizock, B. A. and Troglia, S. (1997). Nutritional support of the hospitalized patient. *Disease of the Month*, **43**, 349–426.

Morita, T., Otani, H., Tsunoda, J., Inoue, S. and Chihara, S. (2000). Successful palliation of hypoactive delirium due to multi-organ failure by oral methylphenidate. *Supportive Care in Cancer*, **8**, 134–137.

Mornhinweg, G. C. and Voignier, R. R. (1995). Music for sleep disturbance in the elderly. *Journal of Holistic Nursing*, **13**, 248–254.

Murray, A. M., Levkoff, S.E, Wetle, T. T., *et al.* (1993). Acute delirium and functional decline in the hospitalized elderly patient. *Journal of Gerontology*, **48**, M181–M186.

Nakamura, J., Uchimura, N., Yamada, S., and Nakazawa, Y. (1997). Does plasma free 3-methoxy-4-hydroxyphenyl(ethylene)glycol increase the delirious state? A comparison of the effects of mianserine and haloperidol on delirium. *International Clinical Psychopharmacology*, **12**, 147–152.

Okamoto, Y., Matsuoka, Y., Sasaki, T., Jitsuiki, H., Horiguchi, J., and Yamawaki, S. (1999). Trazodone in the treatment of delirium. *Journal of Clinical Psychopharmacology*, **19**, 280–282.

O'Keeffe, S. T. and Lavan, J. N. (1999). Clinical significance of dementia subtypes in older people. *Age and Ageing*, **28**, 115–119.

O'Reilly, R., and Rusnak, C. (1990). The use of sedative-hypnotic drugs in a university teaching hospital. *Canadian Medical Association Journal*, **142**, 585–589.

Rahkonen, T., Eloniemi-Sulkava, U., Paanila, S., Halonen, P., Sivenius, J., and Sulkava, R. (2001). Systematic intervention for supporting community care of elderly people after a delirium episode. *International Psychogeriatrics*, **13**, 37–49.

Resnick, N. M. (1995). Urinary incontinence. *Lancet*, **346**, 94–99.

Resnick, N. M. and Marcantonio, E. R. (1997). How should clinical care of the aged differ? *Lancet*, **350**, 1157–1158.

Richardson, J. and Bresland, K. (1998). The management of postsurgical pain in the elderly population. *Drugs and Aging*, **13**, 17–31.

Rothschild, A. J. (1992). Disinhibition, amnestic reactions, and other adverse reactions secondary to triazolam: a review of the literature. *Journal of Clinical Psychiatry*, **53** (Suppl.), 69–79.

Schor, J. D., Levkoff, S. E., Lipsitz, L. A., *et al.* (1992). Risk factors for delirium in hospitalized elderly. *Journal of the American Medical Association*, **267**, 827–831.

Seneff, M. G. and Mathews, R. A. (1995). Use of haloperidol infusions to control delirium in critically ill adults. *Annals of Pharmacotherapy*, **29**, 690–693.

Shapiro, B. A., Warren, J., Egol, A. B., *et al.* (1995). Practice parameters for intravenous analgesia and sedation for adult patients in the intensive care unit: an executive summary. Society of Critical Care Medicine. *Critical Care Medicine*, **23**, 1596–1600.

Sipahimalani, A. and Masand, P. S. (1997). Use of risperidone in delirium: case reports. *Annals of Clinical Psychiatry*, **9**, 105–107.

Sipahimalani, A., and Masand, P. S. (1998). Olanzepine in the treatment of delirium. *Psychosomatics*, **39**, 422–430.

Sultzer, D. L., Gray, K. F., Gunay, I., Beriford, M. A., and Mahler, M. E. (1997). A double-blind comparison of trazodone and haloperidol for treatment of agitation in patients with dementia. *American Journal of Geriatric Psychiatry*, **5**, 60–69.

Tinetti, M. E., Liu, W. I., and Ginter, S,F. (1992). Mechanical restraint use and fall-related injuries among residents of skilled nursing facilities. *Annals of Internal Medicine*, **116**, 369–374.

Weinbroum, A., Rudick, V., Sorkine, P., *et al.* (1996). Use of flumazenil in the treatment of drug overdose: a double-blind and open clinical study in 110 patients. *Critical Care Medicine*, **24**, 199–206.

Zisselman, M. H., Rovner, B. W., Yuen, E. J., and Louis, D. Z. (1996). Sedative-hypnotic use and increased hospital stay and costs in older people. *Journal of the American Geriatrics Society*, **44**, 1371–1374.

Chapter 8

The prevention of delirium

Shaun O'Keeffe

Delirium is a common condition among older people admitted to hospital and is associated with serious short-term and long-term consequences for patients and with increased health costs (see Chapter 4). Management of delirium can be difficult and, at present, primarily consists of supportive care and relief of symptoms. Many patients do badly even with optimum management. Thus, the potential benefits of preventing delirium are substantial for patients and also for health care systems.

Delirium is a multifactorial syndrome. In recent years, there have been substantial advances in our understanding of the multiple risk factors for delirium and how they interact in older people to produce delirium. The recognition that many episodes of delirium occur only after hospitalization has focused attention on the hazards of hospitalization, many of which are potentially preventable. There remain many questions to be answered about the most effective measures to prevent delirium and how to implement preventative strategies. Nevertheless, the preventative era is now upon us.

Preventable risk factors for delirium

In the past, it was usual to describe the acute illness that led to the patient's admission as the 'cause' of delirium and to note that the causes of delirium covered the entire range of medicine. There are two problems with this. First, it ignores the fact that many episodes of delirium develop only after admission to hospital, despite the institution of effective therapy for the illness that led to admission. Indeed, in those studies in which initial assessments for delirium were conducted shortly after admission, most episodes of delirium developed after admission (Levkoff *et al.* 1992; O'Keeffe and Lavan 1997). The second problem is that regarding the acute illness as the cause of delirium may lead to preventative nihilism, often combined with overzealous investigation of patients with established delirium.

A more sophisticated approach to examining the aetiology of delirium has been to draw a distinction between predisposing factors that increase the vulnerability of the patient to delirium and factors that precipitate delirium, although it should be acknowledged that this distinction is often difficult in clinical practice.

Predisposing factors

Many studies have used stratification or multivariate predictive methods to examine independent risk factors for delirium (Elie *et al.* 1998; Francis 1992) (see Chapter 3). It is striking, and reassuring, how similar the results from different studies are, despite many differences in study populations and methods. Prior cognitive impairment, older age, severity of illness, and psychoactive drug use have consistently emerged as the most important risk factors. Laboratory indices of dehydration or metabolic disturbance, alcohol abuse, and visual impairment have also emerged as important risk factors in some studies. Although nothing can be done about advanced age and little about prior dementia or severe illness at the time of presentation to hospital, many other risk factors are amenable to development of preventative strategies.

Precipitating factors

The most important recent work in this field, not least because it formed the basis for a subsequent seminal trial, was the study by Inouye and Charpentier (1996) from Yale. In a study of older patients (aged 70 or more) admitted to the general medical wards of a teaching hospital, they examined potential precipitating factors for delirium under four headings – immobility, medications, iatrogenic events, and intercurrent illness. Eleven variables were included in the final stepwise relative risk model, and five were included in the final predictive model: use of physical restraints, malnutrition, more than three medications added, use of bladder catheter, and any iatrogenic event (Table 8.1). A validation study confirmed the value of the final model in predicting delirium in hospital patients. Furthermore, examination of the relationship between these precipitating factors and vulnerability factors derived in a previous study (visual impairment, severe illness, cognitive impairment, and blood urea nitrogen (BUN)/ creatinine ratio = 18) showed that they added to the risk of delirium in an independent and cumulative manner. Hence, this study provided convincing confirmation of the hypothesis that the severity of the insult needed to precipitate delirium is inversely related to the pre-existing vulnerability of the patient.

Limitations of risk factor studies

Multivariable regression procedures are very powerful tools for deriving independent predictive variables. However, caution is necessary when interpreting the results of the derived model. For example, very slight differences among the correlations between predictor and outcome variables can lead to major differences in which variables enter the final model using the stepwise approach, and the relative importance of variables is not always reflected by the variables retained in a final stepwise model. Thus, it is not appropriate to say that a particular group of variables are the 'best' or 'most important' or to use a stepwise solution to try and explain a phenomenon such as delirium.

Table 8.1 Precipitating factors for delirium in 196 elderly medical patients: variables included in the final stepwise relative risk model

Risk factor	Relative risk (95% confidence interval)
Immobility	
Use of physical restraints ($n=31$)	3.5 (2.0–6.3)*
Use of bladder catheter ($n=50$)	3.1 (1.7–5.5)*
Use of 3+ immobilizing devices ($n=52$)	1.8 (1.0–3.4)
Out of bed less than once a day ($n=78$)	2.3 (1.2–4.1)
Medications	
2+ psychoactive medications ($n=7$)	4.5 (2.1–9.9)
4+ medications added ($n=18$)	4.0 (2.1–7.3)*
Iatrogenic events	
>12 hour stay in emergency department ($n=57$)	2.1 (1.1–3.7)
Any iatrogenic event ($n=81$)	1.9 (1.0–3.4)*
Intercurrent illness	
Malnutrition ($n=14$)	3.9 (2.0–7.5)*
Respiratory insufficiency ($n=14$)	2.7 (1.2–5.8)
Dehydration ($n=110$)	1.5 (0.8–2.8)

*Indicates variable included in final predictive model.

Adapted from Inouye and Charpentier (1996).

It is understandable that risk factor studies focus on those factors that can be measured. Many psychosocial and environmental factors that might plausibly contribute to the development or expression of delirium are not easily quantified. Nevertheless, nursing interventions based on correcting such factors have proved effective in preventing delirium (Cronin-Stubbs 1996; Britton and Russell 2000). Sensory overload and sleep deprivation caused by the noise of bleeps and monitors or by constant lighting has been proposed as a precipitant of delirium, particularly in intensive care units (O'Keeffe and Ni Chonchubhair 1994). Others have emphasized the sensory deprivation and distortion caused by waterbeds, immobilization by monitoring equipment or by failure to wear spectacles or hearing aids (Williams *et al.* 1985). Frequent room transfers, lack of continuity of staff or use of windowless rooms may contribute to disorientation (Wilson 1972; Tsutsui *et al.* 1996). It is difficult to assess the quality of personal interactions between staff and patients, although intervention studies and accounts of patients who have had delirium suggest that this may also be an important factor (Owens and Hutelmyer 1982; Schofield 1997; Simon *et al.* 1997).

Barriers to prevention of delirium

Systems of care

Hospitalization of older people has deleterious effects distinct from the effects of acute illness (Gillick 1982; Creditor 1993). Iatrogenic complications occur in up 40% of older hospital patients (Steel *et al.* 1981; Becker *et al.* 1987; Brennan *et al.* 1991). These include complications of therapeutic and diagnostic procedures, hospital-acquired infections, dehydration and metabolic disturbances, weight loss, medication toxicity, loss of mobility, falls, and pressure sores. The strange environment and routine of hospitals may precipitate or worsen disorientation. Polypharmacy and inappropriate prescribing are common. Use of urinary catheters in incontinent patients or use of physical restraints or sedative medications in cognitively impaired patients may be more convenient for harassed staff but will exacerbate immobility and functional impairment. Bed-rest continues to be advocated by physicians, although it is rarely indicated medically and is associated with a rapid reduction in muscle power and bone mass (Lazarus *et al.* 1991; Allen *et al.* 2000). Functional dependency is further reinforced if nursing staff are overly concerned about risk of falls or if staff perform rather than supervise daily activities. Social networks may disappear during a long illness, and patients may become demoralized and depressed. The end result is often a cascade of physical and mental decline (Creditor 1993).

The adverse effects and failures of hospital care apply to all of the 'giants of geriatrics' – confusion, instability, immobility, and incontinence. All are common 'atypical' presentations of acute illness in older people (Jarrett *et al.* 1995). All occur as complications of adverse hospital events but also predict adverse hospital events and eventual poor outcome.

Part of the blame for the failings outlined above must fall on doctors and nurses. Excessive focus on procedures and on providing efficient care is often to the detriment of clinical skills and the provision of humane care. However, the system of care in modern hospitals is also a contributor (Inouye *et al.* 1999b). The length of stay in acute hospitals has declined dramatically over recent years. Patients are sicker both on admission and on discharge. In these circumstances, staff numbers may be inadequate to provide the quality of care needed by vulnerable older people, and staff may be put in a situation of having to juggle incompatible demands to provide quality care and to ensure a rapid throughput of patients.

Patients with cognitive impairment are often poorly served by the design of hospitals (Kitwood 1997). Lighting and signposting, particularly of toilets, may be inadequate. Rooms within a ward often contain several beds, and, in some countries, 'Nightingale' wards, in which two long rows of patients face each other, still persist. Hence, one disturbed patient in a ward may disrupt the sleep of many others, and, if space or staffing do not permit isolation of such patients, staff may opt to gather all confused patients in one room, possibly to their mutual detriment. On the other hand, isolation of patients at risk for delirium in rooms where they cannot be easily observed from a central nursing station will tend to encourage use of restraints or psychoactive drugs.

Poor recognition of delirium

If delirium is not regarded as an important health issue in hospitals, it will prove all the more difficult to motivate staff to apply preventative measures and to identify patients at especially high risk. Delirium is often unrecognized in hospitals (Cameron *et al.* 1987; Williams 1988; Lewis *et al.* 1995). Patients with the 'quiet' or 'hypoactive-hypoalert' subtype of delirium are most easily missed or misdiagnosed as depression (Farrell and Ganzini 1995). Prodromal symptoms of delirium may include aggression and irritability with staff (Morse and Litin 1971). Failure to recognize the significance of such symptoms may lead staff to label a patient as 'uncooperative' or 'difficult' or to respond in kind, thereby exacerbating the situation.

Outside of specialist units, a cursory or non-existent assessment of cognitive function is often the rule. Even if a patient is noted to have cognitive impairment, 'confusion' is a commonly employed catch-all diagnosis, and little attempt may be made to determine the extent to which there is a reversible component (Simpson 1984). Indeed, doctors and nurses spend less time with confused than with non-confused patients (Armstrong-Esther 1986). Cognitive impairment is often worse at night, particularly if delirium is present. However, Treloar and Macdonald (1995) found that night staff only identified 6 of 34 cognitively impaired subjects. They suggested that nurses may try to avoid causing distress by not asking questions that would test cognition.

Assessing interventions to prevent delirium

Possible interventions to prevent delirium are summarized in Table 8.2, and trials assessing interventions to prevent delirium are shown in Table 8.3. It is apparent that relatively few interventions have been evaluated and supported by good quality clinical trials. In a systematic review including many of these studies, Cole and colleagues (1996) noted the frequent methodological shortcomings of most prevention studies. Many studies are small, non-randomized, and do not have blinded outcome measures. There are substantial differences in the methods used to ascertain whether delirium has developed. Delirium is often poorly defined, even allowing for the changes in definitions over the years.

Outcome measures differ greatly between studies. The incidence of delirium is the measure reported in Table 8.3, but this was not always the primary outcome of the studies. Some studies examined the occurrence of individual symptoms of delirium rather than delirium itself (Chatham 1978), or examined occurrence of agitation (Egbert *et al.* 1990; Bruera *et al.* 1995) or the need for sedative medications (Schindler *et al.* 1989). Some studies included a treatment component (Gustafson *et al.* 1991; Wanich *et al.* 1992). Many of the surgical trials reported rates of delirium using different anaesthetic or analgesic regimens but were not explicitly designed to assess prevention of delirium (Egbert *et al.* 1990; Mann *et al.* 2000).

Table 8.2 Potential interventions to prevent delirium

Risk Factor	Intervention
Cognitive impairment	Routine assessment of cognitive function (B)
	Education regarding delirium – local (A) and national (C)
	Orientation measures: regular verbal communication; provide clock, calendar, familiar artefacts, reassurance and explanation of any procedure; avoidance of ward or room transfers; continuity of care (A)
	Cognitively stimulating activities (A)
Dehydration/electrolyte disturbance	Early recognition: fluid balance charts; biochemical screening (C)
	Nursing measures: fluids accessible to patient; encouragement of oral fluids (A)
	Adequate staffing; use of volunteers, family (A)
	Hypodermoclysis if oral intake inadequate (B)
Sensory overload/sleep deprivation	Non-pharmacological sleep promotion (A)
	Sleep enhancement: noise reduction; avoid constant lighting; schedule adjustments (A)
Polypharmacy/use of psychoactive drugs	Education of staff (C)
	Pharmacy liaison: pharmacy rounds; inappropriate drug indicators; use of computer programmes (C)
	Non-pharmacological sleep promotion (A)
	'Start low and go slow' (C)
	Choose drugs with least anticholinergic activity when possible (B)
Malnutrition/vitamin deficiencies	Routine monitoring of weight, (anthropometric indices?) (C)
	Dietician assessment (C)
	Swallow assessment, e.g. stroke (C)
	Assistance with feeding: adequate staffing; use of family (C)
	Nutritional support in selected groups (B)
	Vitamin supplements in selected groups (C)
Alcohol abuse	Screening tests for alcohol abuse (C)
	Benzodiazepines to prevent withdrawal (A)
	Thiamine supplements (B)
Immobilization	Avoid immobilizing : restraint reduction program; protocols regarding catheter use; education regarding hazards of bed-rest (A)
	Early mobilization protocol (A)
	Assessment by physiotherapist, occupational therapist (C)

(continued)

Table 8.2 (continued) Potential interventions to prevent delirium

Risk Factor	Intervention
Visual and hearing impairment	Screening for visual and hearing impairment (A)
	Provision of visual and hearing aids (A)
	Adequate lighting; use of nightlights (B)
Hospital-acquired infections	Infection control measures: hand-washing; antibiotic protocols (C)
	Avoidance of catheters if possible (C)
Perioperative measures	Optimize medical condition preoperatively (B)
	Preoperative visit by anaesthetist (B)
	Postoperative assessment by physician (B)
	Adequate analgesia (C); patient-controlled analgesia if possible (A)
	Prevent operative hypotension/hypoxaemia (B)
	Monitor for postoperative hypoxaemia (?)
	Keep postoperative haematocrit >30% (?)
Inadequate recognition of delirium	Educate patient at risk (B)
	Educate family (B)
	Educate staff (B)
	Routine assessment of cognitive function (B);
	Use of delirium screening tests (?)
Inadequate hospital care/ systems failure	Education of staff regarding delirium and other geriatric syndromes – local (B) and national measures (C)
	Develop strategies and clinical guidelines to change harmful practice patterns: restraint use; polypharmacy; overuse of psychoactive medications; unnecessary catheters; use of bed-rest (C)
	Promote delirium as quality indicator in hospitals (C)

Grades of recommendation refer to the evidence-based level of confidence with which measures can be recommended to prevent delirium: A, substantial confidence; based on high quality randomized controlled trials: B, moderate confidence, based on non-randomized controlled trials, cohort or case-control studies: C, expert opinion, clinical experience, descriptive studies, indirect evidence: ?, no or conflicting evidence.

Reducing the incidence of delirium is good of itself, given that delirium is a very unpleasant experience for patients. However, it is even more important for patients and for the health-care system that the long-term complications of delirium – functional decline, increased admission to institutional care, prolonged hospital stay, and long-term cognitive decline – should be prevented. Wanich *et al.* (1992) did examine functional status, and Schindler *et al.* (1989) measured length of stay, but otherwise these outcomes have received little attention in prevention studies to date. Rockwood (1999) has suggested that an individualized outcome measure, such as Goal Attainment

Table 8.3 Summary of trials examining interventions to prevent delirium in hospital patients

Trial	Study population	Design	Intervention	Number of patients		Delirium (%)	
				Treat	Control	Treat	Control
Consultation							
Lazarus & Hagens (1968)	Cardiac surgery	NR, NB	Psychiatric assessment and support, pre-+postop	21	33	14	33
Layne & Yudofsky (1971)	Cardiac surgery	NR, NB	Psychiatric assessment, preop	42	19	10	22
Schindler et al. (1989)	Cardiac surgery	R, NB	Psychiatric assessment and support, pre+post-op	16	17	13	0
Nursing care							
Owens & Hutelmyer (1982)	Cardiac surgery	R (unbalanced), B	Education of patient by nurse	32	32	59	78
Williams et al. (1985)	Elderly hip fracture	Before/After Historical control	Special nursing care	57	170	44	52
Nagley (1986)	Elderly medical	NR, NB	Special nursing care	30	30	3	0
Wanich et al. (1992)	Elderly medical	NR, NB	Special nursing care	135	100	19	22
Hospital care							
Inouye et al. (1999)	Elderly medical	Prospective matching, B	Medical and nursing care protocols applied by multidisciplinary team	426	426	10	15
Palliative care							
Bruera et al. (1995)	Terminal cancer	Before/After Historical control	Routine cognitive monitoring, opioid rotation, hydration (hypodermoclysis)	117	162	26	10

Perioperative care

		Before/After Historical control		103	111	48	61
Gustafson et al. (1991)	Elderly hip fracture	Before/After Historical control	Medical and anaesthetic care: pre- and postop geriatric assessment; supplemental oxygen	103	111	48	61
Day et al. (1988)	Elderly hip fracture	R, NB	IV thiamine preop	28	32	39	38
Egbert et al. (1990)	Elderly major elective surgery	R, NB	Patient controlled i.v. (PCA) vs. i.m. analgesia (IM)	43 (PCA)	40 (IM)	2 (PCA)	18 (IM)
Hole et al. (1980)	Elderly, hip replacement	NR, NB	Regional (RA) vs. general (GA) anaesthesia	29 (RA)	31 (GA)	0 (RA)	23 (GA)
Berggren et al. (1987)	Elderly hip fracture	R, B	Regional (RA) vs. general (GA) anaesthesia	28 (RA)	29 (GA)	50 (RA)	38 (GA)
Chung et al. (1987)	Elderly urology	R, B	Regional (RA) vs. general (GA) anaesthesia	20 (RA)	24 (GA)	0 (RA)	7 (GA)
Williams-Russo et al. (1992)	Elderly bilateral knee replacement	R, B	IV fentanyl (IV) vs. epidural analgesia (Epi)	25 (IV)	26 (Epi)	44 (IV)	38 (Epi)
Mann et al. (2000)	Elderly major abdominal surgery	R, B	Patient-controlled analgesia with IV morphine (IV) vs. epidural opioid (Epi) postop	35 (IV)	35 (Epi)	24 (IV)	26 (Epi)

R/NR, Randomized/non-randomized; B/NB, blinded/non-blinded assessment of outcome.

Scaling (Rockwood *et al.* 1993), may be particularly helpful in assessing delirium, in view of the considerable heterogeneity of the study populations.

Comprehensive interventions to prevent delirium

The multifactorial nature of delirium suggests multiple potential interventions to prevent delirium. It also suggests that multicomponent interventions will be more useful than narrowly focused interventions, and there is evidence that this is indeed the case.

Yale-New Haven study of delirium prevention

The major exception to the criticisms outlined earlier is the landmark controlled trial conducted by Inouye and colleagues (1999a) at the Yale-New Haven hospital. They studied 852 patients aged 70 years or more admitted to acute medical units of a teaching hospital (Inouye *et al.* 1999a). Subjects did not have delirium on admission. A pilot study indicated that randomization to different units would not be feasible. Instead, patients from one intervention unit and two usual-care units were enrolled using a prospective matching strategy in which patients were matched according to age and sex and, using the model previously developed by Inouye and Charpentier (1996), by intermediate or high baseline risk of developing delirium. Many patients had dementia, with 25% of patients having a Mini-Mental State Examination score of 20 or less.

The intervention consisted of standardized protocols for the management of six risk factors for delirium: cognitive impairment, sleep deprivation, immobility, visual impairment, hearing impairment, and dehydration. Interventions were implemented by a trained multidisciplinary team supplemented by trained volunteers. Patients were assessed daily until discharge for delirium.

Delirium developed in 9.9% of the intervention group and in 15.0% of the control group [odds ratio 0.60, 95% confidence interval (CI) 0.39–0.92]. In other words, providing the intervention strategy to 19 (95% CI 10–134) patients prevented one patient from developing delirium. The total number of days with delirium (105 versus 161, $P=0.02$) and the number of episodes of delirium (62 versus 90, $P=0.03$) were lower in the intervention group. However, the severity of delirium and the frequency of recurrence did not differ between intervention and control groups. The greatest benefit was seen in patients at intermediate baseline risk for delirium.

The overall rate of adherence to intervention protocols was 87%, and the total number of targeted risk factors per patient was significantly reduced in the intervention group. There was a significant improvement in orientation scores among patients with cognitive impairment at baseline, and use of sedative medications was significantly reduced in the intervention group as a whole. The average cost of the intervention was US$327 for each of the 426 patients in the intervention group, and the cost of intervention per case of delirium prevented was US$6341. A recent economic analysis of this study found that the intervention was cost-effective for those at intermediate risk of developing delirium, but not those at high risk (Rizzo *et al.* 2001).

This trial demonstrates convincingly, for the first time, that delirium can be prevented by a multicomponent strategy. It remains to be seen if the effectiveness of this strategy can be replicated in other settings and what effect reducing the incidence of delirium may have on outcomes such as admission to long-term care and long-term cognitive function. Many of the interventions are relatively straightforward and could readily be applied in other units. Others, such as use of relaxation tapes and back massage to promote sleep and provision of cognitively stimulating activities three times a day to improve cognitive function, will be more difficult to apply. Of course, the relative importance of the component protocols is uncertain, and this is an obvious topic for future research.

Special nursing care

Nursing interventions used in the prevention and management of delirium derive from anecdotal reports and observations and from the reasonable, if unproven, suspicion that psychosocial and environmental factors may contribute to the development and maintenance of delirium (Cronin-Stubbs 1996). The nursing strategies used in prevention studies share many features with those employed in the Yale-New Haven study (Inouye *et al.* 1999a) and in the management trials by Cole *et al.* (1991) and Simon *et al.* (1997). These strategies include careful attention to the physical environment, education of staff to recognize symptoms of delirium, and instruction of staff regarding communication with the delirious or potentially delirious patient. The need for a quiet environment without excessive noise or light is emphasized in most studies. Measures to aid orientation, such as a clock or a calendar, are often employed. Familiar possessions, such as photographs, may be placed on the bedside locker. Staff are asked to communicate slowly and clearly, to make eye contact and to ensure that spectacles and hearing aids are available to patients. Frequent reassurance, explanation, and orientation are advised. Reassurance is particularly important if uncomfortable procedures are performed. Family members are asked to stay with the patient if he or she is confused or frightened. Continuity of care is encouraged. Patients are mobilized as early as possible.

A number of studies have examined whether providing such care to patients might prevent delirium (Table 8.3). In a study of hip fracture patients, Williams *et al.* (1985) reported that 'interpersonal and nursing interventions' to minimize environmental stresses reduced the incidence of delirium from 51.5% in a historical control group to 43.9% in the intervention group. Components of the care provided included repeated orientation and explanation, ensuring that spectacles and hearing aids were worn, provision of adequate analgesia, improved continuity of nursing care, and meticulous attention to bowel and urinary problems. Another recent study of hip fracture patients compared a nurse-led interdisciplinary intervention against usual care (Milisen *et al.* 2001). The intervention involved nurse education, systematic cognitive screening, consultation with specialist psychiatric and nursing staff, and use of a scheduled pain protocol. The intervention did not reduce the incidence of delirium; the duration and severity of delirium was less in the intervention group. A randomized trial of 64 cardiac patients reported that educating the patient preoperatively (Owens and Hutelmyer 1982) about the nature of postoperative delirium and about measures to maintain orientation and function reduced the incidence of delirium from 79% in the control group to 59% in the intervention group. Patients in the intervention group reported feeling comfortable or in control even during delirium. Although delirium was assessed in a blinded manner, there were major baseline differences between the two groups.

Other reports also support these interventions. In a treatment study by Budd and Brown (1974), repeated orientation resulted in a decrease in post-cardiotomy delirium. A randomized study by Chatham (1978) noted fewer symptoms of post-cardiotomy delirium when family members were educated about the importance of eye contact, frequent touch, and verbal orientation. Wanich and colleagues (1992) noted improved functional status (but not confusion) in patients who were mobilized and received orientation and sensory and environmental modifications.

All these studies were flawed: numbers were generally small; few were randomized or had blinded assessment of outcomes. Nevertheless, it is reasonable to conclude that nursing measures do seem useful for preventing delirium in orthopaedic and cardiac surgery patients (Cole 1999). It is more difficult to draw conclusions from the two studies in older medical patients: in the study by Nagley (1986), only one of 60 patients studied became delirious, and in the study by Wanich et al. (1992), 80% of cases of delirium were diagnosed on admission and hence were not amenable to prevention.

It is possible to place too much emphasis on the importance of evidence-based practice. It is obviously appropriate and humane to explain to sick patients where they are and what is happening if they seem uncertain, and to ensure that spectacles and hearing aids are available so that effective communication is possible, irrespective of whether or not there is clear evidence that these measures prevent or improve delirium. Although simple environmental strategies have long been recommended for the management of patients with delirium, a study by Meagher et al. (1996) suggests that these measures are often ignored in favour of psychoactive medications.

Special medical care

Gustafson et al. (1991) examined the incidence of delirium in older hip fracture patients before and after a series of interventions based on changing risk factors. They reported that a joint geriatric-anaesthetic approach reduced the incidence of delirium from 61% in a historical control group to 48% in the intervention group. Episodes of delirium in the intervention group were milder and of shorter duration than those in the control group. Also, complications such as pressure sores, falls, and urinary retention were reduced in the intervention group, and the mean duration of stay on the orthopaedic ward was reduced from 17 to 12 days. Interventions consisted of preoperative and postoperative geriatric assessment, oxygen therapy during surgery and for the first postoperative day, prevention and treatment of perioperative hypotension, and early detection and treatment of postoperative complications. The use of a historical control group in this study means that some caution is needed in interpreting the results. Nevertheless, demographic and clinical features were similar in the control and intervention group, and the authors note that nursing practices remained the same during the two studies.

Delirium is also particularly common in patients with terminal cancer. Dehydration and opioid toxicity, often occurring together, are common potentially reversible risk factors (Lawlor *et al.* 2000). Bruera and colleagues (1995) reported a reduction in 'agitated impaired mental status' in terminal cancer patients in their palliative care unit from 26% in a historical control group to 10% following introduction of a regimen of routine cognitive monitoring, opioid rotation, and careful attention to maintenance of hydration.

Specific interventions to prevent delirium

In the following sections, possible interventions are discussed in terms of the scope for prevention (determined by the frequency of the problem and whether it is practical to intervene) and whether there is any evidence that intervention is effective.

Dehydration

Dehydration is an important cause of hospitalization and increased hospital-associated mortality in older people. For example, in 1991, 6.7% of Medicare hospitalizations had dehydration listed as one of the five reported diagnoses, and about 50% of elderly Medicare beneficiaries hospitalized with dehydration died within a year of admission (Warren *et al.* 1994). Dehydration itself is multifactorial in sick older people; risk factors include the age-associated decline in thirst drive as well as swallowing problems, cognitive impairment, and misuse of diuretics (Weinberg and Minaker 1995). Dehydration has been identified as both a predisposing and a precipitating factor for delirium (Inouye *et al.* 1993; Inouye and Charpentier 1996).

The quality of nursing care is important in the prevention of dehydration. In one study of elderly hospital patients, the most important factor preventing patients taking a drink when asked by a researcher was that the cup was out of reach; even when a cup was within reach, it often contained no fluid (Spencer *et al.* 1999). Careful monitoring of the fluid intake is the best way to recognize the patient who is at risk for dehydration. Physical signs of dehydration have poor sensitivity and specificity in older people (Weinberg and Minaker 1995). Biochemical abnormalities should be monitored and acted upon but may be hard to interpret in older people. Bedside swallow tests are helpful when aspiration is suspected.

Without adequate staffing, there is little point in making hopeful recommendations that patients should be encouraged to drink more when they are ill. For example, volunteers were used to implement the dehydration protocol in the Yale-New Haven study (Inouye *et al.* 1999a). In particular, patients with cognitive impairment may be unable to comply with requests to increase fluid intake and may resist physical help from nursing staff. Family members may be better able to coax a patient into taking fluids (and food). Intravenous cannulation can be very difficult if a patient is unable to cooperate because of cognitive impairment. Subsequently, close supervision is often needed to maintain the drip. Use of subcutaneous infusions (hypodermoclysis) is a valuable alternative to intravenous fluids for prevention and treatment of mild dehydration (O'Keeffe and Geoghegan 2000). In a study of patients with dementia or delirium, subcutaneous fluids were as effective as intravenous fluids at maintaining adequate hydration and were associated with significantly less distress and agitation (O'Keeffe and Lavan 1996).

Dehydration is a particularly important cause of delirium in patients with terminal cancer (Lawlor *et al.* 2000). The issue of hydration in this population is controversial (Fainsinger and Bruera 1997). Nevertheless, hypodermoclysis, as a relatively low-intensity and well-tolerated intervention, may be useful in prevention (and treatment) of delirium (Bruera *et al.* 1995).

Sensory impairment

Visual and hearing impairment are among the most common chronic conditions in older people, although many sufferers remain undetected and untreated. Visual and hearing impairment have also been identified as risk factors for delirium (Inouye *et al.* 1993).

There are many simple measures that could improve vision and hearing among hospital patients. The Yale-New Haven study used readily applicable vision and hearing protocols (Inouye *et al.* 1999a). A standard bedside test for visual impairment was performed, and visual aids and adaptive equipment were provided for patients with less than 20/70 visual acuity. Another bedside test – the Whisper test – was used to assess hearing, and portable amplifying devices and, if appropriate, earwax removal, provided if impairment was identified. It is common to find that spectacles and hearing aids have been left at home when people are admitted urgently to hospital. It is important to ensure that spectacles are clean and that there are working batteries in hearing aids. Knowledge and understanding of visual and hearing loss are often poor among hospital staff; hence, this may also be a suitable subject for educational interventions (Skelly and Millar 1999).

Avoidance of inappropriate prescribing

Inappropriate prescribing is a common problem in older community, nursing home, and hospital patients (McLeod 2000). In studies of elderly hospital patients, drugs have been reported as the cause of delirium in 11–30% of cases (Moore and O'Keeffe 1999). Psychotropic agents and those with significant anticholinergic activity account for a large proportion of inappropriate medications in all settings, and these are also the agents most likely to be associated with delirium (Francis *et al.* 1990). The total burden of anticholinergic drugs may be a more important risk for delirium rather than any single agent (Tune and Egeli 1999). Polypharmacy is particularly associated with the development of delirium, and the risk of drug-induced confusion increases with the number of drugs prescribed (Inouye and Charpentier 1996).

These findings suggest several possible strategies to reduce the frequency of drug-induced delirium (Carter *et al.* 1996; Gray *et al.* 1999; Moore and O'Keeffe 1999). Non-essential drugs should be kept to a minimum in elderly people. Less toxic drugs should replace more toxic drugs whenever possible. This requires education of health-care professionals and of elderly people themselves. Special care is needed for people with pre-existing cognitive impairment. In particular, psychoactive drugs and those with anticholinergic activity should be avoided whenever possible. The adage about prescribing in the elderly, 'start low and go slow', is important in the prevention of confusion and other adverse effects. Blood levels of medications can be useful as a guide to safe prescribing for agents with a narrow therapeutic index, such as digoxin, theophylline, anticonvulsants, and lithium. However, delirium has been reported with all these agents despite serum levels well within the normal limits (Moore and O'Keeffe 1999). Thus, a high index of clinical suspicion is necessary to detect early drug-induced confusion and to prevent further decline.

Greater liaison between pharmacists and clinicians will also improve the appropriateness of prescribing in older patients. In a randomized controlled trial, a clinical pharmacist providing pharmaceutical advice care for elderly primary care patients receiving multiple medications significantly improved appropriateness of medication use; there was a non-significant improvement in the frequency of adverse drug reactions (Hanlon *et al.* 1996). Benefits were also reported in a cohort study in which a computerized drug utilization review database was linked to a telepharmacy intervention (Monane *et al.* 1998).

Sedative medications, particularly benzodiazepines, are the most commonly prescribed psychoactive drugs in hospital patients (Foy *et al.* 1995). The Yale HELP programme has demonstrated that non-pharmacological sleep-promoting techniques can be used to reduce use of benzodiazepines (McDowell *et al.* 1998), although the sleep protocol was also the protocol with the lowest adherence rate in the Yale-New Haven study (Inouye *et al.* 1999a).

Apart from a number of trials of anaesthetic and perioperative interventions (discussed in a later section), there is relatively little direct evidence to support the benefits of medication reduction and monitoring in the prevention of delirium. Nevertheless, some of the agents most associated with delirium are now used less often in clinical practice. For example, the highly anticholinergic agents scopolamine and atropine were traditionally used as premedications before surgery, and delayed or disturbed emergence from anaesthesia and postoperative delirium were common problems (O'Keeffe and Ni Chonchubhair 1994). A reduction in the incidence of postoperative delirium has been reported with the substitution for atropine of the peripherally acting anticholinergic glycopyrronium (Sheref 1985). Studies suggest that about 5% of patients receiving amitriptyline or imipramine, tricyclic antidepressants (TCA) with significant anticholinergic activity, develop delirium (Preskhorn and Jerkovich 1990; Grohmann *et al.* 1999). Many clinicians now prefer to use newer antidepressants such as the selective serotonin reuptake inhibitors (SSRI) or TCAs with relatively little anticholinergic activity, such as desipramine and nortriptyline, in their older patients (Livingston and Livingston 1999).

Opioid toxicity is common in patients with terminal cancer. Some authors (Gagnon *et al.* 1999) have advocated a system of rotation of equianalgesic doses of different opioids to reduce toxicity. In a study with a historical control group, Bruera and colleagues (1995) reported that this contributed to a reduction in agitated confusion in their palliative care unit.

Malnutrition

Although many old people have suboptimal intake of nutrients, clinical evidence of undernutrition is uncommon among older people living in the community (Thomas 1998). On the other hand, undernutrition, defined as a low body mass index or low corrected arm muscle area, is common among older people admitted to hospital, and hospitalization is often associated with a further deterioration in nutritional status. In particular, there is a clear association between low body mass and increased morbidity and mortality in patients with fractured neck of femur (Seymour 1998).

With the exception of vitamin deficiencies, the relationship between delirium and nutritional indices has received little attention. Low serum albumin has been described as a risk factor for delirium (Schor *et al.* 1992), but this more commonly reflects acute and chronic illness than nutritional status. Oral protein and energy feeds may reduce postoperative morbidity in older hip fracture patients, but the evidence is very weak (Avenell and Handoll 2000). While one would expect a reduction in postoperative complications to result in reduced incidence of delirium, this has not been formally evaluated.

Thiamine deficiency

In the Western world, overt thiamine deficiency is usually associated with alcoholism. However, biochemical thiamine deficiency has been frequently found in elderly populations. The reported prevalence in the UK ranges from 8 to 31% for elderly people living in the community and from 23 to 40% for people living in extended nursing care (O'Keeffe 2000). Biochemical thiamine deficiency has also been reported in 48% of patients admitted to an acute geriatric unit (O'Keeffe *et al.* 1994). Reduced dietary intake of thiamine in older people seems the most likely explanation (Wilkinson *et al.* 2000).

Thiamine deficiency is associated with a diffuse decrease in cerebral glucose metabolism and in cholinergic neurotransmission, both important pathogenic mechanisms in the production of delirium (Gibson *et al.* 1991). Autopsy studies have consistently shown a higher incidence of Wernicke–Korsakoff syndrome than was recognized in life (Harper *et al.* 1986). Isolated delirium, without eye signs or ataxia, was the most common feature in cases that were not diagnosed clinically before death. In a study of 36 patients admitted to an acute geriatric unit, delirium was present in 13/17 (76%) patients with thiamine deficiency (only one of whom had a full Wernicke's syndrome) and 6/19 (31%) patients without thiamine deficiency (O'Keeffe *et al.* 1994). Thiamine deficiency is also common following surgery for hip fractures in elderly patients and was associated with postoperative confusion in one study (Older and Dickerson 1982).

Thiamine supplements are clearly indicated in alcoholic patients. Intravenous supplements may be needed in such patients because oral absorption is impaired in alcoholism (Holzbach 1996). The studies quoted above suggest that thiamine deficiency as a cause of delirium may be missed if there is undue focus on alcohol abuse as a risk factor or if diagnosis is only considered when the full-blown clinical picture is present. However, a double-blind randomized controlled trial failed to show that thiamine supplements given preoperatively prevented delirium (Day *et al.* 1988).

Alcohol abuse

Problem drinking has been identified in up to 5% of people aged 65 years or more in the community and in 8–21% of older hospital patients (Seymour and Wattis 1992). Several studies have identified alcohol abuse as a risk factor for delirium; indeed, one study noted that alcohol use greater than three units a week before surgery was associated with a twofold increase in the incidence of delirium (Williams-Russo *et al.* 1992). Alcohol-withdrawal syndrome is associated with a particularly high mortality rate in older patients (Kraemer *et al.* 1997).

Benzodiazepines are effective in reducing delirium (and seizures) in patients withdrawing from alcohol. For example, in a meta-analysis of 65 controlled trials on alcohol withdrawal, benzodiazepines were associated with an absolute risk reduction of 6.6% compared with placebo; this means that 16 patients (95% CI 10–39) need to be treated with benzodiazepines to prevent one episode of delirium (Mayo-Smith 1997). Neuroleptic agents were significantly less effective for reducing delirium (or seizures) in this population. Other agents such as β-blockers and clonidine can reduce withdrawal symptoms but have not been shown to reduce delirium or seizures.

Prevention of the consequences of alcohol withdrawal requires identification of the problem, since alcohol abuse may be successfully hidden from doctors and carers. The CAGE four-question screening test has excellent sensitivity and specificity among older patients; even one affirmative response is highly suggestive of problem drinking in this population (Buchsbaum *et al.* 1992). A modified elder-specific version of Michigan Alcoholism Screening Test (MAST-G) also seems useful for screening older patients (Dufour 1998). The impact of using such tests in preventing delirium has not been examined.

Restraint use

In studies on acute medical and surgical wards in the USA, between 7% and 17% of patients are restrained by cloth or leather devices at some stage during their hospital stay (Evans and Strumpf 1989; Marks 1992). Use of bedrails is even more frequent and is regarded as standard care for elderly people in many hospitals. By contrast, restraints and bedrails are used more sparingly in many other countries (O'Keeffe et al. 1996; Hanger et al. 1999). Patients with cognitive impairment are most likely to be restrained (Marks 1992). However, restraints are particularly unsuitable for such patients since they are liable to increase agitated behaviour, distress, and falls, and there is little evidence of benefit (Frengley 1999). Use of physical restraints was noted as a precipitating factor for delirium in one study (Inouye and Charpentier 1996).

Studies of restraint reduction programmes have found no increased risk of falls or injuries with restraint removal (Evans et al. 1997; Guttman et al. 1999). Minimizing restraints was one component of the successful Yale-New Haven study (Inouye et al. 1999a). Alternative strategies for at-risk patients include use of low adjustable beds, placing such patients close to the nursing station, allowing restless patients to walk around under supervision and placing the mattress on the floor.

Prevention of delirium in the surgical patient

Delirium is common in surgical patients (O'Keeffe and Ni Chonchubhair 1994; Dyer et al. 1995; Parikh and Chung 1995). Prospective studies have found consistently high rates of delirium following hip fracture repair and, to a lesser extent, after elective joint replacement surgery. High rates of postoperative delirium have also been noted after cardiac and transplant surgery and after abdominal aortic aneurysm repair. Delirium occurs in up to 40% of patients admitted to intensive care units. The risk factors for postoperative delirium are generally similar to those noted in delirium in acute medical patients (Marcantonio et al. 1994), although blood loss (Marcantonio et al. 1998) and postoperative pain (Lynch et al. 1998) may be significant additional factors.

Unlike delirium in medical patients, delirium in the surgical patient usually follows a planned insult. This improves the opportunities for instituting effective preventative measures and facilitates research. The benefits of multicomponent interventions involving special nursing care (Williams et al. 1985) or a joint approach by the geriatrician and anaesthetist (Gustafson et al. 1991) have been discussed earlier. A number of studies have examined the benefits of more specific perioperative interventions (see Table 8.3).

Preoperative measures

It is essential to optimize the medical condition of the patient before surgery whenever possible. This will reduce perioperative morbidity and mortality and is very likely to reduce the incidence of delirium. For example, chest infection is a common cause of postoperative delirium. A recent randomized trial has shown that prophylactic chest physiotherapy can reduce the number of patients undergoing elective abdominal surgery who develop radiological and clinical pneumonia; only five patients need be treated to prevent one chest infection (Fagevik Olsén et al. 1997). The study by Gustafsson *et al.* (1991) of a joint approach by the anaesthetist and geriatrician supports the value of a preoperative assessment by the geriatrician.

Preoperative explanation and discussion by the anaesthetist can reduce the need for postoperative analgesia and, hence, the risk of medication toxicity (O'Keeffe and Ni Chonchubhair 1994). It is probably wise, and certainly kind, to warn vulnerable patients and their families about the possibility of transient confusion after surgery. There have been three studies of the effects of preoperative psychiatric assessment and advice on the incidence of postoperative confusion, albeit in predominantly middle-aged cardiac patients (Lazarus and Hagens 1968; Layne and Yudofsky 1971; Schindler *et al.* 1989). The non-randomized studies showed absolute risk reductions in the incidence of delirium of 19% (Lazarus and Hagens 1968) and 12% (Layne and Yudofsky 1971). Schindler *et al.* (1989) performed a randomized study of a structured psychiatric interview to allow patients undergoing coronary artery bypass surgery to express their fears and concerns. There was decreased postoperative morbidity and length of hospital stay but also a 13% greater incidence of delirium in the intervention group.

Perioperative measures

The most important operative features that may promote delirium are use of deliriogenic drugs and impairment of the cerebral oxygen supply. It is dangerous to assume that postoperative delirium is entirely caused by the effects of surgery or anaesthesia. In studies of delirious general surgical patients, postoperative medical or surgical complications were identified in up to 90% of cases (O'Keeffe and Ni Chonchubhair 1994). Nevertheless, it has been hoped that improvements in anaesthetic techniques might lead to a reduction in the incidence of delirium.

Hole *et al.* (1980) suggested that regional anaesthesia was less likely to cause delirium than general anaesthesia: they noted delirium in none of 29 patients receiving extradural anaesthesia and in seven of 31 patients receiving general anaesthesia for hip replacement. However, standardized criteria and mental tests were not used in this study and comparison between techniques was not blinded. Subsequent randomized studies with blinded assessments of outcome failed to demonstrate any difference between the two techniques in the incidence of delirium (Berggren *et al.* 1987; Chung *et al.* 1987) or, except perhaps during the first 24 hours after surgery, in the results of psychometric tests (Jones *et al.* 1990; Williams-Russo *et al.* 1995).

Prevention and treatment of operative hypotension and hypoxaemia are regarded as very important in the management of the older surgical patient. Williams-Russo *et al.* (1999) conducted a randomized, controlled clinical trial in 235 older adults (mean age 72 years) with co-morbid medical illnesses undergoing elective total hip replacement with epidural anaesthesia. Patients were randomly assigned to one of two levels of intraoperative mean arterial blood pressure management: a markedly hypotensive mean arterial blood pressure range of 45–55 mmHg or a less hypotensive range of

55–70 mmHg. There were no significant differences in the incidence of early or long-term cognitive dysfunction (measured using neuropsychological tests) or in the incidence of delirium between the two blood pressure management groups. While this study does suggest that controlled hypotension can be well tolerated in selected elective elderly surgical patients, studies in elderly hip fracture patients support the benefit of avoiding hypotension (Gustafson *et al.* 1991).

A number of studies have examined the effects of different analgesic techniques on the incidence of delirium. In one randomized trial, 'significant confusion' developed in 18% of patients given intramuscular morphine for postoperative pain and 2% of patients given a similar dose via patient-controlled analgesia (Egbert *et al.* 1990). The authors attributed this difference to higher peak concentrations of morphine in the first group. Williams-Russo *et al.* (1992) conducted a randomized controlled trial to compare the effect of postoperative analgesia using epidural versus intravenous infusions on the incidence of delirium after bilateral knee replacement surgery in 60 elderly patients. The overall incidence of acute delirium was 41%, with no difference between types of postoperative analgesia. Mann *et al.* (2000) recently conducted a randomized study comparing patient-controlled analgesia with intravenous morphine and patient-controlled epidural analgesia using an opioid in combination with a local anaesthetic in 70 patients older than 70 years of age undergoing major abdominal surgery. Although pain relief was better at rest in the epidural group, the incidence of delirium was similar in the two groups.

Postoperative care

Early recognition and treatment of medical and surgical complications may prevent development of delirium. In the successful prevention study by Gustafson and colleagues (1988), patients in the intervention group received several postoperative visits by a geriatrician. Marcantonio *et al.* (1998) noted that, even after adjusting for preoperative risk factors, delirium was associated with a postoperative haematocrit <30%. Gustafson *et al.* (1988) had also noted that the intervention group in their study received more transfusions than the control group, and they postulated that this might have contributed to better cerebral oxygen transport and hence to the reduced duration and severity of delirium. Controlled studies are needed to determine whether transfusion to keep postoperative haematocrit above 30% might indeed reduce the incidence of postoperative delirium.

Hypoxaemia is common in the postoperative period, especially during sleep and after administration of opioids, and it has been reported that supplementary oxygen is an effective treatment for delirium in patients who have had a thoracotomy (Aakerlund and Rosenberg 1994) or major abdominal surgery (Rosenberg and Kehlet 1993). It has been presumed that such patients would benefit from monitoring for hypoxaemia by pulse oximetry. However, the only randomized trial of this approach (albeit in patients with a mean age of 55 years) found no diminution in the incidence of postoperative cognitive impairment in patients monitored by pulse oximetry (Moller *et al.* 1993).

Also, an international multicentre study of 1218 patients aged 60 years and older receiving major non-cardiac surgery under general anaesthesia did not find that hypoxaemia or hypotension was related to short-term and long-term cognitive dysfunction (Moller *et al.* 1998). However, since patients with pre-existing brain damage, may be particularly sensitive to the effects of mild-to-moderate hypoxaemia, these findings do not exclude some role for hypoxaemia in the pathogenesis of delirium in this population.

Another possible approach to the prevention of delirium in surgical patients might be the prophylactic preoperative and/or postoperative use of specific medications in high-risk individuals or groups. There is currently some interest in the preventive potential of drugs such as cholinesterase inhibitors and haloperidol, but to date no trials have been published to support their use in this respect.

Improving hospital care for older people

If modern systems of hospital care are contributing to the development of geriatric syndromes like delirium, the most logical form of prevention is to improve the system of care for older people. This is, of course, a daunting task but a number of studies have demonstrated the potential value of this approach.

Geriatric consultation services

This is the least costly approach to bringing specialist expertise to bear on the problems of older people in hospital. These services involve assessment of patients by a mutidisciplinary team, usually led by a physician. Two randomized trials have failed to find measurable differences between patients receiving geriatric consultation and controls (Winograd *et al.* 1993; Reuben *et al.* 1995). This may reflect difficulties in persuading medical and nursing staff to implement recommendations. In contrast to these negative findings, a recent trial of a proactive approach to geriatric consultation in hip fracture patients found that this reduced the incidence of delirium by one-third, and that of severe delirium by over one-half (Marcantonio *et al.* 2001). Consultations were initiated either preoperatively or within 24 hours of surgery, with the geriatrician visiting daily thereafter to make recommendations based on a structured protocol. The intervention was most effective in those patients without pre-existing dementia or functional impairment. The adherence of the orthopaedic team to the recommendations was relatively high (77%), which may explain the positive findings in this study. While a consultation service may help in the investigation and management of individual patients with delirium, unless its recommendations are consistently acted upon, it is unlikely to have much impact on the broader problem of overall hospital care and practices contributing to the development of delirium.

Geriatric post-acute evaluation units

In a randomized clinical trial, Rubenstein *et al.* (1984) demonstrated that patients transferred to their geriatric evaluation unit had lower mortality, better functional

status and less likelihood of admission to nursing homes than controls over 1 year follow up. Others have reported similar findings (Applegate *et al.* 1990). These results are
very impressive. However, the fact that many episodes of delirium develop early in the
course of a hospital stay will limit the ability of such units to prevent delirium.

Acute geriatric units

Acute geriatric units allow the implementation of good geriatric care in routine practice from the time of admission. The Acute Care of the Elderly (ACE) unit in Cleveland,
Ohio, described by Landefeld *et al.* (1995), was explicitly designed to avoid complications of hospitalization. Elements of the care provided included multidisciplinary
assessment and management aimed at maintaining neurocognitive function, protocols
for dealing with common geriatric problems including delirium, and a physical environment geared towards older patients. A randomized trial of 651 patients, of whom
11% were noted to have acute confusion, showed better functional outcomes and less
nursing home admissions in ACE patients than in controls without any increase
in length of stay or cost. However, there was no effect on function at 3 months after
discharge, perhaps reflecting lack of appropriate community supports.

The outcome of delirium was not specifically evaluated in the Landefeld study.
Studies in acute geriatric units in the British Isles report a similar incidence of delirium, and similarly poor outcomes as a consequence, as do studies conducted in general
medical and surgical units. For example, O'Keeffe and Lavan (1997) noted a 30% incidence of delirium following admission to an acute geriatric unit sharing all of the care
aspects described as part of the Cleveland ACE unit. This may not be a fair comparison, however, since acute geriatric units will in general specifically target those patients
most at risk for delirium and a high incidence of delirium can be predicted on that
basis. Nevertheless, it does suggest that specific interventions and protocols are needed
to prevent delirium (Francis 1997).

Specialized delirium ward

Wahlund and Björlin (1999) have described a specialized 16-bed delirium ward in the
700-bed Huddinge Hospital in Sweden. Over a 17-month period, 637 patients were
admitted to this ward with suspected delirium, of whom 169 (27%) ultimately received
a diagnosis of delirium. Most referrals came from the emergency department. Patients
admitted to the ward were selected and managed by geriatricians. No details were
provided of the nursing care provided or of the physical layout of the ward.

Improving hospital-wide care for older people

The approaches outlined above can only apply to a minority of older patients in any
institution. A more ambitious alternative is to seek to improve standards of geriatric
care throughout the institution. In England, Grimley Evans in Newcastle pioneered
integration of geriatric medicine with general medicine, with the aim of spreading the

principles of good geriatric care throughout the hospital (Grimley Evans 1997). However, no study has ever been conducted to show that spread of good geriatric practice does actually occur (as opposed to spread of bad practices among the geriatricians).

Hospital elder life programme

Inouye and colleagues (1999b) have argued persuasively that the incidence of delirium is a marker of the quality of hospital care and that prevention of delirium requires local, and national, strategies that will also benefit other geriatric syndromes. They recommended routine cognitive assessment and monitoring, development of strategies to change poor practices, use of clinical guidelines, and pathways to manage common problems, improve case management and continuity of care and enhance the provision of skilled nursing and geriatric care at the bedside. The model of care provided in their landmark study on prevention of delirium was based on these principles (Inouye *et al.* 1999a). They have since described in detail how this model Hospital Elder Life Program (HELP) has been successfully extended into a permanent programme serving three 28-bed general medical units in their 800-bed hospital (Inouye *et al.* 2000).

All older patients admitted to this unit are screened for risk factors for delirium, and interventions for these risk factors are implemented by an interdisciplinary team who work in liaison with primary nurses. There is a heavy reliance on community volunteers to assist with some interventions. There is regular monitoring of adherence to the protocols and of patient and carer satisfaction. To date, over 1500 patients have been enrolled, and the overall adherence rate was 89% for at least partial adherence to all interventions. The start-up and maintenance costs are moderate, and preliminary cost-effectiveness analyses suggest that the programme may actually save money.

Improving recognition of delirium

Prevention of delirium requires education of doctors and nurses about the importance of the syndrome as a cause of poor outcomes and about the clinical features and risk factors. Education of nurses about delirium has been an essential component of many intervention studies (Cronin-Stubbs 1996; Britton and Russell 2000). Also, some reports have discussed education of patients (Owens and Hutelmyer 1982) or their spouses (Chatham 1978).

Rockwood (1999) has pointed out that few intervention studies to date have been explicitly designed to meet the standard educational principles of relevance to educational needs, integration of new information, and individual, non-judgemental feedback. He and his colleagues in Halifax, Canada performed a before/after study of an educational intervention to improve recognition and management of delirium aimed at medical staff (Rockwood *et al.* 1994). Delirium was discussed at grand rounds, teaching seminars, and during consults and routine bedside patient care. Diagnosis of delirium (or an acceptable synonym) increased from 3% before to 9% after the intervention ($P<0.01$). The intervention described in this study was incorporated into the hospital's regular educational programme and could readily be applied in other institutions.

Other than in specialist units, it is difficult to get medical and nursing staff to perform formal mental status testing. In the Halifax study, although significantly more patients had their memory assessed after the intervention than before (11% versus 3%, $P=0.01$), 'orientation' continued to be the most commonly assessed cognitive domain (49% versus 53%, $P=0.38$) (Rockwood *et al.* 1994). While assessment of orientation can never substitute for a more complete examination of cognitive function, severity of temporal disorientation is moderately predictive of results on more detailed cognitive testing (O'Keeffe *et al.* 2001). Varney and Shephard (1991) have suggested that serial assessment of temporal orientation may be useful in monitoring change in cognitive status in delirious patients. Thus, encouraging staff to note the actual answers to orientation questions will provide more information than simply reporting orientation as either present or absent, as often happens at present. It may also be helpful to emphasize the fact that impairment of attentiveness is a cardinal symptom of delirium, since assessment of this cognitive domain can be incorporated into routine history-taking. We have found that the overall impression of experienced physicians after a brief conversation with a patient is a valuable guide to attentiveness, and hence to the likelihood that delirium is present (O'Keeffe and Gosney 1997).

What limited research there has been to date has focused on local efforts at improving knowledge of delirium and its significance. Inouye *et al.* (1999b) have emphasized the need for system-wide or national initiatives to improve awareness of delirium and of interventions that may impact on delirium. These include changes to the training curriculum for medical, nursing, and paramedical staff and the development of systems to monitor delirium as an indicator of the quality of in-patient care.

Improving care for older people outside hospitals

It is well established that there are considerable unmet medical and social needs among older people living in the community or in residential care. However, it has been harder to prove the effectiveness of preventative assessment programmes, and implementation strategies will depend on the nature of the health service.

Prevention of delirium is but a small aspect of the potential benefits of preventative measures for older people. Nevertheless, there are some measures one would expect to impact on the frequency of delirium. For example, chest infection is among the most commonly identified acute illnesses associated with delirium. Influenza vaccination reduces the incidence of hospitalization and of mortality, although the take-up rate in older populations is often disappointingly low (Gross *et al.* 1998). Although there have been reports that cholinesterase inhibitors may be beneficial in the treatment of delirium (Wengel *et al.* 1998), the possible effects of treating demented patients with these agents on the incidence of delirium have not yet been examined.

Cognitive impairment is particularly common in nursing home residents, and these patients have a high risk of developing delirium in hospital (Levkoff *et al.* 1992). Measures that might be helpful to prevent delirium in nursing home residents include pharmacy interventions to reduce polypharmacy with anticholinergic compounds (Blazer *et al.* 1983; Tollefsen *et al.* 1991) and, particularly in nursing homes that cannot provide intravenous therapy, use of hypodermoclysis to prevent dehydration during acute illness.

One approach to preventing complications of hospitalization is to reduce length of stay or even avoid admission to hospital altogether. Hospital at-home schemes provide, in a patient's own home, care that is usually available only in hospital (for example, observation, administration of drugs, support, nursing care, and rehabilitation). A recent randomized trial of older patients in Leicester, England confirmed earlier reports that this approach costs less than standard hospital care and results in equivalent health status outcomes (Wilson *et al.* 1999). Although almost a third of patients enrolled had some cognitive impairment, the effect on the frequency of delirium was not examined.

Carers are more likely to detect prodromal features of delirium than hospital staff. Chest and urinary tract infections often repeatedly present with delirium. In such cases, it may be useful to provide a reliable carer with a supply of antibiotics for use when they detect early symptoms of increased confusion.

Conclusions

Many risk factors for delirium are potentially preventable or avoidable. This is particularly true for those risk factors arising during hospitalization. Thus delirium can be regarded as a marker of the quality of hospital care. The Yale-New Haven study has provided convincing evidence that delirium can be prevented using a systematic strategy aimed at promoting orientation and mobility, use of non-pharmacological treatments to promote sleep, early recognition and management of dehydration, and use of measures to manage visual and hearing impairment (Inouye *et al.* 1999a). Although many other studies on prevention of delirium have suffered from a variety of methodological flaws, the weight of evidence supports the benefits of nursing interventions aimed at reorienting and reassuring the patient in preventing delirium (Cronin-Stubbs 1996).

Postoperative delirium has been the subject of many studies. There is evidence that meticulous preoperative and postoperative care by the geriatrician and anaesthetist working together can reduce delirium in hip fracture patients (Gustafson *et al.* 1991). Patient-controlled analgesia seems less likely to cause delirium than regular fixed-dose analgesia in older surgical patients (Egbert *et al.* 1990). On the other hand, general anaesthesia is no more likely to cause delirium than regional anaesthesia, provided both are administered in an expert manner (Berggren *et al.* 1987).

There is much that remains uncertain. Although delirium has been shown to be preventable by a multicomponent strategy in a clinical trial, replication of these results in other settings is needed. Further work is needed to determine how best to implement preventative strategies in everyday clinical practice. This may require not only education of medical and nursing staff to appreciate the importance of delirium, but also a change in the culture of hospitals. If far-reaching changes are to be recommended, the cost-effectiveness of interventions to prevent delirium, and other geriatric syndromes, must be determined. This will require examination not only of the effects of interventions on the incidence of delirium but also what effect reducing the incidence of delirium may have on outcomes such as admission to long-term care and long-term cognitive function.

Since delirium is a multifactorial syndrome, it is understandable that systematic multicomponent interventions are most likely to prove effective. Nevertheless, there is also a need to examine the role of specific interventions in the prevention of delirium. For example, it is uncertain as yet whether nutritional and vitamin supplements, greater liaison between pharmacists and clinicians, or use of hypodermoclysis can prevent delirium. It is important that future studies have sufficient power to answer such questions definitively. This will be facilitated by use of standardized assessment instruments to diagnose delirium and to measure its severity and by targeting of high-risk populations.

References

Aakerlund, L. P. and Rosenberg, J. (1994). Postoperative delirium: treatment with supplementary oxygen. *British Journal of Anaesthesia*, **72**, 286–290.

Allen, C., Glasziou, P., and Del Mar, C. (2000). Bed rest: a potentially harmful treatment needing more careful evaluation. *Lancet*, **354**, 1229–1233.

Applegate, W. B., Miller, S. T., Graney, M. J., Elam, J. T., Burns, R., and Akins, D. E. (1990). A randomized, controlled trial of a geriatric assessment unit in a community rehabilitation hospital. *New England Journal of Medicine*, **322**, 1572–1578.

Armstrong-Esther, C. A. (1986). The influence of elderly patients' mental condition on nurse-patient interaction. *Journal of Advanced Nursing*, **11**, 379–387.

Avenell, A. and Handoll, H. H. (2000). Nutritional supplementation for hip fracture aftercare in the elderly. *Cochrane Database of Systematic Reviews*, **2**, CD001880.

Becker, P. M., McVey, L. J., Saltz, C. C., Feussner, J. R., and Cohen, H. J. (1987) Hospital-acquired complications in a randomized controlled trial of a geriatric consultation team. *Journal of the American Medical Association*, **257**, 2313–2317.

Berggren, D., Gustafson, Y., Eriksson, B., *et al.* (1987). Postoperative confusion after anaesthesia in elderly patients with femoral neck fractures. *Anesthesia and Analgesia*, **66**, 497–504.

Blazer, D. G., Federspiel, C. F., Ray, W. A., *et al.* (1983). The risk of anticholinergic toxicity in the elderly: a study of prescribing practices in two populations. *Journal of Gerontology*, **38**, 31–35.

Brennan, T. A., Leape, L. L., Laird, N. M., *et al.* (1991). Incidence of adverse events and negligence in hospitalized patients. *New England Journal of Medicine*, **324**, 370–376.

Britton, A. and Russell, R. (2000). Multidisciplinary team interventions for delirium in patients with chronic cognitive impairment. *Cochrane Database of Systematic Reviews*, **2**, CD000395.

Bruera, E., Franco, J. J., Maltoni, M., Watanabe, S., and Suarez-Almazor, M. (1995). Changing pattern of agitated impaired mental status in patients with advanced cancer: association with cognitive monitoring, hydration, and opioid rotation. *Journal of Pain and Symptom Management*, **10**, 287–291.

Buchsbaum, D. G., Buchanan, R. G., Welsh, J., *et al.* (1992). Screening for drinking disorders in the elderly using the CAGE questionnaire. *Journal of the American Geriatrics Society*, **40**, 662–665.

Budd, S. and Brown, W. (1974). Effect of a reorientation technique on postcardiotomy delirium. *Nursing Research*, **23**, 341–348.

Cameron, D. J., Thomas, R. I., Mulvihill, M., and Bronheim, H. (1987). Delirium: a test of the Diagnostic and Statistical Manual III criteria on medical inpatients. *Journal of the American Geriatrics Society*, **35**, 1007–1010.

Carter, G. L., Dawson, A. H., and Lopert, R. (1996). Drug-induced delirium. Incidence, management and prevention. *Drugs and Safety*, **15**, 291–301.

Chatham, M. A. (1978). The effect of family involvement on patients' manifestations of postcardiotomy psychosis. *Heart Lung*, **7**, 995–999.

Chung, F., Meier, R., Lautenschlager, E., Carmichael, F. J., and Chung, A. (1987). General or spinal anesthesia: which is better in the elderly? *Anesthesiology*, **67**, 422–427.

Cole, M. G. (1999). Delirium: effectiveness of systematic interventions. *Dementia and Geriatric Cognitive Disorders*, **10**, 406–411.

Cole, M. G., Fenton, F. R., Engelsmann, F., and Mansouri, I. (1991). Effectiveness of geriatric psychiatry consultation in an acute hospital: a randomized controlled trial. *Journal of the American Geriatrics Society*, **39**, 1183–1188.

Cole, M. G., Primeau, F., and McCusker, J. (1996). Effectiveness of interventions to prevent delirium in hospitalized patients: a systematic review. *Canadian Medical Association Journal*, **155**, 1263–1268.

Creditor, M. C. (1993). Hazards of hospitalization of the elderly. *Annals of Internal Medicine*, **118**, 219–223.

Cronin-Stubbs, D. (1996). Delirium intervention research in acute care settings. *Annual Review of Nursing Research*, **14**, 57–73.

Day, J. J., Bayer, A. J., McMahon, M., Pathy, M. S. J., Spragg, B. P., and Rowlands, D. C. (1988). Thiamine status, vitamin supplements and postoperative confusion. *Age and Ageing*, **17**, 29–34.

Dufour, M. C. (1998). Alcohol: use and abuse. In: *Principles and Practice of Geriatric Medicine*, 3rd edn, pp. 175–182. John Wiley & Sons, Chichester.

Dyer, C. B., Ashton, C. M., and Teasdale, T. A. (1995). Postoperative delirium. A review of 80 primary data-collection studies. *Archives of Internal Medicine*, **155**, 461–465.

Egbert, A. M., Parks, L. H., Short, L. M., *et al.* (1990). Randomized trial of postoperative patient-controlled analgesia vs intramuscular narcotics in frail elderly men. *Archives of Internal Medicine*, **150**, 1897–1903.

Elie, M., Cole, M. G., Primeau, F. J., and Bellavance, F. (1998). Delirium risk factors in elderly hospitalized patients. *Journal of General Internal Medicine*, **13**, 204–212.

Evans, L. K. and Strumpf, N. E. (1989). Tying down the elderly. A review of the literature on physical restraint. *Journal of the American Geriatrics Society*, **36**, 65–74.

Evans, L. K., Strumpf, N. E., Allen-Taylor, S. L., Capezuti, E., Maislin, G., and Jacobsen, B. (1997). A clinical trial to reduce restraints in nursing homes. *Journal of the American Geriatrics Society*, **45**, 675–681.

Fagevik Olsén, M., Hahn, I., Nordgren, S., Lönroth, H., and Lundholm, K. (1997). Randomized controlled trial of prophylactic chest physiotherapy in major abdominal surgery. *British Journal of Surgery*, **84**, 1535–1538.

Fainsinger, R. L. and Bruera, E. (1997). When to treat dehydration in a terminally ill patient? *Supportive Care in Cancer*, **5**, 205–211.

Farrell, K. R. and Ganzini, L. (1995). Misdiagnosing delirium as depression in medically ill elderly patients. *Archives of Internal Medicine*, **155**, 2459–2464.

Foy, A., O'Connell, D., Henry, D. D., *et al.* (1995). Benzodiazepine use as a cause of cognitive impairment in elderly hospital patients. *Journal of Gerontology*, **50**, M99–M106.

Francis, J. (1992). Delirium in older patients. *Journal of the American Geriatrics Society*, **40**, 829–838.

Francis, J. (1997). Outcomes of delirium: can systems of care make a difference? *Journal of the American Geriatrics Society*, **45**, 247–248.

Francis, J., Martin, D., and Kapoor, W. N. (1990). A prospective study of delirium in hospitalized elderly. *Journal of the American Medical Association*, **263**, 1097–1101.

Frengley, J. D. (1999). Bedrails: do they have a benefit? *Journal of the American Geriatrics Society*, **47**, 627–628.

Gagnon, B., Bielech, M., Watanabe, S., Walker, P., Hanson, J., and Bruera, E. (1999). The use of intermittent subcutaneous injections of oxycodone for opioid rotation in patients with cancer pain. *Supportive Care in Cancer*, **7**, 265–270.

Gibson, G. E., Blass, J. P., Huang, H-M., and Freeman, G. B. (1991). The cellular basis of delirium and its relevance to dementias including Alzheimer's disease. *International Psychogeriatrics*, **3**, 373–396.

Gillick, M. R., Serrell, N. A., and Gillick, L. S. (1982). Adverse consequences of hospitalization in the elderly. *Social Science and Medicine*, **16**, 1033–1038.

Gray, S. L., Lai, K. V., and Larson, E. B. (1999). Drug-induced cognition disorders in the elderly: incidence, prevention and management. *Drugs and Safety*, **21**, 101–122.

Grimley Evans, J. (1997). Geriatric medicine: a brief history. *British Medical Journal*, **315**, 1075–1077.

Grohmann, R., Rüther, E., Engel, R. R., and Hippius, H. (1999). Assessment of adverse drug reactions in psychiatric inpatients with the AMSP drug safety programme: methods and first results for tricyclic antidepressants and SSRI. *Pharmacopsychiatry*, **32**, 21–28.

Gross, P. A., Hermogenes, A. W., Sacks, H. S., Lau, J., and Levandowski, R. A. (1995). The efficacy of influenza vaccine in elderly persons. A meta-analysis and review of the literature. *Annals of Internal Medicine*, **123**, 518–527.

Gustafson, Y., Bergrren, D., Brannstrom, B., *et al.* (1988). Acute confusional states in elderly patients treated for femoral neck fractures. *Journal of the American Geriatrics Society*, **36**, 525–530.

Gustafson, Y., Brannstrom, B., Berggren, D., *et al.* (1991). A geriatric-anaesthesiologic program to reduce acute confusional states in elderly patients treated for femoral neck fractures. *Journal of the American Geriatrics Society*, **39**, 655–662.

Guttman, R., Altman, R. D., and Karlan, M. S. (1999). Council on Scientific Affairs, American Medical Association. Use of restraints for patients in nursing homes. *Archives of Family Medicine*, **8**, 101–105.

Hanger, H. C., Ball, M. C. and Wood, L. A. (1999). An analysis of falls in the hospital: can we do without bedrails? *Journal of the American Geriatrics Society*, **47**, 529–531.

Hanlon, J. T., Weinberger, M., Samsa, G. P., *et al.* (1996). A randomized, controlled trial of a clinical pharmacist intervention to improve inappropriate prescribing in elderly outpatients with polypharmacy. *American Journal of Medicine*, **100**, 428–437.

Harper, C. G., Giles, M. and Finlay-Jones, R. (1986). Clinical signs in the Wernicke-Korsakoff complex. *Journal of Neurology, Neurosurgery and Psychiatry*, **49**, 341–345.

Hole, A., Terjesen, T., and Breivik, H. (1980). Epidural versus general anaesthesia for total hip arthroplasty in elderly patients. *Acta Anaesthesia Scandanavica*, **24**, 279–287.

Holzbach, E. (1996). Thiamine absorption in alcoholic delirium patients. *Journal of Studies in Alcohol*, **57**, 581–584.

Inouye, S. K. and Charpentier, P. A. (1996). Precipitating factors for delirium in hospitalized elderly persons. Predictive model and interrelationship with baseline vulnerability. *Journal of the American Medical Association*, **275**, 852–857.

Inouye, S. K., Viscoli, C. M., Horwitz, R. I., *et al.* (1993). A predictive model for delirium in hospitalized elderly medical patients based on admission characteristics. *Annals of Internal Medicine*, **119**, 474–481.

Inouye, S. K., Bogardus, S. T. Jr, Charpentier, P. A., *et al.* (1999a). A multicomponent intervention to prevent delirium in hospitalized older patients. *New England Journal of Medicine*, **340**, 669–676.

Inouye, S. K., Schlesinger, M. J., and Lydon, T. J. (1999b). Delirium: a symptom of how hospital care is failing older persons and a window to improve quality of hospital care. *American Journal of Medicine*, **106**, 565–573.

Inouye, S. K., Bogardus, S. T., Baker, D. I., Leo-Summers, L., and Cooney, L. M. (2000). The hospital elder life program: a model of care to prevent cognitive and functional decline in older hospitalized patients. *Journal of the American Geriatrics Society*, **48**, 1697–1706.

Jarrett, P. G., Rockwood, K., Carver, D., Stolee, P., and Cosway, S. (1995). Illness presentation in elderly patients. *Archives of Internal Medicine*, **155**, 1060–1064.

Jones, M. J. T., Piggott, S. E., Vaugans, R. S., *et al.* (1990). Cognitive and functional competence after anaesthesia in patients aged over 60: controlled trial of general and regional anaesthesia for elective hip or knee replacement. *British Medical Journal*, **300**, 1683–1687.

Kitwood, T. (1997). *Dementia reconsidered*. Open University Press, Buckingham.

Kraemer, K. L., Mayo-Smith, M. F., and Calkins, D. R. (1997). Impact of age on the severity, course, and complications of alcohol withdrawal. *Archives of Internal Medicine*, **157**, 2234–2241.

Landefeld, C. S., Palmer, R. M., Kresevic, D. M., Fortinsky, R. H., and Kowal, J. (1995). A randomized trial of care in a hospital medical unit especially designed to improve the functional outcomes of acutely ill older patients. *New England Journal of Medicine*, **332**, 1338–1344.

Lawlor, P. G., Gagnon, B., Mancini, I. L., *et al.* (2000). Occurrence, causes, and outcome of delirium in patients with advanced cancer: a prospective study. *Archives of Internal Medicine*, **160**, 786–794.

Layne, O. L. and Yudofsky, S. C. (1971). Postoperative psychosis in cardiotomy patients. The role of organic and psychiatric factors. *New England Journal of Medicine*, **284**, 518–520.

Lazarus, B. A., Murphy, J. B., Coletta, E. M., McQuade, W. H., and Culpepper, L. (1991). The provision of physical activity to hospitalised elderly patients. *Archives of Internal Medicine*, **151**, 2452–2456.

Lazarus, H. R. and Hagens, J. H. (1968). Prevention of psychosis following open-heart surgery. *American Journal of Psychiatry*, **124**, 1190–1195.

Levkoff, S. E., Evans, D. A., Liptzin, B., *et al.* (1992). Delirium: the occurrence and persistence of among hospitalized elderly patients. *Archives of Internal Medicine*, **152**, 334–340.

Lewis, L. M., Miller, D. K., Morley, J. E., Nork, M. J., and Lasater, L. C. (1995). Unrecognized delirium in ED geriatric patients. *American Journal of Emergency Medicine*, **13**, 142–145.

Livingston, M. G. and Livingston, H. (1999). New antidepressants for older people? *British Medical Journal*, **318**, 1640–1641.

Lynch, E. P., Lazor, M. A., Gellis, J. E., Orav, J., Goldman, L., and Marcantonio, E. R. (1998). The impact of postoperative pain on the development of postoperative delirium. *Anesthesia and Analgesia*, **86**, 781–785.

Mann, C., Pouzeratte, Y., Boccara, G., *et al.* (2000). Comparison of intravenous or epidural patient-controlled analgesia in the elderly after major abdominal surgery. *Anesthesiology*, **92**, 433–441.

Marcantonio, E. R., Juarez, G., Goldman, L., *et al.* (1994). The relationship of postoperative delirium with psychoactive medications. *Journal of the American Medical Association*, **272**, 1518–1522.

Marcantonio, E. R., Goldman, L., Orav, E. J., Cook, E. F., and Lee, T. H. (1998). The association of intraoperative factors with the development of postoperative delirium. *American Journal of Medicine*, **105**, 380–384.

Marcantonio, E. R., Flacker, J. M., Wright, R. J., and Resnick, N. M. (2001). Reducing delirium after hip fracture: a randomized trial. *Journal of the American Geriatrics Society*, **49**, 678–679.

Marks, W. (1992). Physical restraints in the practice of medicine. Current concepts. *Archives of Internal Medicine*, **152**, 2203–2206.

Mayo-Smith, M. F., for the American Society of Addiction Medicine Working Group on Pharmacological Management of Alcohol Withdrawal (1997). Pharmacological management of alcohol withdrawal. A meta-analysis and evidence-based practice guideline. *Journal of the American Medical Association*, **278**, 144–151.

McDowell, J. A., Mion, L. C., Lydon, T. J., and Inouye, S. K. (1998). A nonpharmacologic sleep protocol for hospitalized older patients. *Journal of the American Geriatrics Society*, **46**, 700–705.

McLeod, P. J. (2000). A complex conspiracy against the elderly: inappropriate prescribing. *Canadian Journal of Clinical Pharmacology*, **7**, 85–86.

Meagher, D. J., O'Hanlon, D., O'Mahony, E., and Casey, P. R. (1996). The use of environmental strategies and psychotropic medication in the management of delirium. *British Journal of Psychiatry*, **168**, 512–515.

Milisen, K., Foreman, M. D., Abraham, I. L., *et al.* (2001). A nurse-led interdisciplinary intervention program for delirium in elderly hip-fracture patients. *Journal of the American Geriatrics Society*, **49**, 680–681.

Moller, J. T., Svennild, I., Johannsessen, N. W., *et al.* (1993). Perioperative monitoring with pulse oximetry and late postoperative cognitive dysfunction. *British Journal of Anaesthesia*, **71**, 340–347.

Moller, J. T., Cluitmans, P., and Rasmussen, L. S. (1998). Long-term postoperative cognitive dysfunction in the elderly ISPOCD1 study. *Lancet*, **351**, 857–861.

Monane, M., Matthias, D. M., Nagle, B. A., and Kelly, M. A. (1998). Improving prescribing patterns for the elderly through an online drug utilization review intervention: a system linking the physician, pharmacist, and computer. *Journal of the American Medical Association*, **280**, 1249–1252.

Moore, A. R. and O'Keeffe, S. T. (1999). Drug-induced cognitive impairment in the elderly. *Drugs and Aging*, **15**, 15–28.

Morse, R. M. and Litin, E. M. (1971). The anatomy of a delirium. *American Journal of Psychiatry*, **128**, 111–116.

Nagley, S. J. (1986). Predicting and preventing confusion in your patients. *Journal of Gerontological Nursing*, **12**, 27–31.

O'Keeffe, S. T. (2000). Thiamine deficiency in elderly people. *Age and Ageing*, **29**, 99–101.

O'Keeffe, S. T. and Geoghegan, M. (2000). Subcutaneous hydration in the elderly. *Irish Medical Journal*, **93**, 197–199.

O'Keeffe, S. T. and Gosney, M. A. (1997). Assessing attentiveness in older hospital patients: global assessment versus tests of attention. *Journal of the American Geriatrics Society*, **45**, 470–473.

O'Keeffe, S. T. and Lavan, J. N. (1996). Subcutaneous fluids in elderly hospital patients with cognitive impairment. *Gerontology*, **42**, 36–39.

O'Keeffe, S. and Lavan, J. (1997). The prognostic significance of delirium in older hospital patients. *Journal of the American Geriatrics Society*, **45**, 174–178.

O'Keeffe, S. T. and Ní Chonchubhair, A. (1994). Postoperative delirium in the elderly. *British Journal of Anaesthesia*, **73**, 673–687.

O'Keeffe, S. T., Tormey, W. P., Glasgow, R., and Lavan, J. N. (1994). Thiamine deficiency in hospitalized elderly patients. *Gerontology*, **40**, 18–24.

O'Keeffe, S. T., Jack, C. I. A., and Lye, M. (1996). Use of restraints and bedrails in a British hospital. *Journal of the American Geriatrics Society*, **44**, 1086–1088.

O'Keeffe, S . T., Crowe, M., Gustau, B., and Pillay I. (2001). Interpreting errors in temporal orientation in older hospital patients. *Journal of Clinical Geropsychology*, **7**, 47–52.

Older, M. W. J. and Dickerson, J. W. T. (1982). Thiamine and the elderly orthopaedic patient. *Age and Ageing*, **11**, 101–107.

Owens, J. F. and Hutelmyer, C. M. (1982). The effect of preoperative intervention on delirium in cardiac surgical patients. *Nursing Research*, **31**, 60–62.

Parikh, S. S. and Chung, F. (1995). Postoperative delirium in the elderly. *Anesthesia and Analgesia*, **80**, 1223–1232.

Preskorn, S. H. and Jerkovich, G. S. (1990). Central nervous system toxicity of tricyclic antidepressants: phenomenology, course, risk factors, and role of therapeutic drug monitoring. *Journal of Clinical Psychopharmacology*, **2**, 88–95.

Reuben, D. B., Borok, G. M., Wolde-Tsadik, G., *et al.* (1995). A randomized trial of comprehensive geriatric assessment in the care of hospitalized patients. *New England Journal of Medicine*, **332**, 1345–1350.

Rizzo, J. A., Bogardus, S. T., Leo-Summers, L., Williams, C. S., Acampora, D., and Inouye, S. K. (2001). Multicomponent targeted intervention to prevent delirium in hospitalised older patients: what is the economic value? *Medical Care*, **39**, 740–752.

Rockwood, K. (1999). Educational interventions in delirium. *Dementia and Geriatric Cognitive Disorders*, **10**, 426–429.

Rockwood, K., Stolee, P., and Fox, R. A. (1993). Use of goal attainment scaling in measuring clinically important change in the frail elderly. *Journal of Clinical Epidemiology*, **46**, 1113–1118.

Rockwood, K., Cosway, S., Stolee, P., *et al.* (1994). Increasing the recognition of delirium in elderly patients. *Journal of the American Geriatrics Society*, **42**, 252–256.

Rosenberg, J. and Kehlet, H. (1993). Postoperative mental confusion—association with postoperative hypoxemia. *Surgery*, **114**, 76–81.

Rubenstein, L. Z., Josephson, K. R., Wieland, G. D., English, P. A., Sayre, J. A., and Kane, R. L. (1984). Effectiveness of a geriatric evaluation unit. A randomized clinical trial. *New England Journal of Medicine*, **311**, 1664–1670.

Schindler, B. A., Shook, J., and Schwartz, G. M. (1989). Beneficial effects of psychiatric intervention on recovery after coronary artery bypass graft surgery. *General Hospital Psychiatry*, **11**, 358–364.

Schofield, I. (1997). A small exploratory study of the reaction of older people to an episode of delirium. *Journal of Advanced Nursing*, **25**, 942–952.

Schor, J. D., Levkoff, S. E., Lipsity, L. A., *et al.* (1992). Risk factors for delirium in hospitalized elderly. *Journal of the American Medical Association*, **267**, 827–831.

Seymour, D. G. (1998). Surgery and anesthesia in old age. In: *Brocklehurst's textbook of geriatric medicine and gerontology* (eds R. Tallis, H. M. Fillit, and J. C Brocklehurst), 5th edn, pp. 235–254. Churchill Livingston, Edinburgh.

Seymour, J. and Wattis, J. P. (1992). Alcohol abuse in the elderly. *Reviews in Clinical Gerontology*, **2**, 141–150.

Sheref, S. E. (1985). Pattern of CNS recovery following reversal of neuromuscular blockade. Comparison of atropine and glycopyrollate. *British Journal of Anaesthesia*, **57**, 188–191.

Simon, L., Jewell, N., and Brokel, J. (1997). Management of acute delirium in hospitalized elderly: a process improvement project. *Geriatric Nursing*, **18**, 150–154.

Simpson, C. J. (1984). Doctors' and nurses' use of the word confused. *British Journal of Psychiatry*, **142**, 441–443.

Skelly, R. and Millar, E. (1999). Hearing aids: are our knowledge and training adequate? *Age and Ageing*, **28** (supplement 2), 49.

Spencer, B., Pritchard-Howarth, M., Lee, T., and Jack, C. (1999). Can't drink, won't drink. *Age and Ageing*, **28** (supplement 2), 47.

Steel, K., Gertman, P., Crescenzi, C., and Anderson, J. (1981). Iatrogenic illness on a general medical service at a university hospital. *New England Journal of Medicine*, **304**, 638–642.

Thomas, A. J. (1998). Nutrition. In: *Brocklehurst's textbook of geriatric medicine and gerontology* (eds R. Tallis, H. M. Fillit, and J. C Brocklehurst), 5th edn, pp. 899–912. Churchill Livingston, Edinburgh.

Tollefsen, G. D., Montague-Clouse, J., Lancaster, S. P., *et al.* (1991). The relationship of serum anti-cholinergic activity to mental status performance in an elderly nursing home population. *Journal of Neuropsychology and Clinical Neuroscience*, **3**, 314–319.

Treloar, A. J. and Macdonald, A. J. (1995). Recognition of cognitive impairment by day and night nursing staff among acute geriatric patients. *Journal of the Royal Society of Medicine*, **88**, 196–198.

Tsutsui, S., Kitamura, M., Higashi, H., Matsuura, H., and Hirashima, S. (1996). Development of post-operative delirium in relation to a room change in the general surgical unit. *Surgery Today*, **26**, 292–294.

Tune, L. E. and Egeli, S. (1999). Acetylcholine and delirium. *Dementia and Geriatric Cognitive Disorders*, **10**, 342–344.

Varney, N. R. and Shephard, J. S. (1991). Predicting short term memory on the basis of temporal orientation. *Neuropsychologica*, **5**, 13–16.

Wahlund, L-O. and Björlin, G. A. (1999). Delirium in clinical practice: experiences from a specialized delirium ward. *Dementia and Geriatric Cognitive Disorders*, **10**, 389–392.

Wanich, C. K., Sullivan-Marx, E. M., Gottlieb, G. L., and Johnson, J. C. (1992). Functional status outcomes of a nursing intervention in hospitalized elderly. *Image – The Journal of Nursing Scholarship*, **24**, 201–207.

Warren, J. L., Bacon, W. E., Harris, T., McBean, A. M., Foley, D. J., and Phillips, C. (1994). The burden and outcomes associated with dehydration among US elderly. *American Journal of Public Health*, **84**, 1265–1269.

Weinberg, A. D. and Minaker, K. L. Council on Scientific Affairs, American Medical Association. (1995). Dehydration. Evaluation and management in older adults. *Journal of the American Medical Association*, **274**, 1552–1556.

Wengel, S. P., Roccaforte, W. H., and Burke, W. J. (1998). Donepezil improves symptoms of delirium in dementia: implications for future research. *Journal of Geriatric Psychiatry and Neurology*, **11**, 159–161.

Wilkinson, T. J., Hanger, H. C., George, P. M., and Sainsbury, R. (2000). Is thiamine deficiency in elderly people related to age or co-morbidity? *Age and Ageing*, **29**, 111–116.

Williams, M. A. Confusion: testing versus observation. (1988). *Journal of Gerontological Nursing*, **14**, 25–30.

Williams M. A., Cambell, E. B., Raynor, W., Mlynareznk, S. M., and Ward, S. E. (1985). Reducing acute confusional states in elderly patients with hip fractures. *Research in Nursing and Health*, **8**, 329–337.

Williams-Russo, P., Urquhart, B. L., Sharrock, N. E., *et al.* (1992). Post-operative delirium: predictors and prognosis in elderly orthopedic patients. *Journal of the American Geriatrics Society*, **40**, 759–767.

Williams-Russo, P., Sharrock, N. E., Mattis, S., Szatrowski, T. P., and Charlson, M. E. (1995). Cognitive effects after epidural vs general anesthesia in older adults. A randomized trial. *Journal of the American Medical Asssociation*, **274**, 44–50.

Williams-Russo, P., Sharrock, N. E., Mattis, S., *et al.* (1999). Randomized trial of hypotensive epidural anesthesia in older adults. *Anesthesiology*, **91**, 926–935.

Wilson, A., Parker, H., Wynn, A., Jagger, C., Spiers, N., Jones, J., and Parker, G. (1999). Randomised controlled trial of effectiveness of Leicester hospital at home scheme compared with hospital care. *British Medical Journal*, **319**, 1542–1546.

Wilson, L. M. (1972). Intensive care delirium. The effect of outside deprivation in a windowless unit. *Archives of Internal Medicine*, **130**, 225–226.

Winograd, C. H., Gerety, M. B., and Lai, N. A. (1993). A negative trial of inpatient geriatric consultation. Lessons learned and recommendations for future research. *Archives of Internal Medicine*, **13**, 2017–2023.

Chapter 9

The role of families, family caregivers, and nurses

Ingalill Rahm Hallberg

The effective counselling and support of family members of elderly people in a delirious state requires knowledge of recognition, causes, and available treatments (Hallberg 1999). This knowledge has been provided in the previous chapters. It is not enough, however, to know about the antecedents and treatment of the delirium. It is also necessary to know what it means for people to have a close family member be acutely confused, and what it means for the patient. In addition, one must know about problems which caregivers (families or nurses) face in providing care for a delirious individual.

Surprisingly, there is hardly any empirical research addressing the effects of having a family member in a temporary or persistent delirious state, its impact on family members, or the importance to the patient of their presence. Nor is there much systematic information on the reaction of nursing care staff to caring for a delirious patient. We also lack evidence-based knowledge of how to approach a family member in a delirious state (Hallberg 1999). Even more surprising, there are few descriptions of the inner life of the person while he or she is in a state of delirium (Foreman 1993). This is striking because having such knowledge would be of value to the family for at least two reasons:

- first, the family members may play an important role in reaching out to their delirious relative;

- second, it is likely to be distressing for close family members to see a loved one in a state of confusion.

From a nursing perspective, it is important because providing care for the person may be distressing, because it is often difficult to communicate effectively (nurse and patient or family member and patient), and because the staff may have to undertake potentially harmful interventions in caring for the person (Ludwick and O'Toole 1996). Foreman (1993) found from an extensive literature review that there was a lack of intervention studies of the prevention and management of delirium, and this also influences the kind of advice or suggestions that can be given to families dealing with a delirious relative.

The families' situation

Intriguingly, Fratiglioni and colleagues have recently reported that the density of a social support network is correlated with the risk of dementia (Fratiglioni *et al.* 2000). The social network plays an important role in protecting people in difficult life situations (Cohen and Syme 1985). This effect is thought to operate through the extent to which social support (the resources provided by others) can be obtained from the social network. The relationship between social network and social support is not fully understood, although a social network of some kind is obviously needed to obtain social support. The closest and perhaps most important network is the family (Boss *et al.* 1993). Across patient groups, social support is central to people's health, well-being, and ability to cope with difficult life situations (Cohen and Syme 1985). Social support may also have negative effects on health, for instance, by limiting others' space and risk-taking, and thereby hindering the potential to develop.

There are two competing hypotheses about the way social support works. The *direct effect hypothesis* suggests that social support contributes to health irrespective of the level of stress the person is under. An individual's confidence that others are at hand if needed, and that the social network is stable and predictable, are key factors in this respect. The *buffering hypothesis* suggests that social support is beneficial in stressful situations, as it protects the person from the negative effect of the stress involved in the situation. Others may help out, for instance, by reducing or even eliminating the negative appraisal of the situation (Cohen and Syme 1985).

Clearly, people share and ease each other's burdens, so that a harmful situation to one person is likely also to be harmful to those close by. Such harm arises from threats to the family dynamics, the intimacy between family members, and the family's goals and balance. The converse is also true, in that social support from family members eases the burden and helps them to cope with difficult life situations. There is no reason to believe that people with delirium or their family members are any exception to this reciprocity and the importance of the social network as an important resource in dealing with difficult life situations.

Delirium, as stated in Chapter 6, is often a concomitant to other more or less severe conditions, especially in elderly people. The overall vulnerability, physically as well psychologically, of a person is perhaps one of the most important signs that he or she is at risk of developing delirium. The strength of the external stressor is also important. Young, previously healthy people may well be delirious if they are under heavy influence of stress, for instance, those in an intensive care unit (ICU) after major traumatic injuries (Granberg 2001). The strain on the family members is not only due to an elderly relative or spouse being delirious but also to the underlying disease or trauma in the context of which delirium develops. Research focusing on family members *per se* is lacking, but in some studies their reactions are touched upon. For instance, delirium or confusion has been described in relation to the end of life as a strain on family members that is often neglected (Boyle *et al.* 1998; Harris 1995). It has been recognized as one reason for emergencies in palliative care, perhaps because families are not well prepared for the development of delirium during the last phase of life (Smith 1994). Similar findings have been reported from critical care. In a review of the literature on the occurrence, risks, and consequences of delirium in this setting by Tess (1991), the impact of family involvement is emphasized, and it is suggested that family and friends could assist in orienting the patient and thus counteracting the development of delirium. Patients demonstrate better orientation and less confusion when a family member uses touch, eye contact, and repeated information regarding time, place, and person. It is also suggested that standardized teaching and audio-visual aids to educate patient and families about the ICU environment might hinder the development of delirium.

These findings accord with the theories of social support. The studies mainly demonstrate the importance of families to a person with delirium, but they also touch on the negative effect on families. Tess, however, presented only two studies on this topic, each of which was small and consisted more of clinical observations than of generalizable empirical research findings. Nevertheless, the studies point to the importance of families in comforting the patient, and that it is necessary to counsel the families in their roles as caregivers, as well as to relieve them of strain.

Other areas from which delirium and the families' reactions and role have been reported are: severely burned patients (Davidson 1973; Goodstein 1985), patients undergoing bone marrow transplantation (Bryant *et al.* 1997), patients in sudden cardiac arrest (Dougherty 1994), and patients treated on ICU units for various reasons (Granberg 2001). Goodstein (1985) examined the reactions of nursing staff and families to burns victims and found that, apart from the strain caused by the experience of a family member being severely burned, they felt frustrated and anxious about the patient's being delirious or behaving regressively. The importance of information, education, and providing the opportunity to verbalize feelings and fears were emphasized. In the study of cardiac arrest (Dougherty 1994), it was evident that the episode caused not only short-term worries but also long-term adjustment difficulties and anxiety, in which families tended to adjust less well than the patient, mainly because of worries about the future and possible relapses. Thus the entire experience, including the person having been delirious, meant that marital adjustment was threatened on a long-term basis because of worry of the spouse.

From these few studies it is evident that, depending on the severity of the disease or injury, the delirium may be more or less in the foreground for family members. Family counselling in situations such as severe traumatic injuries, or severe conditions like leukaemia or cardiac arrest, needs to be adapted to these particular situations, but it also needs to include information about delirium. It seems justified to say that, for the family, delirium adds to the burden of the main reason for hospital treatment and may in some instances, if the family is unprepared, lead to unnecessary emergency visits or strains on the marriage, or an extra burden on the family.

Family caregiving for a person in a delirious state

Family caregiving has been well studied, particularly in the context of dementia (Rolland 1994; Nolan *et al.* 1996). Here, observations are limited to families caring for those in a temporary or persistent delirious state. However, it is not possible to draw any strong conclusions from these studies because they are scarce, sometimes too small, and/or have a design that does not allow generalizable conclusions to be drawn. While caregiving can be stressful and burdensome, and can result in health problems in the caregiver, very few studies have highlighted the positive effects upon families of providing care to an elderly person in need of help. Caregiving in itself is rewarding, is an important aspect of a long-term relationship, and even maintains some kind of intimacy. Nevertheless, some care situations seem to be more distressing than others. Episodes of delirium often complicate the care of people with dementia, and it has been reported that delirium in the cared-for person means more strain on the caregiver (Gregory 1991; Adams 1994). England (1996) reported that the caregiving burden of adult children caring for a neurologically impaired parent was significantly higher in adult offspring caring for a confused parent than for those who cared for a lucid parent. Exhaustion associated with more than 3.5 hours of caregiving per day placed the caregiver at greater risk of negative impact on perceived health; the length of caregiving per day perhaps reflects the patient's cognitive ability. People who are delirious may need someone close by all the time to keep them from harming themselves.

Given such stress, the question of abuse arises. Phillips (1987) has suggested a greater risk of abuse if the family care recipient is confused because the delirium violates the family dynamics. Moreover, communication difficulties arise from impaired orientation. Such difficulties normally also mean loss of the previous intimacy. A study of elder abuse by Saveman (1994) appears to confirm these suggestions. She found that in cases of family abuse, in particular those where the care recipient was delirious, the burden of care had become overwhelming to the family caregiver who, out of exhaustion, did things that harmed the other. In some cases it was neglect rather than abuse, but in others it was outright abuse and the family caregiver was aware of the situation. Thus the family caregiver and the patient were trapped in a mutually abusive situation. Phillips (1987) has stressed that the caregiver needs to have a logical disease-based explanation for their relative's behaviour, the opportunity to verbalize his or her thoughts and feelings, and support to maintain normality in daily life. She also emphasized the need for respite care, and for supporting family caregivers to consider other ways to fulfil their responsibility to the delirious family member. The fact that caregiving also involves positive aspects, for instance, that the family makes it possible for the elderly to remain in his/her own surroundings, keeping up the relationship, and bringing the family together, is often forgotten (Gregory 1991). This increases the demands on professionals to actively support and counsel family members in approaching a person in a delirious state, and to help them deal with the most difficult problems, such as interpretation of the patient's behaviour, encountering and protecting them, as well as explaining the state and its causes to the family members. Several authors point out the need for a family-oriented approach to nursing people who are chronically confused, and there are such models, although not tested (Phillips 1987; Boss *et al.* 1993; Adams 1994; Opie 1991a). The studies reported here have shortcomings in that it is not always clear whether the patients had dementia, delirium, or a combination of the two. Studies that distinguish these states are needed.

Caring for older people is often a responsibility that is shared by families and health-care professionals (Hellström and Hallberg 2001). This shared responsibility increases demands on the professionals to treat family members as collaborators. The family has knowledge and makes observations that staff do not have or cannot do. They often have contextual knowledge that professionals cannot readily obtain. A collaborative approach to the family caregiver requires that their views are taken into consideration when making decisions about treatment, discharge, or other matters that have an impact on the caregivers' and the cared-for person's lives. Unfortunately, this is often not the case. Based on interviews with patients, families, and nurses, Congdon (1994) found that they often had rather opposite views of, for instance, discharge readiness. Moreover, the families supported the patient but were not offered any support themselves. In general, patients and families were not involved in decision-making, and they felt that the team was not coordinated in its approach to the family and patient. Although this study did not report on patients' cognition, it seems reasonable to believe that it is even more important to keep up a close relationship for a family caregiver who is going to take on the responsibility of an elderly person in a delirious state, or at risk of developing one. Also, collaboration is needed about when and how caregiving can be handed over to the family caregiver.

Opie (1991a, 1991b) has emphasized partnership as essential in family caregiving for confused older people, as a result of a programme called 'Research with elders and carers at home'. She argued that professionals were not aware and did not systematically explore the stress family caregivers were under, and suggested an open discussion to keep them informed about the formal care available, and to discuss cut-off points for family caregiving. Acknowledgement of the family caregiver was believed to be essential in the relationship between formal and informal caregivers. Opie found, however, that this did not happen, especially in the physician–family relationship. Family caregivers must feel confident in the services available, as their wider social network is likely to shrink when a family member takes on caregiving. In the absence of informal support, the responsibility increases on professionals to support them to maintain their social network, and also to provide social support to family members. Family caregivers also reported that nursing care staff lacked training and knowledge of confusion and also lacked influence on decisions that they had to carry out or live with (Opie 1991a, 1991b). Thus, there still seems to be a long way to go to develop partnerships in caring for delirious individuals.

Families participating in interventions

Theories of social support can be traced in some intervention studies, mainly intended to intervene in the state of delirium, but also to relieve patients of the anxiety and stress they are under when delirious. Some authors put forward the idea of family involvement without further elaboration, for example, as part of non-pharmacological treatment (Simon *et al.* 1997). Standards of nursing care for delirious patients have been outlined by Zimberg and Berenson (1990). Reassuring family members and family participation are emphasized. It is suggested that the family's knowledge of a patient's previous emotional/behavioural patterns should be assessed, that information about the patient's condition should be given, and that they should be encouraged to participate in the care according to their ability. Instructions should be given to families to interact with the patient in a simple, clear, and concise manner, to orient the patient as regards time, place, and the purpose of the treatment, and hospital stay. In cases where restraints were used, the staff should discuss their indication with families as well as the patient. It is recommended that the knowledge deficits of the families, as indicated in emotional distress, questions, and misapprehensions about nursing care, are assessed. Intervention strategies in this respect were to educate the family about causes and the pattern of interaction with the patient, to clarify the families' concern, and to structure families' interactions with the nursing staff in a simple manner (Zimberg and Berenson 1990). This approach has not to my knowledge been evaluated, and there is not enough evidence available for some of its components (for instance, in the approach to the patient). Also, the notion of structuring families' interaction with nursing staff is perhaps contradictory to the idea of partnership and collaboration with the family.

Very few studies have reported results from interventions to prevent or alleviate delirious episodes (Wanich *et al.* 1992; Foreman 1993; Foreman and Zane 1996), and no studies to date have explicitly reported findings from family counselling programmes. There are, however, some intervention studies that have included families as part of the intervention. These are mainly based on the idea that it is reassuring to the frail elderly person if a family member is present. However, this mainly takes the perspective of the fragile elderly person and not the family member *per se*. Family members themselves can also benefit if they are actively involved in the elderly person's care, and if they are given the opportunity to receive first-hand information about their elderly relative. Burnside and Moehrlin (1980) state that families need regular support, and that staff need to obtain some idea of how family members view the confusion in the elderly person. Among other things, this is so that they can understand how they feel about it, to help them to comprehend and obtain a valid view of the state.

More active family involvement has been evaluated in a rooming-in study involving 24 patients (13 intervention and 11 control) (Wells and Baggs 1997). The intervention consisted of a family member staying overnight with the patient for 4 or more days of the first 7 days after surgery. They arrived at 10 p.m. and slept in the patient's room.

They were not responsible for any nursing care and were instructed to use the bell if the patient required assistance. They were free to leave in the morning. The design of this intervention was based on a literature review indicating that delirium typically occurred within the first 6 days of the hospital stay. No rationale was given for rooming-in taking place only at night. No significant differences were found between the two groups with respect to confusion, complication rate, or length of stay. The families who roomed in were, however, very satisfied with the experience. It seems reasonable not to reject the idea that rooming-in is of value for the patient's state, the occurrence of delirium, or the length of stay. Instead, it seems fair to say that this study needs to be repeated under more scientifically rigorous circumstances, with sample sizes based on power calculation, and elaborating the intervention in various ways.

Other studies have explored a larger role for family involvement. For instance, Miller (1991, 1996) has reported on 'environmental optimization' interventions. These have several components, including meaningful sensory input. This component included orientation about the hospital and services the family could rely on, making available such things as wheelchairs so they could go out and take a stroll, inviting them to ask about anything they were concerned or unclear about, encouraging them to stay, showing them appreciation, and explaining the importance of their presence and participation. The intervention also included aspects such as acting as a role model to the families by using touch, orientation, and information to the patient in their interaction with the elderly person. The staff were supposed to encourage families to stick to their usual pattern of communication with the elderly. The component also included such things as supporting families to rest and take time off in order to maintain their well-being. Staff were also supposed to help the patient call families in moments of anxiety and ask them to help in orienting and calming the patient, or/and leaving handwritten letters at the ward that staff could read aloud to the patient in situations of strain. Nevertheless, the results of the entire intervention showed that involving families was the component that was used the least. This was because nurses forgot to implement it or because no families paid visits. Thus, despite the opportunity to do so, families were not effectively invited to participate. The reasons for this are not clear, but may reflect a staff perception that family involvement was not important. Alternatively, professionals may feel hesitant about asking families.

Wanich et al. (1992) also tested an intervention that included family involvement. Families or any other significant person were contacted within the first 24 hours and asked to visit frequently, call daily, and bring in familiar things from the elderly person's home. It is not clear from this study to what extent the family part of the intervention actually was applied, but there were no significant differences between the groups apart from a slightly better functional status at the follow-up. The sample was small, and there may be other confounding issues that make it difficult to draw any conclusions about the effects of such an intervention. More stringent and powerful studies are needed to establish the importance of the presence of family members for the patients or for themselves.

The meaning of being delirious from the perspective of the patient

Communication difficulties pose problems in delirium. Andersson *et al.* (1993) reported from a case study that communication between nurses and a delirious elderly woman who had had acute surgery because of a hip fracture broke down totally, ending up in her being given an intramuscular injection and held in her bed until she fell asleep. The breakdown of communication arose from the woman using her previous life experience to speak about her present situation, while staff interpreted her metaphoric communication as nonsense and used reality orientation (telling her facts about the fracture, surgery, and hospital) to bring her into their world. The situation started with the woman asking for a telephone and her telephone book. It was obvious from this request that she had displaced herself to her home, since she pointed somewhere in the room and asked the staff to take the telephone book on the shelf over there. When the staff did not respond to this request but tried to orient her, the patient tried to get out of bed, following which the staff held her and she was given a tranquillizer. When lucid again, the patient was able to explain the things she had spoken about and thus she was able to make sense of her behaviour when she had been delirious. She wanted to get in touch with her sister because she felt threatened and trusted her a great deal. She felt humiliated and disrespectfully treated by the staff, and she feared that she was in danger. She spoke about war during the delirium and could afterwards explain that she and her family were very much involved in rescuing people during the Second World War and that it was a frightening period in her life. Thus, it seemed that a memory from the past that resembled the present came into her mind during the delirious state.

In this case, the situation ended up with the use of force. Sadly, the use of pharmacological and non-pharmacological restraint seems to be a common intervention in care for people in delirium. In one study (Ludwick and O'Toole 1996), nurses in hospital-based medical and surgical wards frequently came into contact with confused elderly people, approximately three such patients a week, and restraints were the major treatment. Indeed, 84% of the nurses reported that the last patient they provided care for was restrained. This may indicate that nurses are limited in their intervention strategies and have to resort to a method that is well known to be ethically and emotionally difficult for both nurses and patients. This shortage of intervention strategies in professional care may also mean that families are short of methods to reach out to the elderly in a delirious state. Families do, however, have contextual knowledge of the patient's life and a more solid relationship than professionals. This could be useful in understanding the reactions of a person in delirium.

The very few studies that report on the patient's experiences of being confused are mainly from ICUs, and it is not always clear that the patient is delirious according to formal diagnostic criteria. However, the findings are of interest because they provide some information about the patient's inner life during the state and may yield some knowledge about how to approach the patient while he or she is delirious. Granberg *et al.* (1998, 1999) reported that patients (19 of whom had been intubated) recalled their experiences as being in a state of chaos, persistent tension, feeling extremely emotionally instable, vulnerable, and fearful, and that trivial events could trigger changes in either direction, toward greater or lesser tension and fear. Increased fear in turn was said to aggravate unreal experiences and produce yet more fear. Trust and confidence in the carer or other persons close to the patient seemed to reduce the feelings of unreal experiences, as described afterwards. Similar findings were reported from a study including ten patients telling about their experiences of confusion after having had coronary artery bypass surgery (Laitinen 1996). The patients remembered being confused, and that this was a significant, incomprehensible, and frightening experience for them. Patients were interpreted as being on the borderline of awareness of space and time and, interestingly enough, they spoke about being both conscious and unconscious at the same time, which was frightening and provoked great anxiety. They also said that the rapid pace of the unit tended to draw them into a vicious circle, aggravating their state of confusion. The presence of a nurse in whom they felt trust and confidence tended to affect them in a positive direction, making them feeling safe and secure (Laitinen 1996). In these studies, some patients did not want to talk about their experiences while delirious. This may indicate that it was even more frightening to them or that they had no means of handling their emotional reactions.

Very few studies address what actually takes place during the delirium, by trying to obtain an understanding of the lived experience. Andersson *et al.* (2001a) followed a sample of elderly people from admission to hospital because of a hip fracture or for elective surgery for hip or knee replacement ($n=505$), and those who became delirious and lucid again ($n=51$) were followed with non-participant observations while in the state of delirium and afterwards interviewed. As expected, more of those with a hip fracture became delirious, and the more frail the patient, the earlier the delirium developed and the longer it lasted, with more episodes of delirium emerging during the hospital stay. The observational study (Andersson *et al.* 2001b), including the 51 patients that became delirious and lucid again, provided some new and thought-provoking findings. As with the findings reported by Laitinen (1996), there was a strong indication that the patients, whilst in the middle of the delirium, were well aware of themselves being delirious, for example:

> Some strange element that had come and taken over reality, I mixed things up, it was a mess, confused thoughts. I mistook things and repeated what others said. Something strange happened.

It was also obvious from these extensive observations of the patients' verbal and motor expressions that most exhibited behaviour and verbal expressions indicating fear, anger, or irritation, or being restless or uneasy in other ways. On the other hand, some patients had a happier experience, while others had an emotionally indifferent experience during delirium. The most striking finding, however, when more of an inside perspective on the patients' actions was taken, was that 'struggling to understand and taking control when being confused and viewing oneself being confused' stood out as the overarching theme. Patients at some level were aware that they were confused and that they could not control their condition. It was also clear from their statements that they tried very much to get this confusion under control and tried to understand what was happening to them. In this struggle to obtain control and understand what was going on, they used various strategies. They tried to make a whole of the present by piecing together a seemingly sensible story using fragments from their life prior to the fall and fracture or to obtain clarity, for instance, by asking others or withdrawing to get peace and quiet. Also, they apparently attributed meaning to the present by using their life story and/or events from their earlier life that came into their minds (Andersson *et al.* 2001b; Andersson *et al.* 2002). Thus the findings strongly indicate that the patients, although the situation was out of their control, understood that something was wrong with their minds and tried to regain a grasp on themselves and reality. This indicates the importance of not regarding their verbal and motor activity as nonsense behaviour, but as a functional attempt to get back to 'normal', and therefore there are communicative messages within what seems to be nonsense.

Families have an important role in helping to translate these expressions into the current situation, because of their knowledge of the patient's past and of material from their current life. A sensible use of confirmation in combination with reality orientation adapted to what is taking place at that particular moment is perhaps a more valid way of approaching patients than just one or the other way. It seems to be a matter of striking a balance between bringing in the outer reality, interpreting and responding to the emotional quality of the patient's inner life, and trying to translate that into the patient's current situation. Other authors have made similar suggestions, although they tend to favour either reality orientation or validating (Kelly 1995) without any solid empirical research basis for the one or the other. McCaffrey *et al.* (1998) suggests that:

> Reassurances and making calm, orienting suggestions are beneficial. Rather than trying to reason or argue with the patient, attend to the meaning behind the misinterpretations. (p. 1342)

Although these findings in most cases stem from people's narratives after they have been in a state of confusion, they provide us with several important pieces of knowledge. Most patients are extremely emotionally strained and frightened; those who are especially frightened may need to be more closely monitored. Contrast this approach with the use of restraints. In addition, delirious patients feel that they are between being conscious and unconscious. In these cases, patients commonly strive to gain control over their situation. If families or nurses could cling on to that straw, they may be able to avoid the common confrontation between them and the delirious person. Finally, it is noteworthy that the presence of a person they have confidence in seems to ease the burden for them. This is a very important thread to follow, clinically as well as in research. The study in which rooming-in for the elderly was used is one step forward (Wells and Baggs 1997).

Supporting the family

Counselling or providing social support to family members can be addressed from several perspectives. There is the temporal perspective, meaning that support and counselling can be provided before a person enters into a delirious state, and there is the counselling and support needed while the person is in such a state. Lastly, there is the after-care or follow-up care when the person has become lucid again.

Another perspective relates to the content of the counselling or social support provided. This, of course, must be adapted to varying contexts, e.g. a family caregiver who has a long-term carer's role in relation to the patient, compared with a relationship in which the expectation is that the parties will go back to mutual independence.

A third perspective concerns whom to address in these matters. If staff are unaware of the importance of counselling and social support to family members, then they will not apply it. There have been successful attempts to increase staff knowledge of delirium (Rapp *et al.* 1998). However, whether or not it actually resulted in altered staff behaviour was not reported. Such findings have been reported, although rarely (Rockwood 1999). Sometimes, nurses' awareness of the importance of a family-oriented approach can be enhanced so that they are more motivated to apply it. It is notable that viewing a family as a social unit that needs to be given information, sometimes together and sometimes separately, can conflict with the view of patients as autonomous individuals (Rolland 1994). Applying a family-centred approach means acknowledging the fact that each family is a unique relational system, including members having different roles in this system and also various expectations of each other (Minuchin 1975). Significant family members in such situations should routinely have a family consultation in the crisis phase, which, among other things, can help the family to normalize their expectations of the situation and allow them to reduce feelings of helplessness (Rolland 1994).

It may seem odd to suggest interventions before the person has developed delirium, and this may be regarded as putting families under unnecessary stress. However, viewing it from the perspective of control and empowerment, it makes sense. The concept of empowerment was originally developed within community work to increase the inhabitants' involvement in the community decisions and work. More recently, it has more often been discussed as a useful concept for health care because it emphasizes the power and control of the care recipient or family, rather than doctors or other health-care staff as the experts. According to Gibson (1991), empowerment is easier to understand by its absence than through its presence. The absence is demonstrated in a sense of powerlessness with overall feelings of distress, restrictions, and having limited or no support, which also indicates some sort of alienation. Empowering means:

> a helping process whereby groups or individuals are enabled to change a situation, given skills, resources, opportunities and authority to do so. It is a partnership, which respects and values self and others, aiming to develop a positive belief in self and the future. (Rodwell 1996, p. 309)

If people in vulnerable situations are told about the risk of developing delirium, for instance, after surgery or in relation to severe diseases, injuries, or demanding treatments, it may be less frightening should such a condition develop. This is likely to be so for the family members but it may well be so for the patient too. Studies (Laitinen 1996; Granberg *et al.* 1998, 1999; Andersson *et al.* 2002) reporting patient experiences indicate that patients were simultaneously aware and unaware, perhaps indicating that information may comfort the patient while delirious. It does in fact show that it is not a matter of understanding or not. Information to families (and patients) needs to include aspects such as risk factors, signs and expressions of being delirious, preventive, protective, and intervening steps that can be taken, as well as the need to process the experience while lucid again. It seems particularly important to eliminate the view of the state in terms of insanity and nonsense. Perhaps staff also need to include more narrative information on what it is like to be delirious. It may be easier for people to identify with narratives than with paradigmatic information. It is likely to make a difference if people are told that what takes place during the state probably has a communicative meaning, although professionals are not always able to interpret it correctly, and that families play an important role because they have historical and contextual knowledge that the staff do not.

The concept of social support is perhaps useful in outlining the content of counselling or supporting the family before as well as while the person is in a state of delirium. This concept comprises several components, including tangible support, emotional support, and informational support (Cohen and Syme 1985). Tangible or instrumental support means providing assistance with tasks of various kinds. This could be helping out with transportation, household matters, looking after pets or other things that take time and energy from the, at that time, more important matter of focusing attention on the person in a delirious state. In cases where the family member is also the caregiver, there may be other practical matters to consider. From the perspective of professionals, it means making sure that the family member has the practical support needed to focus on the more important matters. In cases of family caregiving, it means helping the caregiver to obtain and organize the help needed. As noted, staff are sometimes insufficiently focused on informing families about available services. Thus, one component to consider in supporting families is to assess and help out in obtaining tangible support, either through the service system or through their social network.

Informational support means providing knowledge about various aspects of the situation. This can be guidance, factual knowledge, or advice. Such information should include aspects such as risk factors, symptoms and signs, preventive, protective, and interventional measures, and the need to process the experience while lucid again. The importance of the informational support has perhaps been underestimated in delirium, with the result that it is inadequately studied in this condition, even though it is well recognized in other types of care.

It has been said that to find meaning and reduce uncertainty, three components are important:

- to understand the symptom pattern;
- to create familiarity with the event; and
- to provide congruence (Mishel 1988).

This is very much what patient and family education is about. There are several meta-analyses of studies on patient education (Mazzuca 1982; Mumford *et al.* 1982; Devine and Cook 1983). The findings indicate that educational/psychoeducational interventions and psychological interventions do result in a positive outcome in various respects. The studies show that pure education in the form of lectures or the like are not as effective as when the participants have the opportunity to share, narrate, or express their own situation. This indicates that it is not having the knowledge *per se* that is effective but having the opportunity to process the feelings, worries, and thoughts that go along with the experience.

This component of informational support is interrelated with the component of emotional support, which means understanding and closeness, love, and empathy. Emotional support is sometimes called esteem support because the stress situation concerns touching on or revealing what could be regarded as negative aspects of the self (Cohen and Syme 1985). Emotional support is commonly obtained in mutual and respectful relationships where people feel free to confide in each other. To the family member of patients in a delirious state, this means that staff members provide them with an opportunity to verbalize their feelings or fears, and that the other listens attentively, and offers understanding, sympathy, and reassurance. The fact that another person shows acceptance and approval and shares the person's inner feelings and thoughts is supposed to contribute to one's self-esteem and evaluation. Emotional support is often part of informational support. This may be an explanation as to why informational support in the form of lectures seemingly is not as effective as when more expressional components are included.

The importance and the content of emotional support can be understood from a narrative gerontological perspective. The narrative approach is more consistent with the way people are supposed to process their life and experiences. Bruner (1986, 1996) suggests that there are two 'modes of thought' which people use to make sense of their life situation, the paradigmatic and the narrative mode. The paradigmatic mode is the one nursing and medicine rely on in most cases, and also the one put forward when discussing how to inform people about their disease or related problems. The models used in medicine, psychology, and nursing are based on the paradigmatic mode to explain various phenomena. The diagnostic system, descriptions of symptoms, treatment, information about diagnosis and prognosis and treatment use this mode to convey knowledge to students, patients, and families and to communicate professionally. For instance, in the way crisis reactions are described according to a phase model, theories explaining stress and stress reactions or psychodynamic models for interpreting and understanding people in various life situations are all paradigmatic ways of describing phenomena. This is, of course, useful scientifically and clinically, and perhaps also in understanding the world, but only to a limited extent.

The more common way for people to process their life experiences is the narrative mode. People conduct themselves, and interpret and understand themselves, others, and events by storying and re-storying, and by telling and further listening to their own and others' stories. Understanding another person therefore requires that health-care staff participate in the person's inner story of the events (Bluck and Levine, 1998; Kenyon and Randall, 1999; Randall, 1999). It is perhaps the story and not the facts that are most important in informing staff about patients' and families' experiences. It may well be that what seems to be the human drive to make a coherent story out of difficult life situations, in this case being in a delirious state, also operates during a delirious episode (Andersson 2002). It is perhaps the case that making sense of events does not necessarily mean that the event is meaningful, but that the person can make a sensible story out of it and integrate the events into her/his life story. The latter assumption has significant implications for after-care for people who have been delirious, and for their families. Information is normally presented in a paradigmatic manner, telling about facts, causes, frequencies, prognosis, and so on. Often this is not sufficient to achieve good communication. Families and patients, especially after they become lucid again, need narrative information as well. This is perhaps best provided by giving time and space to them to narrate their experiences, and also to listen to others who have been in similar situations (Hallberg 2001).

For health-care staff it is an everyday task to encounter people in difficult life situations. Such familiarity can mean that they lose sight of the uniqueness of each person and their needs in these situations (Hallberg 2001). During the last few years, cognitive theories have received increasing interest, and informing and educating patients as well as encouraging 'positive thinking' have become more emphasized. Such theories are helpful, but they do not emphasize the novelty of each person's individual experience. Rather, they give a generalized image of people. It is possible that the staff member approaching a person in a difficult life situation recognizes someone who has lost orientation or is delirious, and the response to this is a medical reaction without personal meaning. While this is preferable to viewing the problems as somehow the patient's fault, it is nevertheless important to understand that person's attempt to make sense of the delirious situation in his or her own way. The results presented by Andersson *et al.* (2001b, 2002) may well reflect the patient's attempt to put together a sensible story from this disruptive experience. It seems as if the basic human drive to make a coherent story out of the present and use one's previous life experience is not lost during the delirious condition. For families and for patients, it may be easier to come to terms with a state of delirium if it is to a certain extent understandable.

Follow-up care is perhaps as important as counselling while the patient is delirious. This is so because this is the time when family members, as well as the patient, process the entire experience. The aim of this process is to put the story of one's life back together again and to make sense of it. Being successful at making a coherent story of 'my life' is also a platform for trust in the future. Perhaps the narrative mode for processing is even more important during this phase. This means providing time and space for families and patients to narrate their memories, feelings, and thoughts at that time as well as currently. It is extremely value-laden to have a view of oneself as having been 'insane'. This may decrease a person's self-confidence, trust, and self-esteem and needs to be addressed in a more valid way.

Future research

Given the frequency and clinical importance of delirium, it is surprising that so little research has been done to highlight the situation of families, family caregivers, or the patients themselves. We urgently need to obtain more knowledge about the impact on family members and on the family dynamics of having someone close being delirious, and to acquire more insight into the experience of being delirious. Understanding people's experience is the basic foundation of family counselling as well as of patient counselling. That understanding is not available yet.

References

Adams, T. (1994). The emotional experience of caregivers to relatives who are chronically confused – implications for community mental health nursing. *International Journal of Nursing Studies*, **31**, 545–553.

Andersson, E. (2002). *Acute Confusion in Orthopaedic Care. With the Emphasis on the Patients' View and the Episode of Confusion*. Lund University Medical Dissertations, Bulletin No 10, The Department of Nursing, The Medical Faculty.

Andersson, E., Knutsson, I., Hallberg, I. R., and Norberg, A. (1993). The experience of being confused. A case study. A breakdown in communication between a confused patient and a nurse may have everything to do with the nurse's point of view. *Geriatric Nursing*, **14**, 242–247.

Andersson, E., Gustafson, L., and Hallberg, I. R. (2001a). Acute confusional state in elderly orthopaedic patients: Factors of importance for detection in nursing care. *International Journal of Geriatric Psychiatry*, **16**, 7–17.

Andersson, E., Norberg, A., and Hallberg, I. R. (2001b). Acute confusional episodes in elderly orthopaedic patients. The patients' actions and speech. *International Journal of Nursing Studies*, **39**, 303–317.

Andersson, E., Hallberg, I. R., Norberg, A., Edberg, E.-K. (2002). The meaning of acute confusional state from the perspective of elderly patients. *International Journal of Geriatric Psychiatry*. (in press).

Bluck, S. and Levine, L. J. (1998). Reminiscence as autobiographical memory: a catalyst for reminiscence theory development. *Ageing and Society*, **18**, 185–208.

Boss, P. G., Doherty, W. J., LaRossa, R., Schumm, W. R., and Steinmetz, S. K. (1993). *Sourcebook of Family Theories and Methods. A Contextual Approach*. Plenum Press, New York.

Boyle, D. McC., Abernathy, G., Baker, L., Wall, A. C. (1998). End-of-life confusion in patients with cancer. *Oncology Forum*, **25**, 1335–1343.

Bruner, J. (1986). *Actual Minds, Possible Worlds*. Harvard University Press, Cambridge, MA.

Bruner, J. (1996). *The Culture of Education*. Harvard University Press, Cambridge, MA.

Bryant, L. H., Heiney, S. P., Henslee-Downey, P. J., and Corwell, P. (1997). Proactive psychosocial care of blood and marrow transplant patients. *Cancer Practice*, **5**, 234–240.

Cohen, S. and Syme S. L. (1985). *Social Support and Health*. Academic Press Inc., London.

Congdon, J. G. (1994). Managing incongruities: the hospital discharge experience for elderly patients, their families and nurses. *Applied Nursing Research*, **7**, 125–131.

Davidson, S. P. (1973). Nursing management of emotional reactions of severely burned patients during the acute phase. *Heart and Lung*, **2**, 370–375.

Devine, E. C. and Cook, T. D. (1983). A meta-analytic analysis of effects of psychoeducational interventions on length of postsurgical hospital stay. *Nursing Research*, **32**, 267–274.

Dougherty, C. M. (1994). Longitudinal recovery following sudden cardiac arrest and internal cardioverter defibrillator implantation: survivors and their families. *American Journal of Critical Care*, **3**, 145–154.

England, M. (1996). Caregiver burden, strain and perceived health of adult children caring for a neurologically impaired parent. *Geriatrician*, **14**, 11–19.

Foreman, M. D. (1993). Acute confusion in the elderly. In: *Annual review of nursing research* (eds Fitzpatrick, J. and Stevenson, J.), pp. 3–30. Springer Publishing Co., New York.

Foreman, M., Zane, D. (1996). Nursing strategies for acute confusion in elders. *American Journal of Nursing*, **4**, 45–57.

Fratiglioni, L., Wang, H., Ericsson, K., Maytan, M., and Winblad, B. (2000). Influence of social network on occurrence of dementia: a community-based longitudinal study. *Lancet*, **355**, 1315–1319.

Gibson, C. H. (1991). A concept analysis of empowerment. *Journal of Advanced Nursing*, **16**, 354–361.

Goodstein, R. K. (1985). Burns: an overview of clinical consequences affecting patient, staff and family. *Comprehensive Psychiatry*, **26**, 43–57.

Granberg, A. (2001). *The Intensive Care Unit Syndrome/Delirium, Patients Perspective and Clinical Signs*. Lund University Medical Dissertations, Department of Anesthesiology and Intensive Care, Faculty of Medicine.

Granberg, A., Bergbom Engberg, I., and Lundberg, D. (1998). Patients' experience of being critically ill or severely injured and cared for in an intensive care unit in relation to the ICU-syndrome. Part 1. *Intensive and Critical Care Nursing*, **14**, 294–307.

Granberg, A., Bergbom Engberg, I., and Lundberg, D. (1999). Acute confusion and unreal experiences in intensive care patients in relation to the ICU syndrome. Part II. *Intensive and Critical Care Nursing*, **15**, 19–33.

Gregory, S (1991). Stress management for carers. *British Journal of Occupational Therapy*, **54**, 427–429.

Hallberg, I. R. (1999). Impact of delirium on professionals. *Dementia and Geriatric Cognitive Disorders*, **10**, 420–425.

Hallberg, I. R. (2001). A narrative approach to nursing care of people in difficult life situations. In: *Narrative Gerontology: Theory, Research, and Practice* (eds Kenyon, GM., Clark, P., and de Vries, B.). Springer Publishing Company.

Harris, J. (1995). A heart-breaking lesson. *Nursing Times*, **91**, 48–49.

Hellström, Y. and Hallberg, I. R. (2001). Perspectives of elderly people receiving home help on health, care and life quality. *Journal of Health and Social Care in the Community*, **9**(2), 61–71.

Kelly, J. S. (1995). Validation therapy. A case against. *Journal of Gerontological Nursing*, **21**, 41–43.

Kenyon, G. M. and Randall, W. L. (1999). Narrative Gerontology. *Journal of Aging Studies*, **13**, 1–5.

Laitinen, H. (1996). Patients' experience of confusion in the intensive care unit following cardiac surgery. *Intensive and Critical Care Nursing*, **12**, 79–83.

Ludwick, R. and O'Toole, A. W. (1996). The confused patient. Nurses' knowledge and interventions. *Journal of Gerontological Nursing*, **22**, 44–49.

Mazzuca, S. (1982). Does patient education in chronic disease have therapeutic value? *Journal of Chronic Disease*, **35**, 521–529.

Miller, J. (1991). A *Clinical Study to Pilot Test the Environmental Optimization Interventions Protocol.* UMI Dissertation Services. Bell & Howell Company, Michigan.

Miller, J. (1996). A clinical project to reduce confusion in hospitalized older adults. *Medsurg Nursing*, **5**, 436–460.

Minuchin, S. (1975). *Families and Family Therapy.* Harvard University Press, Cambridge.

Mishel, M. H. (1988). Uncertainty in illness. *IMAGE Journal of Nursing Scholarship*, **20**, 225–232.

Burnside, I. M. and Moehrlin, B. A. (1980). Health care of the confused elderly at home. *Nursing Clinics of North America*, **15**, 389–401.

Mumford, E., Schlesinger, H. J., and Glass, G. V. (1982). The effects of psychological intervention on recovery from surgery and heart attacks: an analysis of the literature. *American Journal of Public Health*, **72**, 141–151.

Nolan, M. R., Grant, G., and Keady, J. (1996). *Understanding Family Care. A Multidimensional Model of Caring and Coping.* Open University Press, Milton Keynes.

Opie, A. (1991a). The informal caregivers of the confused elderly and the concept of partnership: a New Zealand report. *Pride Institute Journal of Long Term Home Health Care*, **10**, 34–40.

Opie, A. (1991b). Social policy and community care for confused older people. *Community Mental Health in New Zealand*, **6**, 2–27.

Phillips, L. R. (1987). The relationship between confusion and abuse. In: *Alzheimer's Disease Problems, Prospects and Perspectives* (ed. Altman, H. J.), pp. 219–223. Plenum Press, New York.

Randall, W. L. (1999). Narrative intelligence and the novelty of our lives. *Journal of Aging Studies*, **13**, 11–28.

Rapp, C. G., Onega, L. L., Tripp-Reimer, T., Mobily, P., Wakefield, B., Kundrat, M., *et al.* (1998). Unit-based acute confusion resource nurse: an educational program to train staff nurses. *The Gerontologist*, **38**, 628–632.

Rockwood, K. (1999). Educational interventions in delirium. *Dementia and Geriatric Cognitive Disorders*, **10**, 426–429.

Rodwell, C. M. (1996). An analysis of the concept of empowerment. *Journal of Advanced Nursing*, **23**, 305–313.

Rolland, J. S. (1994). *Families, Illness and Disability. An Integrative Treatment Model.* Basic Books, New York.

Saveman, B. I. (1994). *Formal Carers in Health Care and the Social Services Witnessing Abuse of the Elderly in their Homes.* Umeå University Medical Dissertations New Series No. 403.

Simon, L., Jewell, N., and Brokel, J. (1997). Management of acute delirium in hospitalized elderly: A process improvement project. *Geriatric Nursing*, **18**, 150–154.

Smith, A. M. (1994). Emergencies in palliative care. *Annals of Academy of Medicine*, **23**, 186–190.

Tess, M. M. (1991). Acute confusional states in critically ill patients. A review. *Journal of Neuroscience Nursing*, **23**, 398–402.

Wanich, C. K., Sullivan-Marx, M. S., Gottlieb, G. L., and Johnson, J. C. (1992). Functional status outcomes of a nursing intervention in hospitalized elderly. *IMAGE Journal of Nursing Scholarship*, **24**, 201–207.

Wells, N. and Baggs, J. G. (1997). Rooming in for elderly surgical patients. *Applied Nursing Research*, **10**, 72–79.

Zimberg, M. and Berenson, S. (1990). Delirium in patients with cancer: nursing assessment and intervention. *Oncology Nursing Forum*, **17**, 529–538.

Chapter 10

Education about delirium

Kenneth Rockwood

For many years articles were written and lectures given with a title such as: 'the confusion about confusion', or 'delirium: a confusing matter'. The intent was to signal that the routine management of the delirious patient was poorly done and that education was an important remedy. After more than 20 years of experience with such presentations, however, I do not think that we can use the term 'confusion' in relation to delirium management any longer. The problem is so pervasive and so chronic that our failure to come to grips with delirium must be considered a form of dementia.

In earlier chapters we have seen why this might be. There is no doubt that aspects of our nosology, terminology, and practice have been confusing. Any dispassionate reader must also agree that a lot of the textbook writing on delirium has served no good end other than, perhaps, the expansion of the writers' resumés and the acknowledgement of their friends and colleagues through sometimes dubious citations. The latter has been especially harmful in my view, particularly when coupled with the 'my differential diagnosis is longer than yours' impetus that appears to have driven many authors. In consequence, our education about delirium is much more confusing than is reasonable.

This chapter briefly outlines the evidence with respect to educating people about delirium. In addition, the outline of a remedy is proposed, to which my co-editor colleagues, and the other authors, see this book as potentially making a useful contribution.

Inquiry into education about delirium is motivated by many observations. The first is that, in the absence of systematic pharmacological interventions, it is the education of health-care professionals to implement what is known to be beneficial which underlies our chief means of coming to grips with this syndrome and its adverse consequences. In addition, the clear thinking needed for effective education is one way out of the terminological chaos that has characterized much of the modern publication about delirium. Moreover, developing education and practice guidelines about delirium inevitably points to gaps in what we wish we knew, or what we wish we knew to be effective. This in turn has motivated additional inquiries, including inquiry into how to educate people about delirium.

As discussed elsewhere, it is time for educational interventions in delirium to explicitly take into account principles of adult learning (Rockwood 1999). Some principles which seem to be particularly important in this regard are:

- making the programme relevant to the learners;
- providing a context in which they can learn information incrementally; and
- providing them opportunities to judge whether the practices arising from their education are useful to them.

Unfortunately, few educational interventions to date have explicitly incorporated these principles. In consequence, we next turn to describing how each might be carried out.

Relevance

For individuals to take the time to learn something new with the intent that their practice should change requires a high degree of motivation. Such motivation is best if it comes from within. To avoid the trap of circularity (by only teaching those who already know they want to know), a number of techniques can be used to make evident the relevance of the material to learn. One method is to ask them to share their experience in the management of delirious patients. This can be undertaken by a variety of means, depending on the context. For example, in preparing for teaching for practising physicians, it is now a widely accepted practice to have a questionnaire circulated beforehand as part of a needs assessment (see Appendix A). While it must necessarily be brief, a good deal of information can be put into appropriately worded questions. Another practice, common in some areas, is to sample, from a list of all possible participants, a few who can serve as a focus group. At the focus group, specific patient scenarios can be presented, and the participants' comments elicited. These comments can be presented to the group at the outset, and the attending participants asked to indicate whether the comments of their colleagues have resonance for them. Relevance has also been established through the use of eye-catching posters aimed at nurses, which describe the importance of correct and early diagnosis of delirium (Milisen *et al.* 2001).

A traditional way of establishing relevance is by the presentation of a representative case. The traditional didactic presentation, however, is often too passive, and it can be very much enhanced by asking for feedback from the audience about various points of the case and management. Of course it requires a delicate touch to ensure that this engages the audience without being heavy-handed.

Another means of encouraging prospective learners to see the relevance of information about delirium is by the presentation of the information through art. This can be accomplished through the use of artistic portrayals of delirium, either using material accessible in the public domain, or even, as we have done with great success, by commissioning artistic pieces such as paintings, plays, and dance. In this way it is possible to take off the mask of professionalism that so often undermines effective teaching about delirium.

The mask of professionalism undermines teaching, because it is our selective use of this mask which is a key failing of health-care professionals in their approach to patients with delirium. When a patient calls out, or is uncooperative, or even is physically aggressive, it is not usually the case that this behaviour reflects orneriness. Rather, in the settings in which we encounter patients, it is more likely that their behaviour occurs because they are ill and still more so the case if such bad behaviour occurs acutely. It seems an incredible thing to the lay public, but an important challenge in teaching health professionals about delirium is to persuade them that a patient who was well oriented and an attentive member of the family a few days ago and who presently is now angry and disoriented, is likely to be ill. But too often health-care professionals take off the mask of professionalism when encountering such a patient, and instead react as though they take personal offence. The use of the term such as 'gomers' or 'train wrecks' or even the more benign 'poor historian' reflects our attempt to distance ourselves, and we do so not just at the patient's peril but also at our loss of being effective health-care providers. So in the author's experience, it is often useful to explore the emotions that people feel when they encounter patients with delirium and then present these feelings as barriers to effective care that can be overcome with education. This works very well in establishing relevance.

Relevance is also powerfully made by testimonial. It is often best, if one is to retain a necessary distance in teaching, that the testimonial comes from someone else. Sometimes unplanned testimonials can have powerful impacts. The author recalls giving a Continuing Medical Education (CME) lecture at a regional hospital to a large group of physicians and nurses. Towards the end of the presentation one of the physicians in the audience stood up to endorse the view that the delirious patient is often badly managed, and pointed to the care of his own father, who, at that moment, was hospitalized at the same hospital in which the CME was being carried out. This was a powerful and compelling moment, and one that, to the author's certain personal knowledge, changed the practice of a number of physicians and nurses. Of course, this cannot be counted upon, but it is often worth asking members of the audience to share their perspective to increase the relevance of the information being provided about the need to overcome the barriers to effective care of patients with delirium.

Integration

An important component of the efficiency of expert learners in acquiring new information in their own field is their ability to integrate the information into an existing framework. When addressing the management of delirium in an elderly patient, it is helpful to provide context for the material to be mastered, so that it can readily be integrated into what is known and thus does not overwhelm the learner. It can be helpful in teaching a variety of health-care professionals to have them consider the question of why the atypical disease presentations in elderly people who are frail are delirium, falls, and immobility, and not other problems, such as shortness of breath, or diarrhoea, or rash. With minimal coaching, learners typically will rapidly come to the conclusion that maintaining attention and staying upright are higher-order functions. If we accept that frailty is the failure to integrate diverse organ systems and the social network in the face of environmental stress, then it is easy for most people to accept that failure of such a complex system will manifest itself as failure of its highest-order functions. In consequence, the atypical disease presentations are the ones that arise from the failure of these higher-order functions. A balance beam analogy can be helpful here, to point out that health assets can be countered by underlying deficits and by new insults (see Figure 6.1). When the assets are overwhelmed (when the balance is tipped in favour of deficits), delirium results. This makes clear to most people the idea of predisposing and precipitating events, and to the extent that it incorporates a variety of each, and is dynamic, it appears to be not that bad an analogy. The balance beam analogy can also often be extended to consider delirium in another context. For example, most people will recognize that even fit athletes can become delirious in the intensive care unit, and one can therefore make the case that strong deficits can overwhelm even strong assets.

In some ways, recent successful trials reinforce the need to develop specific strategies to integrate information, so that it can be used (Inouye *et al.* 1999; Marcantonio *et al.* 2001). For example, in a randomized controlled trial of geriatric consultation at a single institution that successfully reduced the incidence of delirium after hip fracture, the consultation included manoeuvres that, in essence, were educational. The suggestions to treat pain, ensure adequate nutritional intake, mobilize early, and provide appropriate environmental stimuli each constitute information transfer that could be generalized to other patients. As the authors noted, however:

> based on our experience performing consultations in the intervention group, there was no evidence that our management principles were being systematically integrated into routine care....' (Marcantonio *et al.* 2001, p. 521)

A useful adjunctive context for considering delirium is that of stupor and coma (Plum and Posner 1980). As the medical differential diagnosis in delirium is not conceptually distinct from the approach to stupor and coma, I have found it useful, particularly with health-care professionals, to situate the approach to delirium in that context. Briefly, physicians are asked to recall the traditional teaching that disorders of consciousness arise chiefly in the following settings:

- as a result of focal neurological insults, affecting either both hemispheres or a single lesion in the brain stem reticular activating system;
- in the setting of meningeal infection; or
- as a consequence of toxic or metabolic insults.

In consequence, this approach requires that they must rule out focal or lateralizing neurological signs, above and below the tentorium, must rule out meningismus (admittedly a more difficult task in elderly patients with a cervical osteoarthritis and spondylosis), and then consider toxic and metabolic causes. As this screening level of neurological examination can typically be carried out very quickly, it also provides a review that many physicians welcome.

In teaching about delirium, it can be useful to make the point that, as with coma, toxic and metabolic causes predominate in most medical series. Here it can be useful to contrast a useful approach to recalling the differential diagnosis of delirium in elderly people with a more usual textbook approach, and to make it a habit to present, in rapid succession, several detailed lists of potential causes of delirium, taken from a standard medical textbook. It is then easy to point out both that this list is impossible for an individual to remember with any degree of efficiency, and that such lists simply indicate that in patients who are so predisposed, any illness or medication can potentially give rise to delirium. This can be contrasted with a short useful approach to the differential diagnosis of delirium (Table 10.1).

The point of Table 10.1 is to illustrate that the usual differential diagnosis is easy to learn, that a meticulous approach to medications can be undertaken with a high yield, that more than one cause can be present, and that if considering each of these common conditions does not yield a cause, a more broad differential diagnosis must be considered. Still, the latter can wait until the others have been investigated. This approach is meant to help avoid injury from promiscuous investigations. Examples of such investigation-induced injury include falls from dehydration from a bowel preparation in the investigation of anaemia, or extrapyramidal side effects from neuroleptics prescribed to sedate a delirious, claustrophobic patient who is having a CT head scan, or simply anaemia from repeated phlebotomy.

Integration of information can also be carried out when talking to lay people or those with only notional health education. Many people have experience with a child who has become delirious. They understand it to be an emergency, and one that should prompt a careful approach by a physician. The analogy can be made to an older patient, as a means of helping learners understand delirium is a disease presentation and

Table 10.1 A useful approach to the differential diagnosis of delirium

- Medications (prescribed)
- Medications (over the counter)
- Medications (alcohol and illicit drugs)
- Infection
- Heart failure/myocardial infarction
- Metabolic causes
- Some combination
- Something else

Adapted from Rockwood, K. and MacKnight, C. (2001), and used with permission.

one which, in most circumstances, is expected to largely settle with treatment. Sometimes it is helpful to provide context by asking the learners to consider how a delirious patient makes them feel. Often, he or she makes them feel irritable or anxious. Again, the analogy can be made with depression, where a useful clinical teaching point is that, for a healthcare professional with no mood disorder, the induction, by interacting with a patient, of feelings of sadness in the interviewer often signals that the patient is depressed.

Feedback

According to standard educational theories, feedback should include not just tests of knowledge, which have been traditional in medical education, but should also attempt to evaluate attitudes. Ideally, the feedback should let learners know how their attitudes compare with those of others. Most importantly, it should include information on how their actions might be expected to have changed as a consequence of learning. Feedback seems particularly useful, and particularly likely to result in behavioural change when it includes follow-up to see how their practices actually have changed, and how that change compared with their peers. Some CME organizations have formalized this to the extent of having learners sign a 'contract for change', in which learners agree to submit, within 3 months of the programme, evidence from charts of how their own practices have changed as a consequence of the information. Short of this ideal, it is worthwhile providing learners with the opportunity to not just respond to examination-style questions, but also to have their responses compared with others. A particularly effective way is to have answers read out, often anonymously, and have other group members comment on the answer. These can be strong inducements to changing behaviour.

It is often the case that the integration of new information, particularly that of learners' attempts to change their behaviour, result in new learning issues being identified. The use of the World Wide Web provides an opportunity for follow-up at times and distances removed from the original CME; *Internet Mental Health* has a useful website on delirium: http://www.mentalhealth.com/dis/p20–or 01.html. Through the use of chat rooms, structured feedback sessions or even web-based conference calling, learners can have the opportunity to apply their new knowledge, provide feedback to the teachers on aspects that were confusing, and raise additional questions about the real world application of the new information.

Overview of existing evidence

As reviewed elsewhere, the target of educational intervention studies has included physicians, nurses, and patients' spouses (Rockwood 1999). The content of the teaching has included both pharmacological and non-pharmacological management, the details of which are provided in the relevant chapters elsewhere in this book. The interventions have been evaluated based both on their ability to change knowledge and attitudes, but also on their ability to reduce functional disability, length of stay, and even death.

As also noted elsewhere, the methodological rigor of many of these studies is suspect (Cole *et al.* 1996). In addition, many have not conformed to the usual principles of adult education (Rockwood 1999). What seems clear, however, is that systematic educational efforts, when evaluated with care, can point to reproducible benefits in the management of delirium (Engle and Graney 2001). Such interventions need to be carefully planned and to embrace the complexity of the patients and their components, i.e. they must be multidimensional. Ironically, as Inouye has pointed out, this very multidimensionality has been criticized by those of a rigorous evidence-based approach as a 'fatal flaw', presumably because it does not allow each link in a causal chain of effectiveness to be established (Inouye 2001). In addition, the outcome measures must be chosen with care; in some settings, traditional outcome measures, such as length of stay, are now so dictated by practice guidelines that they require patients to be discharged even when delirious.

Future directions

This chapter has argued for an approach to learners about delirium that emphasizes comprehensibility of the information to be acquired, and which explicitly discusses the 'social reaction' of many health-care professionals who see patients with delirium. It has advocated the development and evaluation of education packages that conform with principles of adult education. In addition, such packages should be individualized. They should cover the range of people who encounter delirium, including health-care professionals, other workers in health-care environments, and patients' families.

Given the extent to which the presence of delirium, particularly incident delirium, is seen as an indicator of poor health-care delivery, delirium and its management should be evaluated as a form of quality assurance indicator (Inouye *et al.* 1999). In this way, through systematic, responsive feedback about what we do and how we do it, we can hope to achieve better outcomes for patients suffering from delirium.

In addition, future interventions should also permit targeting of groups (e.g. frail individuals with dementia) and situations (e.g. hip fracture) where the risk of developing delirium is high, and where specific intervention and evaluation strategies need to be adopted. Most importantly, we need to educate health-care providers that acquiring and putting into practice the skill needed to care for patients with delirium demonstrates the best features of our professions.

References

Cole, M. G., Primeau, F., and McCusker, J. (1996). Effectiveness of interventions to prevent delirium in hospitalized patients: a systematic review. *Canadian Medical Association Journal*, **155**,1263–1268.

Engle, V. F. and Graney, M. J. (2001). Designing a study for success. *Journal of the American Geriatrics Society*, **49**, 523–532.

Inouye, S. K. (2001). Delirium after hip fracture: to be or not to be? *Journal of the American Geriatrics Society*, **49**, 678–679.

Inouye, S. K., Schlesinger, M. J., and Lydon, T. J. (1999). Delirium: a symptom of how hospital care is failing older persons and a window to improve quality of care. *American Journal of Medicine*, **106**, 565–573.

Milisen, K., Foreman, M. D., Abraham, I. L., *et al.* (2001). A nurse-led interdisciplinary intervention program for delirium in elderly hip-fracture patients. *Journal of the American Geriatrics Society*, **49**, 680–681.

Marcantonio, E. R., Flacker, J. M., Wright, R. J., and Resnick, N. M. (2001). Reducing delirium after hip fracture: a randomized trial. *Journal of the American Geriatrics Society*, **49**, 678–679.

Plum, F. and Posner, J. B. (1980). *The diagnosis of stupor and coma*, 3rd edn. F. A. Davis, Philadelphia.

Rockwood, K. (1999). Educational interventions in delirium. *Dementia and Geriatric Cognitive Disorders*, **10**, 426–429.

Rockwood, K. and MacKnight, C. (2001). *Understanding dementia: a primer of diagnosis and management*. Pottersfield Press, Halifax.

Appendix A

We are planning an educational programme to potentially include information about delirium. Please take a few minutes to answer this questionnaire so that we can better plan the session.

Needs Assessment Questionnaire for Family Physicians

1 Approximately what proportion of your patients are aged 65 years or older?

  <10%   11–20%   21–30%   31–50%   more

2 Do you attend patients in hospital?   Yes/No

3 How confident are you in your ability to recognize delirium?

  1 2 3 4 5 (1 being 'Not at all confident'; 5 being 'Very confident')

4 How long since you last diagnosed delirium in an elderly patients?

  Within the week; Within the month; 1–3 months ago; 3–6 months ago; longer

5 What was the cause of the delirium?

6 How confident are you in your ability to treat delirium?

  1 2 3 4 5 (1 being 'Not at all confident'; 5 being 'Very confident')

7 Considering the last few cases of delirium that you saw in elderly people, which of the following medications did you use?

  lorazepam po; lorazepine IM/IV; haloperidol po; haloperidol IM/IV

  thiordizine; loxapine; risperidone; olazapine

  quetiapine; trazadone; oxazepine; diazepam

  donepezil; chlordiazepoxide; donepezil; galantamine

  rivastigmine; other (specify):_____

Chapter 11

The future

James Lindesay, Kenneth Rockwood, and
Alastair Macdonald

As all investors are constantly warned, the future cannot be predicted from the past, but a better future can be facilitated by the careful use of history, and the bulk of this chapter is therefore autistic [wish-fulfilling, in Bleuler's terms (1970)] rather than attempting too much in the way of crystal-gazing. However, a cautionary note must be sounded by what appears to be a waning of interest in delirium, judging by the numbers of references to empirical studies. In 1970, there were 203 MEDLINE (National Library of Medicine 2001) references to delirium (2.5% of all mentioning patients or subjects), but this had only risen to 243 references by 2000 (0.2% of all mentioning patients or subjects). The disorder's claim to interest as a boundary issue (its rich basic science, clinical, psychiatric, physical, social, and health service importance) may also be responsible for it being considered as peripheral by many disciplines and central to none. Claims by any one discipline to a dominant role [e.g. old age psychiatry (Meagher 2001)] must – with the possible exception of geriatric medicine – be rejected, but this lack of clear 'ownership' also makes it difficult to obtain funding for high-quality, large-scale research. It seems to us self-evident that delirium is a perfect subject for interdisciplinary research, including the biological, psychiatric, psychological, medical (including palliative care), nursing, and social sciences. Our primary desire, then, is to see delirium research increase in volume and quality to match its importance and relevance, and the intellectual challenge it poses.

The concept of delirium

Continuing research into the conceptualization of delirium is needed, because it is by no means clear that the current diagnostic constructs in ICD-10 and DSM-IV fully capture the unique, defining aspects of this disorder, especially in relation to dementing disorders like Alzheimer's disease and Lewy body dementia. We would hope that the diagnostic distinction of delirium from other states of cognitive impairment in older, ill patients will be increasingly empirically based rather than continuing to rely on expert consensus (currently held as the lowest form in the hierarchy of evidence).

In the absence of clear biological markers, the criteria against which these distinctions can be made are not immediately obvious, but strong candidates are:

- reversibility, and
- mortality independent of underlying physical illness severity.

We would also expect that, in a rational world, the 'lumper/splitter' issue of subtypes of delirium would await the better empirical distinction of the syndrome itself rather than, at present, being addressed with contradictory results.

Another distinction that needs urgent, careful exploration is that between delirium as a potentially reversible complication of medical illness and delirium as a terminal event. It may well be that the pathophysiology and management of the two states (even at a symptomatic level) will be different.

Instrumentation of delirium

Being pragmatic, we clearly cannot wait for any major transformations in our conceptual understanding of delirium, and so research will continue to be based upon current diagnostic criteria. There is currently a wide range of published instruments and scales for screening and for measurement of the severity of delirium, for the most part derived from ICD-10 and DSM-IV definitions of the disorder. Among the screening instruments, the Confusion Assessment Method (CAM) (Inouye *et al.* 1990) is emerging as the most widely used, despite some variability in the results of its application (e.g. Rolfson *et al.* 1999). If it were to become the principal means of identifying patients for research into the full delirium syndrome, this would at least improve comparability between studies. As Johnson *et al.* (1990) have pointed out, case definition requires not only the use of explicit diagnostic criteria, but also explicit and validated means by which these are applied.

There is still much work to be done on improving our understanding of the psychometric properties of delirium rating scales. One important issue that is still insufficiently appreciated is that concepts such as validity and reliability are not inherent attributes of scales, but functions of the context in which they are used. If a scale has good validity and reliability when applied to one population, this does not mean that it will perform as well in other populations, for example, those with different prevalence rates of the disorder. If researchers are using an instrument in a population that is substantially different from that in which the instrument was developed, they need to show that it is appropriate for use in their study.

There are other issues that need to be addressed when developing case-finding instruments for delirium. While many instruments rely on patient-generated responses (i.e. they are tests), others incorporate the judgement of the rater. Given the importance of professional judgement in the clinical diagnosis of delirium, this seems reasonable, but it does raise important methodological issues. For example, when judgements are invoked, the distinction between the inter-rater reliability of expert clinicians and convergent construct validity becomes blurred. Consequently, a useful practice when undertaking studies reliant on judgement-based scales would be to incorporate more than one observer for a proportion of the ratings, and to test formally and report on the reproducibility of their independent assessments.

It is likely that instruments designed to identify cases of delirium will not be efficient in measuring its severity, as this requires a more dimensional approach to the disorder. Moreover, should severity assessments only be applied to syndromal cases, or should they reflect clinical reality and extend to sub-syndromal developing, resolving, and partial episodes? Our view is that they should. The validation of measures of change is difficult and complex, and these problems have not yet been fully addressed in relation to the current delirium severity measures. We probably need more input from statisticians and mathematicians to help us model change in this disorder.

Related to this is the issue of the diurnal fluctuation of delirium. Current instruments incorporate this as a global judgement/observation, but we lack valid and reliable means to quantify this phenomenon, based on frequent, repeated observations. In general, research into the specific symptoms of delirium will require the development of more sophisticated measures than are currently available, and this development will in turn need to be grounded in more detailed study of delirium phenomenology. We need to develop better means of asking patients about their experiences, and assessing their performance in specific domains. A good place to start would be with attentional deficits, as these seem to be the aspects of the disorder that most clinicians base their diagnostic judgements upon.

Research into the validity and significance of the hyperactive and hypoactive subtypes of delirium will also require the refinement of current instruments, or the development of new ones. While factor analysis of data collected using a symptom checklist supports the existence of subtypes (Camus et al. 2000), there is currently no validated tool available for their diagnosis or quantification.

Delirium measures are necessary for research, but they are also useful in clinical practice, particularly as a means of improving the currently poor recognition rates in elderly patients. Quick and simple case-finding screens are valuable in this respect, but, in a perfect world, we would be able to reliably identify patients in the earliest stages of delirium, and treat them before the full-blown syndrome appears. Better measures of specific symptoms will contribute to this. Another clinically useful development would be an instrument (self-rated or interviewer-rated) to measure the observations and experiences of lay informants, such as family members and care staff in nursing homes.

Progress in delirium research also requires improvements in instrumentation and measurement in other areas. An example is the measurement of severity of physical illness, which is an important confounding factor in many studies. This is conceptually and methodologically a very difficult issue (e.g. acute versus chronic disease, single-system versus multi-system disease, single versus multiple disorders, etc.), and existing scales [e.g. APACHE II (Knaus et al. 1985)] are relatively crude and insensitive.

Epidemiology of delirium

As Chapter 3 makes clear, the epidemiology of delirium in elderly medical and surgical in-patients has been extensively studied over many years. Do we need more unselected case series? So far as in-patients are concerned, the answer is probably no, unless there are some major changes in patient care or hospital environments that might impact upon prevalence and incidence rates. However, in some populations, such as ethnic minorities and the elderly residents of nursing homes, the occurrence of, and risk factors for, delirium are still relatively unresearched. We also need a better understanding of the risk factors in more specific patient populations, e.g. hip fracture patients as opposed to those with advanced cancer (Zelenik 2001).

Future epidemiological research should focus on longitudinal studies, with longer follow-up periods and shorter intervals between assessments, to characterize better the course of the disorder and its outcomes. Outcome research to date has been largely restricted to relatively 'hard' measures, such as death and institutionalization. Some other factors such as dementia and functional impairment have been studied, but we know little about other potentially important adverse outcomes of delirium. For example, is it associated with higher subsequent rates of other psychiatric disorders, such as depression or post-traumatic stress? Longitudinal studies are expensive, however, and would be supported by the development of assessment methods using telephone interviews, informant-based measures, etc. So far as the study of predisposing and precipitating factors is concerned, unselected case series are insufficiently powered to demonstrate the effect of less prevalent risk factors (e.g. some specific physical and mental disorders, drugs, etc.); there is a need for case-control studies to examine these.

Neuropathophysiology of delirium

As Chapter 4 makes clear, the neuropathophysiology of delirium is not well understood, but current thinking is that the disorder represents a 'final common neural pathway' for its many aetiologies, possibly involving reduced cholinergic and increased serotonergic activity in the brain. The body's stress-response mechanisms may provide an important link between disease and delirium. While there is much supportive evidence for these hypotheses (see Chapter 4), they are difficult to test by direct experiment, for obvious practical and ethical reasons. In this respect, delirium research is no different from that into most other psychiatric disorders.

Methodologically, there are a number of possible ways forward. A good animal model of delirium would be very useful in the study of its underlying mechanisms and the testing of possible treatments; a few rat models have been developed (see Chapter 4), but it is not yet clear to what extent they mimic delirium in humans. There is still much work to be done in this area. Elsewhere, developments in functional neuroimaging may provide us with non-invasive means of studying delirium in human subjects, including patients. The problems here are more to do with the practicalities of investigating elderly delirious patients by this means (Lindesay and Macdonald 1997).

Neuroimaging research in general is also fraught with other methodological problems, such as: unrepresentative selection of study populations, inadequate sample sizes, inappropriate control groups, and ethical constraints. All of these will need to be addressed in research into delirium using these techniques.

Developments in this aspect of delirium research are likely to go hand in hand with basic research into the dementias (particularly Alzheimer's disease) and into the neurobiology of normal ageing. One important unanswered question is whether the pathophysiology of delirium has any direct neurotoxic effects, perhaps *via* immune activation (Broadhurst and Wilson 2001), that result in persistent cognitive impairment (i.e. can delirium cause/exacerbate dementia?). If the answer is 'yes', this would be a powerful stimulus to improving assessment, diagnosis, treatment, and prevention.

Clinical assessment and diagnosis

When all is said and done, the recognition of all but the mildest of delirious states should be easy for most doctors and nurses. It does not represent a major intellectual challenge. All that needs to happen is that the clinician knows the syndrome pattern and becomes aware of the information – from examination of the patient and knowledge of the course – necessary to recognize it. But recognition is an active process, motivated by appreciation of the outcomes likely if the syndrome is not recognized; without this motivation, recognition will not be often achieved. Within health services, there is a continued tension between the need to allow individual professionals freedom to develop and use clinical methods that they find most effective, and the need to insist on protocols and standardization of the assessment process – standardization which can sometimes do more harm than good, both for its overt aim and in terms of the professional self-esteem so necessary for good clinical work. In the case of delirium, we would see this balance as possibly erring to far in the direction of laxity, and would like to see the empirical basis of protocol-based approaches strengthened. Clearly, recognition rates are low, but just how low, and what impact on outcomes there are when recognition rates are increased, with or without educational intervention to improve motivation, needs addressing.

As is emphasized in Chapter 5, some of the diagnostic issues in delirium – its distinction from, or recognition of, its superimposition upon dementing illnesses, or its distinction from other acute disorders such as schizophrenia or depression, can only be resolved with a collateral history. Two conditions have to be met. Someone has to take this collateral history, asking about onset of cognitive and other psychological and behavioural symptoms, and the history must be available to the person assessing the patient with delirium. We would like to see an increase in the former activity, and improvement in systems to facilitate the latter.

Causes of delirium

Undoubtedly, the future will see the emergence of new candidates as possibly causal in delirium. However, as Chapter 6 makes clear, our difficulties in assessing these may be due to the fact that in its complexity delirium takes us beyond the edge of our current capacity to think. The 'single cause' model is desired because it makes choosing the course of action clear, but this is rarely useful in delirium. A flat 'multifactorial' model is also unsatisfactory, for it does not suggest one factor over another. The predisposing/precipitating (and let us not forget the sustaining/restorative) taxonomy is definitely more helpful. However, interactions between causal influences needs further exploration in the future. Medication as a precipitating factor is a case in point. Clearly, much (we dare not say all) medication is given in or for medical conditions. Thus the two (precipitating and predisposing) are irrevocably linked, and this is true of other predisposers and precipitants. We would see a role for the development of more sophisticated models which may ultimately help clinicians decide which possible causal factor to try and influence first, and with what degree of vigour. Studies of well-defined sub-populations of patients would also be useful in this respect (Zelenik 2001). Complexity science (Plsek and Greenhalgh 2001) may (or, like other sweeping ideas whose name begins with a 'C', may not) be helpful when its ramifications are better understood. But the idea of simple causes in medicine definitely needs rooting out. This will take time, since we doctors are simple folk, and the more widespread promulgation of the predisposing/precipitating/sustaining/restorative model is an important intermediate aim.

Management of delirium

Just as our models of causation may not be quite up to the job in delirium, so our management strategies may be constrained by conceptual poverty. Delirium management is, par excellence, a complex intervention in a complex system, and simple ideas, enshrined in the placement of the Randomized Controlled Trial (RCT) at the top of the hierarchy of evidence, are inadequate. There are some surprising gaps, however, even in the drug-efficacy literature; for instance, the virtual absence of RCTs of the use of haloperidol or atypical antipsychotics in delirium. The 'cholinergic theory of delirium' (Chapter 4) suggests that anticholinesterase inhibitors may be of value; at least one trial is underway in the USA. The evidence base for effective management strategies is still very limited; indeed, it is non-existent for some important groups, such as delirium in elderly people with chronic cognitive impairment (Britton and Russell 2001).

Once one moves away from simple, standardized interventions like medication assessed against simple outcomes such as behavioural scores and lengths of stay, normal rules of evidence break down. A strong candidate for a useful theoretical model is 'Realistic Evaluation' (Pawson and Tilley 1997), in which the question posed is not 'what works?' but 'what mechanisms may be modified, thus producing which outcomes in which people?'. This sort of detailed approach, embracing traditional quantitative and qualitative methodologies, allows key issues of generalizability (for both sorts of method) to be addressed by tying results down to particular contexts, which are carefully described. As an example, take the apparent cultural difference in relative use of chemical and physical restraint in disturbed delirious patients between USA/France/Spain and UK/Scandinavia/Australia. There is as yet no empirical evidence on this observation, but were it to be verified, it raises important questions – and these can be expressed in two ways. The traditional, experimentalist question, answered by an RCT, would be: 'is restraint better than risperidone in the management of acute behavioural problems in delirium?' For various reasons, it is never likely to be answered; for instance, it is highly unlikely that the two interventions could be carried out with the same gusto by one team in anything other than a grossly unrepresentative service. Even if a trial were possible, the chances of the results changing practice seem minimal. However, the observationalist question, 'which patients with what sorts of delirium have more reduction of behavioural problems with which type of intervention?', is at least theoretically answerable, and importantly the answer would be much more likely to be useful to clinicians, weighing up the options in a given case. We would like to see more sophisticated, theory-based, iterative work of this nature in the assessment of complex treatment options in delirium, rather than the slavish application of RCTs in all but the simplest interventions. In this regard, individualized outcome measurement techniques, and clinimetric measures that made the bases of clinical judgements explicit might be especially useful (Rockwood *et al.* 2000).

One aspect of the management of delirium that might well drive future change is the possibility that litigation will become a more regular consequence of not recognizing, treating, or explaining delirium properly. This may well have good and bad consequences: more effort will ensue to make sure that these are optimized, but equally there will be an increasing reliance on standardized approaches to assessment and management representing the 'shoal-centre' approach, rather than necessarily the best approach for the patient. Development of more evidence, using complexity-based approaches like Pawson and Tilley's, would help keep the overall balance favourable.

Finally, the counsel of perfection represented in this textbook, and in all future advice, needs to be tempered by the realities of life on public hospital wards in many countries in the developed ward, particularly the UK and USA. This, too, should be a subject of enquiry in its own right. With the increasing use of routine outcomes measurement in medicine and psychiatry, it may well be possible to explore the circumstances in which delirious patients have better or worse outcomes; one key variable may well be the trade-offs achieved between theoretical optimization and pragmatic reality by staff in the units with better outcomes. This is particularly an issue in implementing some of the best evidence-based advice available – that concerning the prevention of delirium.

Prevention of delirium

Interestingly, the evidence base for prevention studies appears stronger than for intervention studies in delirium. In particular, the combination of interventions described by Inouye and colleagues (1999) in their huge RCT represent, to a large extent, a package of optimal nursing and medical care, and, as they suggest, may well have succeeded more because of the failures of care-as-usual than because of any special impact of the interventions. The question now being wrestled with is how to implement a model of optimal nursing care, proven to prevent delirium in at-risk patients, in hospital wards in which suboptimal care for all patients is the norm. Here, the complexity issue is obvious – apparently straightforward translation of research findings from a state-of-the-art RCT is very difficult indeed, particularly because the research itself can say very little about the contexts in which such interventions succeed or do not succeed. It is the experience of many clinicians that medical wards are deliriogenic [compare this idea with Kitwood's (1990) 'malignant social psychology' in dementia care], but they may not be the only parts of the health-care system with this propensity. It follows that whilst we, as clinicians, are comfortable with assessing interventions that may or may not reduce the impact of predisposing and precipitating factors in our patients, the main task may lie in addressing these factors in the ward and hospital culture in which the patients (and we) find ourselves.

Clearly, however, folding our hands and waiting for the chaos of modern publicly funded health care to resolve is not an option, and neither is concentrating our efforts entirely on the mysteries of organizational change. While not neglecting the influence we clinicians can have in shaping the culture and organization of the hospitals we work in and beyond, what we would like to see is the teasing out of the most feasible and effective elements of multicomponent interventions, using appropriate analytic strategies (e.g. Tinetti *et al.* 1996), and the testing out of other pragmatic preventative strategies, like the preventative use of anticholinesterase inhibitors or low-dose antipsychotic medication in vulnerable patients. A key preventative strategy enshrined in the phrase 'intermediate care' in the UK is the possibility of more home management of acute medical illness in older people and, as a likely consequence, reduction in any delirium caused by removal to hospital. For this to succeed, and for many of the beneficial interventions in hospital to succeed, a crucial resource needs development – the family support of people with or at risk of delirium.

Family and carer involvement

There is a startling lack of research into this crucial topic, and yet the importance of family and other carers in the recognition and management of delirium is obvious, whether at home or in hospital. In addition, interventions aimed at educating and counselling relatives so as to minimize their distress and any secondary adverse outcomes, like permanent stigmatization of the patient, or unnecessary fear of hospitalization or medical intervention, are urgently needed, and also need evaluation. Familiarity of circumstances clearly reduces risk of delirium and may attenuate its severity, and the presence of well-prepared and supported relatives is a key part of preventative strategies. This also means that attempts to reduce the rates of hospital admission of medically ill older people – an initiative strongly supported in the UK for mainly financial reasons – may have positive benefits in reducing the burden of delirium added by such admissions. However, if family and carer roles are ignored, there is a strong possibility that such initiatives will fail, and thus their impact on reducing delirium will be lost.

Educating health professionals

Most cautious observers would probably suggest that the recognition, understanding, and management of delirium in the everyday practice of medicine and surgery in older patients in most countries are dismal. There are system-wide problems specific to delirium and also general ones that indirectly affect its outcome. Specific to delirium are failures to recognize its importance (for instance, in its tiny presence in medical school and nursing college curricula, its absence from the indexes of resident/house officer handbooks, and what appears to be a decline in empirical delirium research) and the particular relationship of delirium to preventable but too-common iatrogenic influences, both physical (for example, poor infection control or medication review) and psychological (noise, poor continuity of care, lack of personal communication). More general failures, which affect many other disorders beside delirium, include inadequate time available to gather collateral historical information, poor communication with patients, relatives, other disciplines, and agencies, and a tendency to believe that time spent at the bedside is activity secondary to ordering and analysing the results of investigations, or attaching, servicing, and managing equipment, and only to be indulged in when there is nothing else to do (which means never).

The concept of 'education' – changing the knowledge, skills, and attitudes of staff – needs to be extended to the whole system that deals with delirious older people. However, there is plenty already known about delirium that could be helpful immediately if communicated well to key staff and we would like to see, against the backdrop of changes to the culture in which treatment is delivered to older people in hospital, a continued increase in specific and general educational initiatives. This should mean that the considerable percentage educational intervention effect sizes already achieved can be transformed into higher and higher absolute post-intervention status scores. We look forward to a time when educational and other intervention research in delirium is restricted by ceiling effects.

References

Bleuler, E. (1970). *Autistic undisciplined thinking in medicine and how to overcome it.* Hafner, Connecticut.

Britton, A. and Russell, R. (2001). Multidisciplinary team interventions for delirium in patients with chronic cognitive impairment. (Cochrane Review) In: *The Cochrane Library, Issue 3.* Update Software, Oxford.

Broadhurst, C. and Wilson, K. (2001). Immunology of delirium: new opportunities for treatment and research. *British Journal of Psychiatry,* **179**, 288–289.

Camus, V., Burtin, B., Simeone, I., Schwed, P., Gonthier, R., and Dubos, G. (2000). Factor analysis supports the evidence of existing hyperactive and hypoactive subtypes of delirium. *International Journal of Geriatric Psychiatry,* **15**, 313–316.

Inouye, S. K., van Dyck, C., Alessi, C. A., Balkin, S., Siegal, A. P., and Horwitz, R. I. (1990). Clarifying confusion: the confusion assessment method. A new method for detection of delirium. *Annals of Internal Medicine*, **113**, 941–948.

Inouye, S. K., Bogardus, S. T. Jr, Charpentier, P. A., Leo-Summers, L., Acampora, D., Holford, T. R., and Cooney, L. M. (1999). A multicomponent intervention to prevent delirium in hospitalized older patients. *New England Journal of Medicine*, **340**, 669–676.

Johnson, J.C., Gottlieb, G.L., Sullivan, E., *et al.* (1990). Using DSM-III criteria to diagnose delirium in elderly general medical patients. *Journal of Gerontology*, **45**, M113–M119.

Kitwood, T. (1990). The dialectics of dementia: with particular reference to Alzheimer's disease. *Ageing and Society*, **10**, 177–196.

Knaus, W.A., Draper, E.A., Wagner, D.P. and Zimmerman, J.E. (1985). Apache II; a severity of disease classification system. *Critical Care Medicine*, **13**, 818–829.

Lindesay, J. and Macdonald, A. (1997). Delirium. In: *Neuroimaging and the psychiatry of late life* (eds D. Ames and E. Chiu). Cambridge University Press, Cambridge.

Meagher, D (2001). Delirium: The role of psychiatry. *Advances in Psychiatric Treatment*, **7**, 433–442.

National Library of Medicine (2001). *MEDLINE*. National Library of Medicine, Bethesda, MD.

Pawson, R. and Tilley, N. (1997). *Realistic evaluation*. Sage Publications Ltd, London.

Plsek, P. and Greenhalgh, T. (2001). The challenge of complexity in health care. *British Medical Journal*, **323**, 625–628.

Rockwood, K., Stadnyk, K., Carver, D., *et al.* (2000). A clinimetric evaluation of specialized geriatric care for rural dwelling, frail older people. *Journal of the American Geriatrics Society*, **48**, 1080–1085.

Rolfson, D., McElhaney, J., Jhangri, J., and Rockwood, K. (1999). Validity of the Confusion Assessment Method in detecting postoperative delirium in the elderly. *International Psychogeriatrics*, **11**, 431–438.

Tinetti, M.E., McAvay, G., and Claus, E. (1996). Does multiple risk factor reduction explain the reduction in fall rate in the Yale FICSIT trial? *American Journal of Epidemiology*, **144**, 389–399.

Zelenik, J. (2001). Delirium: Still searching for risk factors and effective preventive measures. *Journal of the American Geriatrics Society*, **49**, 1729–1732.

Index

acetylcholine 60–6
acute geriatric units 174
age 37–8, 74–6
agitated delirium 58
alcohol abuse/withdrawal 35, 38, 39, 40, 67,
        73, 169
    clinical assessment and diagnosis 102, 103, 111
    management of delirium 125
    prevention of delirium 154, 158
Alzheimer's disease 11, 38, 39, 64, 70, 75, 213, 217
anaesthesia 115–16
anticholinergic delirium 76
assessment tools 96–7
auxiliary instruments 11–14

barriers to prevention of delirium 156–7
behavioural control, maintenance of 131–6
Blessed Orientation-Memory-Concentration
        Test 15
brain 52–6
Brief Cognitive Rating Scale 14–15, 97
Brief Psychiatric Rating Scale 17
buffering hypothesis 188

CAGE four-question screening test 169
Canada 29, 36, 175–6
care, improvement of outside hospitals 176–7
case definition 27–8
case finding 28–9
causation, external 4
causes of delirium 101–19, 217–18
    conceptual model 104–6
    diversity in delirium literature 102–4
    prediction models and preoperative risk scores
        117–18
    see also specific causes of delirium
Clinical Assessment of Confusion-A 19
clinical assessment and diagnosis 27, 91–9, 217
    differential diagnosis 97–8
    history 92–3
    mental state, examination of 93–6
    rating scales and assessment tools 96–7
Clock Drawing Test 15, 96
co-morbidity 11, 40, 58, 109, 118
cognitive:
    decline 74–6
    reconditioning programme 140

recovery 41–2
tests 13
common complications, anticipation and
        prevention of 136–9
community 30–1
concept of delirium 104–6, 213–14
Confusion Assessment Method 16–17, 18, 21, 22,
        123, 145, 214
Confusion Rating Scale 16, 18–19
Confusional State Evaluation 20
consultation services, geriatric 173
controversies in conceptualisation of
        delirium 4–5
course of delirium 3
cytokines 54–6

dehydration 165–6
Delirium Assessment Scale 17
Delirium Index 21, 61
delirium with psychomotor agitation 29
Delirium Rating Scale 15, 58, 63, 76, 77, 103
Delirium Severity Scale 21
Delirium Symptom Interview 16, 17–18, 62
delirium tremens 43, 63, 125
dementia 5–6, 10–11, 31, 35, 37–9, 42, 217
    clinical assessment and diagnosis 97–8, 110
    families, caregivers and nurses 188, 190, 191
    management of delirium 123, 131
    neuropathophysiology of delirium 75
    prevention of delirium 162
depression 10, 11, 37, 39, 57, 72, 157, 217
    clinical assessment and diagnosis 98, 105
diagnosis
    differential 97–8
    see also clinical assessment and diagnosis
diagnostic instruments see screening and diagnostic
        instruments
diagnostic manuals 9–10
Diagnostic and Statistical Manual of Mental
        Disorders 11
    -II 36
    -III 2, 4, 15, 17–18
        epidemiology of delirium 27, 30, 34, 35, 36
    -III-R 2, 3, 5, 10, 16, 18, 21
        epidemiology of delirium 27
        neuropathophysiology of delirium 58
    -IV 3, 5, 9, 10, 13, 213, 214
        causes of delirium 102, 104
        epidemiology of delirium 27
        neuropathophysiology of delirium 58

Digit Span 17, 21
direct effect hypothesis 188
diversity in delirium literature 102–4
dopamine 66–70

education about delirium 38, 139–42, 205–12,
    221
  existing evidence, overview of 210–11
  feedback 210
  future directions 211
  integration 207–10
  relevance 206–7
elimination problems 114, 130–1
environmental factors 41, 114–15, 139–40, 155,
    163, 164
epidemiology of delirium 27–43, 216
  case definition 27–8
  case finding 28–9
  outcome 41–3
  prevalence and incidence in various
      settings 30–7
  selection bias 29–30
  study setting 30
evaluation units, geriatric post-acute 173–4

families, family caregivers and nurses 187–201,
    220–1
  family caregiving 190–1
  interventions, families participating
      in 192–3
  patient's perspective on being
      delirious 194–6
  situation of families 188–9
  supporting the family 197–201
family education and support 139–42
final common neural pathway 56–9
fluid balance 128–9
frontal lobe dementia 11
frontotemporal dementia 39
functional needs, support of 139–42
functional recovery 42–3
future prospects 213–21
  causes of delirium 217–18
  clinical assessment and diagnosis 217
  concept of delirium 213–14
  educating health professionals 221
  epidemiology of delirium 216
  family and carer involvement 220–1
  instrumentation of delirium 214–15
  management of delirium 218–19
  neuropathophysiology of delirium 216–17
  prevention of delirium 219–20
general medicine 117–18

geriatric
  consultation services 173
  in-patients 31–2
  post-acute evaluation units 173–4
  units, acute 174
Goal Attainment Scaling 159, 162

historical antecedents and present meanings 1–7
  consciousness level, alteration in 2–3
  controversies in conceptualisation of
      delirium 4–5
  course of delirium 3
  dementia and delirium 5–6
  external causation 4
  thinking, disturbance of 3
history 92–3
hospital care improvement 173–5
Hospital Elder Life programme 175
hospital in-patients 31–6
  medical and geriatric in-patients 31–2, 33
  psychiatric in-patients 35–6
  surgical in-patients 32–5
Hospital-at-home schemes 31, 177
hyperactive delirium 28, 32, 36, 43, 77, 134, 215
  clinical assessment and diagnosis 96, 98,
      103, 104
hypoactive delirium 1, 28, 32, 43, 77, 157, 215
  clinical assessment and diagnosis 96, 103, 104
  management of delirium 134–5
hypoperfusion states 113–14
hypothalamic-pituitary-adrenocortical axis 53–4

illness, severe 52–6, 112
incidence see prevalence and incidence
instrumentation of delirium 9–22, 214–15
  auxiliary instruments 11–14
  coexistence with other disorders 11
  diagnostic manuals 9–10
  recommendations 21–2
  screening and diagnostic instruments 14–19
  severity measuring scales 20–1
International Classification of Diseases 5, 11
    10 5, 6, 9, 10, 13, 27, 213, 214
interventions
  assessment 157–62
  comprehensive 162–5
  specific 165–70

Lewy body dementia 6, 27–8, 63, 111, 134, 213
limbic system 53–4
management of delirium 123–48, 218–19

behavioural control, maintenance of 131–6
common complications, anticipation and
        prevention of 136–9
functional needs, support of and restoring
        function 139–42
medico-legal aspects 143–5
terminal care 142
underlying causes, addressing of 124–31
medical in-patients 31–2, 33
medications 107–11, 124–5, 126–7
medico-legal aspects 143–5
Memorial Delirium Assessment Scale 20–1, 76, 77
mental state, examination of 93–6
Mental Status Questionnaire 14, 96
metabolic causes 112–13
metabolic disorders 128–9
Michigan Alcoholism Screening Test
        (MAST-G) 169
Mini-Mental State Examination 14, 17, 21, 22, 28,
        62, 96, 162
morbidity 43, 118, 168, 170, 171
mortality 42–3, 125, 168, 169, 170, 173, 176, 214
multifactorial model of delirium 106

Neecham Confusion Scale 19, 22
neurological illness 116–17
neuropathophysiology of delirium 51–78, 216–17
    ageing and cognitive decline 74–6
    final common neural pathway 56–9
    severe illness, stress response and the
        brain 52–6
    see also neurotransmission
neurotransmission 59–73
    acetylcholine 60–6
    dopamine 66–70
    neurophysiology of ageing and cognitive
        decline 74–6
    rat models of human delirium 73–4
    serotonin 70–3
    treatment of delirium and relationship to
        neuropathophysiology 76–8
nurses see families, family caregivers and nurses
nursing homes 36–7

Organic Brain Syndrome scale 18
outcome 41–3

pain, severe 129–30
Parkinson's disease 39, 59, 67, 70, 73, 75,
        111, 134
patient's perspective on being delirious 194–6

perioperative measures 171–2
physical illness factors 39–40
populations 102–3
postoperative care 172–3
postoperative delirium 32–5, 39, 40, 42, 43, 118
    clinical assessment and diagnosis 102, 115–16
    neuropathophysiology of delirium 62, 63, 72, 76
    prevention of delirium 163–4, 167, 169, 170, 177
precipitating factors 154–5
prediction models 117–18
predisposing factors 154
preoperative
    delirium 43
    measures 170–1
    risk scores 117–18
prescribing, inappropriate, avoidance of 166–8
prevalence and incidence in various settings 30–7
    community 30–1
    hospital in-patients 31–6
    nursing homes 36–7
    risk factors for delirium 37–41
prevention of delirium 153–78, 219–20
    barriers to 156–7
    care, improvement of outside hospitals 176–7
    hospital care improvement 173–5
    interventions assessment 157–62
    interventions, comprehensive 162–5
    interventions, specific 165–70
    preventable risk factors 153–5
    recognition, improvement of 175–6
    in surgical patients 170–3
process of care, risk factors related to 40–1
psychiatric disorders 37, 39
psychiatric in-patients 35–6
psychological contributors 114–15
psychosis 10, 11, 70, 103
pulmonary compromise 113–14

Randomized Controlled Trial 218, 219, 220
rat models of human delirium 73–4
rating scales 96–7
Realistic Evaluation 218
recognition, improvement of 175–6
research 13–14
restoring function 139–42
restraint use 169–70
risk factors for delirium 37–41
rooming-in study 192–3, 196

Saskatoon Delirium Checklist 17
screening and diagnostic instruments 12–13,
        14–19, 27, 28
    brief cognitive tests 14–15
    Clinical Assessment of Confusion-A 19

screening and diagnostic instruments (*Contd*)
   Confusion Assessment Method 16–17
   Confusion Rating Scale 18–19
   Delirium Assessment Scale 17
   Delirium Rating Scale 15
   Delirium Symptom Interview 17–18
   Neecham Confusion Scale 19
   Organic Brain Syndrome scale 18
   Saskatoon Delirium Checklist 17
selection bias 29–30
serotonin 70–3
severe and persistent delirium 58
severity measuring scales 20–1
Short Portable Mental Status Questionnaire
   14, 96
special medical care 164–5
special nursing care 163–4
specialized delirium ward 174
Specific Activity Scale 40
specific causes of delirium 106–17
   environmental/psychological contributors
      114–15
   hypoperfusion states and pulmonary
      compromise 113–14
   infectious causes 112
   medications 107–11
   metabolic causes 112–13
   neurological illness 116–17
   severe acute illness 112
   substance withdrawal 111–12
   surgery and anaesthesia 115–16
   urinary and faecal retention 114
stress response 52–6
stroke 40, 56–7, 58–9, 64, 103
substance withdrawal 111–12
subtypes of delirium 103–4
   see also hyperactive delirium; hypoactive
      delirium
superimposed delirium 11
surgery 115–16, 117, 118
surgical patients 32–5, 170–3

Sweden 31, 37, 174
systems of care 156–7

terminal care 142
thiamine deficiency 168–9
thyroid hormone metabolism 54
Trail Making Test 15, 96
treatment of delirium 76–8

under-recognition of delirium 28–9, 118, 123, 157
underlying causes, addressing of 124–31
   central nervous system oxygenation, impaired 129
   elimination problems 130–1
   fluid balance and metabolic disorders 128–9
   infections 125, 128
   medications 124–5, 126–7
   pain, severe 129–30
   sensory deprivation 130
United Kingdom 168, 174–5, 177, 219, 220
United States 37, 143, 169, 218, 219
   Acute Care of the Elderly unit (Cleveland,
      Ohio) 174
   Eastern Baltimore Mental Health Survey 30
   Epidemiologic Catchment Area 28, 30
   Yale HELP programme 167
   Yale-New Haven study 162–3, 165, 166, 167,
      170, 177

vascular dementia 6, 11, 38, 59, 64

Whisper test 166